Family Well-Being

Social Indicators Research Series

Volume 49

This new series aims to provide a public forum for single treatises and collections of papers on social indicators research that are long to be published in journal Social Indicators Research. Like the journal, the book series deals with statistal assessments of the quality of life from a broad perspective, It welcomes the research on a wide variety of substantive areas, including health, crime, housing, education, family life, leisure activities, transportation, mobility, economcs, work, religion and environmental issues. These areas of research will focus on the impact of key issues such as health on the overall quality of life and vice versa. An international review board, consisting of Ruut Veenhoven, Joachim Vogel, Ed Diener, Torbjorn Moum, Airjam A.G. Sprangers and Wolfgang Glantzer, will ensure the high quality of the series as a hole.

For further volumes:
http://www.springer.com/series/6548

Almudena Moreno Mínguez
Editor

Family Well-Being

European Perspectives

Springer

Editor
Almudena Moreno Mínguez
Department of Sociology and Social Work
Universidad de Valladolid, Segovia, Spain

ISSN 1387-6570
ISBN 978-94-017-8208-1 ISBN 978-94-007-4354-0 (eBook)
DOI 10.1007/978-94-007-4354-0
Springer Dordrecht Heidelberg New York London

Printed on acid-free paper

Springer is part of Springer Science+Business Media (www.springer.com)

Contents

Contributors

Pamela Abbott University of Aberdeen, Scotland, UK

Ulla Björnberg Department of Sociology, University of Gothenburg, Göteborg, Sweden

Thomas P. Boje Department of Society and Globalisation, Roskilde University, Roskilde, Denmark

Simon Chapple Social Policy Division, OECD, Paris, France

Daniela Del Boca Department of Economics, University of Turin, CHILD Collegio Carlo Alberto, Turin, Italy

Anders Ejrnæs Department of Society and Globalisation, Roskilde University, Roskilde, Denmark

Anna Escobedo Departamento de Sociología y Análisis de las Organizaciones de la, University of Barcelona, Barcelona, Spain

Joris Ghysels Faculty of Humanities and Sciences, Maastricht University, Maastricht, The Netherlands

Bernard Harris Division of Sociology and Social Policy, School of Social Sciences, University of Southampton, Southampton, UK

Frédérique Hoffmann EuropeanCentre for Social Welfare Policy and Research (ECSWPR), World Health Organization (WHO), Vienna, Austria

Manfred Huber European Centre for Social Welfare Policy and Research (ECSWPR), World Health Organization (WHO), Vienna, Austria

Anna Laura Mancini CHILD-Collegio Carlo Alberto, Turin, Italy

ZEW, Mannheim, Germany

Almudena Moreno Mínguez Department of Sociology and Social Work, Universidad de Valladolid, Segovia, Spain

Antonio López Peláez Universidad de Educación a Distancia, Madrid, Spain

Axel Pohl Institute for Regional Innovation and Social Research (IRIS), Tubingen, Germany

Ricardo Rodrigues European Centre for Social Welfare Policy and Research (ECSWPR), World Health Organization (WHO), Vienna, Austria

Sagrario Segado Sánchez-Cabezudo Universidad de Educación a Distancia, Madrid, Spain

Barbara Stauber Institute of Education, Tübingen University, Muenzgasse 22-30, D 72070 Tübingen

Karin Wall Institute of Social Sciences, University of Lisbon, Lisbon, Portugal

Claire Wallace University of Aberdeen, Scotland, UK

Andreas Walther Institute für Social Pedagogy and Adult Education, University of Frankfurt, Frankfurt, Germany

Shirley L. Zimmerman, Ph.D. Family Social Science, University of Minnesota, St. Paul, MN, USA

Chapter 1
Introduction

Almudena Moreno Mínguez

In recent years, there has been extensive research into the subject of changes in the family, particularly into family structures and typologies, demographic and economic dynamics, the repercussions of the progressive entry of women into the workplace and the different family policies enacted by the various welfare states. In fact, the family has taken on a key role in comparative economic and sociological theory since the 1980s (Castles 1998; Esping Andersen 2009; Ferrera 2005). However, the conceptualisation and empirical research into the topic of 'family well-being' (McKeown and Sweeney 2001), within the area of family change and well-being, is a topic which has barely been analysed in sociological and economic treatises on the family (Jordan 2008).

On this basis, an OECD working paper, for example, introduced the concept of equitable and sustainable 'well-being' (Hall et al. 2010). According to this approach, human well-being consists of both individual and social well-being, and it is embedded in culture, the economy and governance (Kroll 2011). Moreover, the human system must always be considered in relation to the ecosystem and its interactions with it. Important cross-cutting themes in determining the well-being of a society also include (a) fair distribution and (b) sustainability with regard to the available resources. It is also important to add that the concept of quality of life is traditionally measured by means of so-called 'objective' and 'subjective' indicators (Noll 2004). The first provide external descriptions of people's conditions of life, while the second is based on direct questioning of people concerning how satisfied they are with their lives overall and with particular aspects (such as work or family). Taking this conceptual basis of well-being as a reference, the general objective of this book is to collate, using different theoretical and methodological approaches,

A. Moreno Mínguez (✉)
Department of Sociology and Social Work, University of Valladolid,
Plaza de Colmenares, s/n, 40001 Segovia, Spain
e-mail: almudena@soc.uva.es

A. Moreno Mínguez (ed.), *Family Well-Being: European Perspectives*,
Social Indicators Research Series 49, DOI 10.1007/978-94-007-4354-0_1,

the various research works currently underway into the quality of life of the individuals who live in families in today's context of family change throughout the various stages of the family cycle. The European comparative approach has been used in order to include the main aspects of family change and its effects on well-being throughout the different stages of the family cycle.

Thus, this volume will focus on the comparative analysis of family and well-being, a dimension which literature has not covered sufficiently till the present in a European perspective. This book collects the studies made in Europe on family well-being comparing family change and well-being in different institutional and cultural contexts. This book takes a deeper look at early evidence of family well-being and a compilation of findings from the main researches on this topic. In this book, we present reasoned arguments on the need to focus upon much more than simply economic interpretations of well-being. Thus, this book covers a broad range of topics, from the theorising of children's well-being to the development of specific measures of family well-being and quality of life.

The book has therefore been structured around three major objectives. In the first place, it introduces and presents the concept of family well-being as a central study objective in economic theory, as people's individual well-being is in part dependent on the well-being of the family. The book thus seeks to define and delimit the term 'family well-being' from a variety of viewpoints in order to be of use in future empirical research. Hence, one of the most important contributions of this book is that it incorporates family well-being into the scientific debate.

In the second place, the book presents the results of the most important current European research into the subject of well-being of individuals at different stages of the family cycle (childhood, adolescence, family formation and the elderly). This family perspective is examined throughout the whole of the life cycle of the family in order to highlight the most significant research currently underway into the well-being of individuals and families in today's society, within a climate of increasing risk and uncertainty.

In the third place, the book takes a look at the effects produced by factors such as immigration and the new family dynamics and structures on people's well-being and quality of life. This is a multidisciplinary approach which is designed to integrate the analysis of family changes with the well-being and satisfaction of the individuals who are themselves the main protagonists of these family changes.

The book also dedicates particular attention to gender issues deriving from the impact of women's entry into the workplace on questions, such as the division of labour within the home, and policies designed to address the work-life balance from a comparative European point of view.

This work therefore offers a comparative macro outlook on family change and the well-being of individuals, and also provides an analysis of specific examples of these changes in particular national contexts. This approach enables the comparative international perspective to be integrated with the specific historical perspective of all the different national contexts analysed in the book.

The book has been structured into various chapters in order to respond to the general objectives of the work. Chapter 2, by Shirley Zimmerman, presents an introduction to the concept of family well-being based on a compilation of the various current theoretical approaches to family change. According to Zimmerman, the application of different conceptual frameworks allows a more holistic and contextual approach to the subject and a closer examination of the implications of the policies enacted by governments that affect families – and almost all policies do, whether directly or indirectly, implicitly or explicitly, intentionally or not. Given the importance of families regardless of their form, not only for individuals but for society and its future, such an examination could facilitate the enactment of family policies that do in fact enhance the well-being of families.

In Chap. 3, Pamela Abbott and Claire Wallace analyse the social quality of families in Europe by focussing upon parents with young children using the European Quality of Life Survey, 2007. It considers the role of employment and unemployment in modifying the quality of life for fathers and mothers in 27 European countries. The aim of the chapter is to test the applicability of the social quality model to this particular group and to look at the variation in European countries.

The book dedicates a second section to an analysis of the impact of family change on well-being and child poverty. The purpose of Chap. 4 written by Daniela Del Boca and Anna Laura Mancini is to examine several dimensions of relative and absolute poverty among children, with a special focus on the Italian case, and to explore its underlying factors mainly related to the nature of the labour market and the structure of the welfare state. Given that child poverty outcomes result from complex interactions between joblessness, in-work poverty and the impact of transfers, the countries achieving the best outcomes are those that are performing well on all fronts, notably by combining strategies aimed at facilitating access to employment and enabling services (childcare, etc.) with income support (social transfers other than pensions).

In Chap. 5, Simon Chapple focusses on research published in the 1990s or later that investigates relationships between child well-being and single-parent family structure in OECD. According to Simon Chapple, in comparison say to some policy-related literatures like the impact of education on earnings or even the employment effects of minimum wages, the empirical literature on the impact of family structure on child outcomes is at an immature stage. The immaturity is signalled by the lack of a consensus regarding the existence of a causal effect of lone parent family structure. The extent to which different welfare regimes across the OECD influence the transmission of causal effects of lone parenthood is extremely difficult to judge, since the causal effects of lone parenthood are so difficult to define. In conclusion, policy makers should be aware that the current immature state of the literature does not allow strong conclusions to be drawn regarding the impact of lone parenthood on child well-being in the absence of additional strong priors.

Karin Wall and Anna Escobedo (Chap. 6) explore the diversity of leave policy models in contemporary European society. Seven empirically based ideal types are identified by looking at data for the 22 countries on leave systems, early childhood services and maternal and couples' employment patterns. They address the complex interplay between leave systems and work family, gender and welfare regimes. The analysis reveals three sets of conclusions, which relate to convergence and divergence in care leave policies across Europe, leave generosity and its linkages to gender equity and family well-being.

The third section of the book refers to the subject of work-family balance and gender. Anders Ejrnæs and Thomas P. Boje (Chap. 7) examine how different welfare policy regimes have influence on the social risks which individuals are confronted in managing and reconciling the relationship between work and family life. This chapter examines how institutional as well as individual dimensions determine the risk of spending more time than wanted outside paid work because of care responsibilities. This study includes both individual and institutional factors in analysing to which extent the individuals are forced to sacrifice their employment career in order to take care of family members or relatives. This question is closely related to the discussion about inequalities in the opportunities or capabilities individuals have in realise their life goals.

Joris Ghysels in Chap. 8 addresses family well-being through a discussion of spousal preferences regarding the task division between partners in a couple. For the empirical analyses of this chapter, Joris Ghysels rely on data of the 2004–2005 Flemish Families and Care Survey (FFCS), which provides a representative sample of families with young children. This chapter shows it to be relatively rare that both spouses agree in their task division preference and are able to get what they want. Particularly, women have trouble to realise their task division preferences. This has much to do with many women having less traditional preferences than men, combined with our gendered care culture which makes women more receptive to care demands in their household than men. According to Joris Ghysels, the data does not sustain that relatively more wealthy spouses would be more likely to realise their task division preferences than the relative poor. Further inquiries, however, suggest limited evidence of monetary compensation for households with an unbalanced preference outcome.

The aim of the study presented in Chap. 9 by Almudena Moreno is to analyse how far institutional and cultural factors linked to a particular family model, as well as individual factors such as education, work situation and occupation, affect a couple's decisions and actions with regard to the WFB, depending on the cultural context of each country, with particular emphasis on the Spanish case. This chapter describes the extent to which the gender stereotypes rooted in a given cultural context and family policies condition the reconciliation strategies adopted by citizens in distinct institutional and cultural contexts. In a second part of this study, the author uses more complex statistical analysis to find out the extent to which individual factors such as professional status, education, and so on, neutralise the impact of culturally assigned gender roles and consequently the expectations and strategies of work-family balance.

In Chap. 10, Bernard Harris attempts to review some of the evidence in relation to a range of European countries in order to examine the extent to which differences in the circumstances of male and female lives during the nineteenth and twentieth centuries were reflected in health statistics. This chapter has explored the extent to which the particular hardships experienced by the female population may have been reflected in the size and shape of women's bodies and in their mortality rates. Although these are important dimensions of welfare in their own right, the chapter has been particularly concerned to examine the extent to which they can be associated with underlying differences in the circumstances of male and female lives.

The final part of the book contains a range of research into youth, the elderly, migration and social work. Andreas Walther, Barbara Stauber and Axel Pohl in Chap. 11 analyse the meaning of success and support in youth transitions from a life course perspective. This has a comparative dimension with regard to different 'transition regimes' and a biographical dimension asking for the subjective views of young men and women. In this chapter, the authors have tried to enlarge a dominant institutional perspective which reduces success in transitions to work and adulthood to entering the labour market, founding a family and avoiding poverty and which informs policy measures aimed at supporting young people in their transitions to work. First, they have shown that assumptions of success and support held as generally valid actually do differ across different contexts and constellations of youth transitions. Second, they have found that successful transitions for them include not only stable and well-paid jobs – although this remains important – but also trajectories they can identify with. Their findings suggest that research which up to now has concentrated on input and output of young people's agency needs to put more stress on analysing the complex interpretation and negotiation processes that underlie individual decision-making.

Chapter 12 written by Frédérique Hoffmann, Manfred Huber and Ricardo Rodrigues, seeks to provide an overview of the challenges facing informal carers today and in the near future, while also presenting a critical appraisal of the public policies in place to support them. The first section of this chapter discusses the division of responsibilities between the family and the state in the provision of care and portrays informal care giving in Europe as being in a state of flux. In the second section, the authors turn to some of the main policies that exist to support carers, namely, cash benefits, care leaves and in-kind benefits and analyse whether they sufficiently meet the challenges caregivers are faced with. The final section concludes by summarising the main findings and policy trends.

Ulla Björnberg in Chap. 13, drawing upon a study of the experiences of asylum-seeking children and their families in Sweden, examines how children cope with their life situations while awaiting their asylum decisions. In the text, the author asks what influences the well-being of asylum-seeking children caught up in a tension between experiences of past and present exclusion and expectations of improvement upon arrival in the host country. The analysis is based on qualitative interviews with 18 children (aged 9–18) and 18 parents (one parent for each child). Among the asylum-seeking families studied, family bonding provided a strong source of resilience for both the parents and the children, in particular in families with many adversities to cope with. Uncertainty about the future was usually accompanied by a desire to appear independent and self-reliant vis-à-vis the environment.

In the last chapter, Chap. 14, Antonio López and Sagrario Segado presents some of the results of their research on family social work and well-being. The authors first analyse the main paradoxes of our societies which influence our ability to live with dignity and achieve our aspirations. They then present the theoretical orientation that has guided our intervention projects, namely, empowerment. Finally, based on the experience they have gained through our projects, they discuss the elements that should be included in a key stage of any family intervention project: the assessment process. In short, the aim of this chapter is to complement other theoretical approaches presented in the chapters of this book by delving deeper into a key issue, namely, how to take the step from describing a reality to actually transforming that reality using a properly designed method of assessment. In this process of constructing social well-being, social work plays a key role.

References

Castles, F. (1998). *Comparative public policy: Patterns of post-war transformation*. Chetlenham: Edwar Elgar.

Esping Andersen, G. (2009). *The incomplete revolution*. London: Polity Press.

Ferrera, M. (2005). *The boundaries of welfare: European integration and the new spatial politics of social protection*. Oxford: University Press.

Hall, J., Giovannini, E., Morrone, A., & Rannuzi, G. (2010). *A framework to measure the progress of societies* (Working Paper No. 34). Paris: OECD Statistics Directorate.

Jordan, B. (2008). *Welfare and well-being: Social value in public policy*. Bristol: Policy Press.

Kroll, C. (2011). *Measuring progress and well-being achievements and challenges of a new global movement*. Berlín: Friedrich-Ebert-Stiftung International Policy Analysis.

McKeown, K., & Sweeney, J. (2001). *Family well-being and family policy: Review of research on benefits and costs*. Dublin: Stationery Office. June.

Noll, H. H. (2004). Social indicators and quality of life research: Background, achievements and current trends. In N. Genov (Ed.), *Advances in sociological knowledge. Over half a century* (Vol. 1, pp. 151–181). Wiesbaden: Verlag für Sozialwissenschaften.

Part I
Approaches to the Study of Family Well-Being

Chapter 2
Conceptualizing Family Well-Being

Shirley L. Zimmerman

Introduction

This chapter focuses on family well-being as a family policy goal. Family policy is defined as all of the actions of governments that affect families, directly or indirectly, explicitly or implicitly, intentionally or not. Three frameworks are presented together with their underlying assumptions and concepts for assessing the extent to which such policies meet the family well-being standard: family systems theory, exchange and choice theories, and family stress theory.

The application of such frameworks allows for a more holistic and contextual approach to the conceptualization of family well-being and the implications of policies that governments enact that affect families. Given the importance of families, not only for individuals but also for society, such an approach is long overdue.

Given trends in family life, how should we think about families and their well-being? This chapter is written from a family policy perspective, providing frameworks that can be used to assess the effects of policies that governments enact that affect families and their well-being, directly or indirectly, intentionally or not, regardless of country. Collectively, such policies are known as family policy (Zimmerman 1988, 1995, 2001), that is, temporarily agreed-upon courses of action consisting of a series of interrelated choices affecting families (Kamerman and Kahn 1978), their goal presumably being to enhance the well-being of families. The frameworks presented in this chapter include family systems theory, exchange and choice theories, and family stress theories. The concepts associated with these frameworks provide criteria that can be used to assess the degree to which

S.L. Zimmerman, Ph.D. (✉)
Family Social Science, University of Minnesota,
St. Paul, MN 55108, USA
e-mail: szimmerm@umn.edu

A. Moreno Mínguez (ed.), *Family Well-Being: European Perspectives*,
Social Indicators Research Series 49, DOI 10.1007/978-94-007-4354-0_2,

different family policies indeed foster family well-being. Frameworks also useful for assessing family well-being but not presented here because of space limitations include symbolic interaction, conflict theory, feminist, and cultural theories; interested readers can find discussion of these frameworks in other venues (Zimmerman 1988, 1995, 2001).

Defining Well-Being

Well-being has been defined in several ways. Webster's dictionary defines it as "the state of being healthy and free from want." The family and sociological literature operationalize it similarly, based on indicators such as income, employment, health status, housing, and so forth, as well as on psychological and interpersonal measures that include satisfaction, self-esteem, affect-balance, and so forth. Campbell et al. (1976), Andrews and Withey (1976), and others (Rettig and Bubolz 1983; Rettig et al. 1991) view it as a composite of satisfactions in such life domains as marriage, jobs, leisure, family, and housing. Inglehart (1990) holds satisfaction to be a part of a broad syndrome of attitudes that people hold toward the world in which they live, positive or negative, which Herzog et al. (1982) regard as the outcome of long-term socialization and developmental processes and concurrent environmental conditions. Griffin (1986), like Webster, defines well-being in terms of basic needs and the degree to which they are met, basic needs referring to that which is essential for survival, health, the avoidance of harm, and proper functioning. Sen (1980, 1985) says the primary feature of well-being can be seen in terms of how a person "functions in the broadest sense" which here extends to families – how families function in the broadest sense. Each of the frameworks and all of the chapters in this publication speak to one or more of these definitions, illustrative of their application across countries (Wallace and Abbott 2012).

What Is Family?

As one of the most important institutions shaping human life (Frankel 1976), the definition of family has broadened in recent years to include a wide variety of family forms and structures. Family(ies) is (are) defined here as two or more people who share the same goals and values, are committed to one another over the long term, and usually live in the same household. According to Charles Frankel (1976), the family is "the most immediate and ineluctable of human settings," linking the generations by involving people in the care of their children and, increasingly, their aging parents. As such, it is the source of social memory, legend, history, and a person's identity. Or as the lead actor in a play titled "Somebody, Nobody," by Jane Martin, shouted in a local performance, "In families, people stick, no matter what." Family groupings include married couple families, single-parent families, blended or stepparent and stepchildren families, adoptive parent and adopted children families, intergenerational families, cohabiting heterosexual or gay couple families, and so forth. Given the many forms families can take, how can the different family frameworks presented here be used to conceptualize their well-being? The following discussion includes the assumptions underlying each of the frameworks together with a presentation of their associated concepts and relevant news illustrations.

Conceptualizing Family Well-Being

Family Systems Theory

The family systems perspective that guides the discussion here is drawn from Reuben Hill's (1971) paper titled "Modern Systems Theory and the Family: A Confrontation." Not surprisingly, because it is more structural than other versions of family systems theory such as Broderick's (1993) and Kantor and Lahr (1975), data to support it are more readily available through public sources such as the Census Bureau. Hill begins with the assumption that all family systems are characterized by four properties:

- The tasks they perform to meet the needs of their members and the environment with which they interact.
- The interdependence of component parts, that is, their members.
- Boundaries and boundary maintenance proclivities that serve to differentiate on family from another and the external environment.
- Equilibrium and adaptive propensities for ensuring system viability.

Family Tasks and Functions

The task performing property of families pertains to the functions families are expected to perform. These include (a) the physical maintenance and care of family members; (b) the addition of new members through procreation or adoption and their relinquishment when they mature; (c) the socialization of children for adult roles, such as spouse, parent, worker, citizen, neighbor, community member; (d) the social control of family members to ensure the maintenance of order within the family and groups external to it; (e) the maintenance of family morale and motivation to ensure the performance of tasks that are central to the family and between the family and its external environment; and (f) the production and consumption of goods and services needed to support and maintain the family as a unit. From a system's perspective, then, and according to Sen (1980, 1985), family well-being can be conceptualized as the capacity of families to perform their various functions.

Here, it is important to note that the ways in which families perform their tasks vary and change over time in conjunction with the family life cycle which is determined not only by the age of family members and their sex but also by families' ethnic and socioeconomic background. Thus, the urgency with which such tasks are performed at different life cycle stages – the establishment, childbearing, school age, adolescent, launching, post-parental, and retirement stages – varies and changes accordingly. Because the sequencing of family life cycle stages has blurred in recent years, the timing of the tasks associated with these stages has changed as well. For example, the retired parents of adolescent children who have children may be required to perform tasks associated with both parenthood and grandparenthood simultaneously. Culture too plays a role in the ways in which families perform their developmental tasks. For example, Hmong children enter adulthood as farmers or soldiers when they are 13 or 14 years old, the concept of teenager being alien to the Hmong culture (Mydans 1994). Nevertheless, from a systems perspective and taking culture into account, family well-being can be conceptualized in terms of the effectiveness with which families perform their various tasks, that is, their socialization, social control, physical maintenance, economic, morale, and membership functions, at different life cycle stages.

Interdependence of Family Roles and Positions

The concepts of interdependence and interrelated positions also may be applied to the conceptualization of family well-being. These concepts refer to the interacting reciprocal positions and roles that make up the family system, such as husband-wife, brother-sister, mother-father, father-son, father-daughter, and so forth. Implicit in such positions are roles that must be performed if the family as a system is to fulfill its functions for its members and the larger society. Based on shared values and normative expectations, a network of family relationships develops that serves to unite members in ways that distinguish one family from other families and groups. These relational networks which vary with social class and culture are likely to persist unless or until disrupted by members who challenge the system's basic values and norms. Such relational networks are able to continue even when members are geographically dispersed, largely because of technological advances in communications and transportation that make meaningful family exchanges and the retention of family identity possible (Litwak 1985). Even in the area of finance, technological advances enable families to perform essential caregiving roles for aging parents living in another community and become ill or disabled. Given the leadership content inherent in the parent role, social/community supports for parents in the form of parent education, family and medical leave, child care, and so forth, take on particular significance in terms of families and their well-being. Because of increased longevity, this same observation can be extended to middle-aged children who are responsible for the care of aging or disabled parents and require social, financial, and community supports to perform essential caregiving tasks.

Structural Deficit and Excess

Structural deficit is characteristic of families with empty or unoccupied family positions, such as female-headed or male-headed households with children. Because tasks associated with particular family positions are important for family functioning, such tasks must be allocated or reallocated to other or remaining family positions. Those positions tend to become overburdened with having too many tasks to perform as heads of single-parent families, both male and female, and grandparent-only families frequently report. Some positions also may become overburdened by having new or additional tasks to perform (e.g., the care of frail elderly parents, a grandchild, or stepchildren in addition to one's own) unrelated to family structure. A different case is families, such as blended or polygamous families, with more than one set of parents that could have too many competing occupants for different family positions. Such families are characterized by structural excess. Family structure, in terms of both deficit and excess, often plays a role in conceptualizing, discussing, and assessing family well-being.

Boundaries and Boundary Maintenance

The boundary of any system, another system property, can be conceptualized as the demarcation line separating the system from other systems in its environment. Family boundaries can be determined by differences in the intensity, frequency, and content of interactions that take place within the family from those that take place between the family and other families with which it interacts and such community institutions as schools, social service agencies, churches, hospitals, workplaces, and so forth. Indeed, because of the intimate functions that families perform for their members, family privacy laws have been enacted to protect families from outside intrusion when their boundaries are threatened – unless the safety of a family member is at stake, such as in the case of domestic and child abuse.

Equilibrium and Adaptive Propensities

The notion of equilibrium assumes a range of possible states within which a system can function and to which it presumably can adapt (Hill 1971). In terms of families, if patterns of interactions develop in conformity with the range of norms that members share, they probably can continue to function and survive as systems. The point at which this range has been exceeded becomes apparent in the behaviors of individuals members, such as when a teenager runs away from home or when one of the marital partners engages in an extramarital affair or risks the financial solvency of the family. John Edwards, US senator and presidential candidate in 2008, whose wife, Elizabeth, subsequently divorced him, comes to mind. She died in 2010.

States of equilibrium and adaptation are made possible through negative and positive feedback processes which can be either negative or positive in their consequences for families (Hill 1971). Families as social systems need information and feedback about their performance in relation to their external environment and internal component parts, that is, their members. Information and feedback incongruent with established family goals become the basis for modifying family behaviors and operations. Such feedback is used as inputs into family decision-making processes. Families, for example, need information about changes in the Social Security program as input into decisions about retirement as well as other information pertinent to their situation, such as the status of their pension fund. In this manner, they may be able to make decisions that will ensure the maintenance and viability of the family once labor force participation is no longer their income source. The same may be said with regard to health care reform in the United States, particularly as it pertains to health care coverage for members with a preexisting health condition.

Feedback about family task performance can be both negative and positive without necessarily being negative or positive in its consequences. Both negative and positive feedback begin with error or a mismatch between system behaviors and internal and external standards or values. Negative feedback differs from positive feedback, however, by acting to reduce the mismatch between information about a system's performance and values, triggering behaviors to bring the two into convergence. In this respect, negative feedback is a change-resistant set of operations, geared toward the status quo or morphostasis. Positive feedback, on the other hand, is a deviation-amplifying rather than a deviation-reduction process. Viewed as instructive and system enhancing, positive feedback is considered essential to the morphogenic process through which systems grow and change. Change that occurs as a result of positive feedback is referred to as morphogenesis. Morphogenesis can take many forms such as a change in system values, purposes, and standards such as can occur during periods of economic downturn when family members may be out of work – or an economic upturn when family fortunes might improve. It also can occur when families move to a different country, adopting the latter's culture as their own, as many immigrant families in fact do.

In addition to changes in system values, purposes, and standards, morphogenesis may take the form of changes in a family's internal and external input operations, such as changes in the ways in which parents communicate with their children – or with each other – at different stages of family development or as a consequence of changes in members' attitudes and knowledge. Illustrative is a mother who reported that she learned how to be a better parent as a result of participating in family education programs. Finally, such change may take the form of the ascendance of members with new and different properties and attributes in the governance and management of the system. Here again, family education programs that teach *both* mothers and fathers how to parent and assume their leadership roles in the family are illustrative.

Integrally related to the concepts of positive feedback and morphogenesis is the idea of "mapping for variety" and the necessity for a continuous flow of varied information, experience, and input into the system – new and different ways of looking at problems or the world in which families live. Here, computer technology and the internet, by making information on a wide variety of subjects instantaneously and readily available to families, are relevant. Also relevant are the disparities in access to such technology among families at different income levels in the United States, accentuating differences in family well-being as well.

The Environment

The environment refers to conditions or influences external to the system that are both system specific and general in nature (Hall 1972). General environmental conditions affecting all systems include weather, economic globalization, technological advances, war, social unrest, and so forth. Examples of environmental conditions specific to families as systems include political and financial support for child care, child care subsidies for working parents, insurance coverage for prescription drugs for elderly family members, access to health care, banking regulations, and so on. Terreberry (1972) characterized the environment in which families live as highly complex, interactive, and turbulent, constantly presenting families and other social systems with sudden and unpredictable changes that continually threaten to upset their equilibrium and capacity to adapt and predict the future and control the consequences of their actions. Thus, families as systems are vulnerable not only to disequilibrium internally induced by their members and their own developmental processes but also are vulnerable to the turbulent nature of their external environment, and threatening to their well-being. The ongoing restructuring of the economy and the uncertainty surrounding health care reform in the United States are but two examples. Terreberry's conceptualization of the environment in terms of systems' transactional interdependencies underscores the importance of the input–output processes connecting families to their environment, such processes facilitated through linkage or liaison roles incorporated into different family positions, such as mother/father. These liaison roles have serious implications for family well-being in terms of facilitating the input–output processes with respect to government policies and programs that affect families, directly or indirectly.

Exchange and Choice Theories

Although based on a different set of assumptions and concepts, exchange and choice theories offer another way of conceptualizing the input–output processes associated with family systems theory and for thinking about family well-being. From the perspective of family systems theory, such exchanges are forms of inputs and outputs which from the perspective of exchange and choice theories are based on choices. Among the assumptions underlying these theories are that:

- Families are made up of members who as human beings are rational, make decisions, and initiate actions (Blau 1964; Ekeh 1974; Gouldner 1960; Levi-Strauss 1966; Nye 1979).
- Within the limits of the information they possess and their ability to predict the future, they are able to assess the rewards and costs of alternative choices (Sabetelli and Shehan 1993).
- Based on their assessment of the costs and rewards of alternative choices, members choose the alternative that promises the greatest rewards at the lowest cost. In other words, they seek to maximize the rewards and minimize the costs of their behaviors and choices and thereby enhance their family's well-being.
- By engaging in one set of behaviors rather than another, families incur costs in the rewards they seek and forego the rewards of alternative choices.
- The values and standards that members hold determine the rewards and costs of alternative choices.
- If other viable choices are available to them and their costs are low, members will not repeat behaviors that were not rewarded in the past.
- In assessing the costs and rewards of different exchanges, norms of reciprocity and fairness take precedence over profitability.

Rewards and Costs

Rewards from the perspective of the exchange and choice frames are defined as pleasures, satisfactions, and gratifications derived from particular statuses, relationships, interactions, relationships, and experiences (Nye 1979). Rewards may include any of the following:

- Social approval in the form of respect, prestige, and admiration
- Autonomy in terms of being able to choose activities, positions, relations, or locales that offer gratification and satisfaction at no or low cost
- Physical security having to do with food, clothing, shelter, health care, physical safety, etc.
- Money for purchasing goods and services that provide pleasure and/or satisfy needs
- Equality based on what the respective parties can offer each other.

Costs are the opposite of rewards. They are defined as statuses, relationships, interactions, and situations that family members regard unpleasant, distasteful, or uncomfortable. Costs also can take the form of rewards foregone as a consequence of choosing a competing alternative, that is, one alternative over another. For example, some adult children, saddled with student loans and out of work, regard the necessity of moving back home with their parents to save money distasteful and unpleasant, in other words, costly. "Living at home absolutely crimps my social life," one adult daughter low on finances said (Roberts 2010). Other adult children deliberately choose to remain at home because of the financial and other benefits it offers. One scuba diver instructor said that while his family's rent-stabilized apartment was a consideration in his decision to live at home, so was his grandmother's age, 90. "The truth is my grandmother is not going to live forever and I want to spend as much time with her as possible with no regrets later," he explained. Indeed, the number of people in the 25–39 age group living at home with their parents increased by almost a third between 2000 and 2008 – before the full effects of the recession in the United States were felt (Roberts 2010), their percentage almost doubling during that period.

Because of the uncertainty involved in the calculation of the costs and rewards of alternative choices, the actual costs and rewards of alternative choices cannot be fully known in advance – health care reform in the United States again being an example – for individuals, families, and government. Therefore, decision-makers – whether parents or policy makers – often experience considerable anxiety and ambivalence when making choices whose outcomes are uncertain. Choices with regard to retirement often are of this nature, involving uncertain calculations with regard to life expectancy, personal investments, the future of Social Security, health status, and health care costs. Many other examples could be cited. Recently, one newly divorced mother of two young boys wrote that based on her experience today and with the recession raising the stakes, fewer mothers in the future may be willing to risk the choice of opting out of the job market to care for children and the financial sacrifices that it entailed (Read 2011).

In general, unpredictability, ambiguity, uncertainty, and anxiety all represent costs that individuals and families – and governments – must bear when making choices. Such costs may prevent consideration of alternatives that could offer rewards exceeding those presently known. This applies to the uncertainty confronting abused wives when trying to decide whether to leave or remain in their present situation, which they already know. It also applies to those who, fearful that health care reform would result in higher taxes, oppose it, placing their health care and economic security in jeopardy.

Profitability

Profitability strives for the most favorable reward-cost ratio. The profitability of alternative choices can be determined by assessing the potential rewards and costs of a sequence of possible actions. A profitable outcome is one that not only absorbs the costs of an alternative choice but also compensates for it. Such was the choice of the scuba diver who decided to live at home in pleasant surroundings where his grandmother also lived rather than live by himself in less pleasant surroundings that would cost him more money. Some polls show that many families would willingly pay more taxes to profit from the rewards of quality education, better police protection, and health care for everyone. Depending on the values they hold relative to particular relationships, statuses, experiences, and objects, individuals and families vary in their perceptions of the rewards and costs of alternative choices, as illustrated by some of the examples already cited. Such differences can be discerned by observing the behaviors of individuals and families and also by asking them what they like and do not like about the alternatives that confront them.

Comparison Level and Comparison Level Alternatives

According to Thibaut and Kelley (1959), comparison level refers to the standard by which families compare the costs and rewards of different choices. The assumption is that those perceiving they are less well off than they think they deserve or would like to be will be angry about the choices that confront them while those perceiving they are better off than they think they deserve will feel guilty. Both anger and guilt represent costs. Illustrative are workers whose jobs are retained while those of coworkers are cut when their companies downsize. Newspaper accounts are replete with stories about the anxiety and guilt remaining employees experience as a result of company layoffs and downsizing.

Individuals and families intuitively compare the costs and rewards of alternative situations and choices, aided sometimes by computer simulations that make more precise comparisons possible. Illustrative are computer analyses of the costs and rewards of alternative tax and health care plans for families in different circumstances, such as the costs of the premiums of different health care plans in 2010 compared to projected costs in 2015 – with and without health care reform. The concept of comparison level alternatives is defined as the comparison of the rewards and costs associated with alternative relationships, statuses, or situations. Clearly, the couple who moved with the 28 children they adopted in Haiti to their home in an abandoned school building in Indiana compared their situation favorably to what it would have been had they not adopted the Haitian children.

Reciprocity

In exchange and choice theories, reciprocity as a norm takes precedence over the norm of profitability or for the most favorable reward-cost ratio (Nye 1979). Reciprocity implies interdependence, a spirit of mutuality, of taking other people into account when making choices. It is based on the assumption that people should help, not hurt others, especially those who have helped them in the past. Based on the norm of reciprocity, individuals and families often make choices accordingly, as illustrated again by the couple cited above who adopted the 28 children in Haiti. No-smoking ordinances and the 55-mile-per-hour speed limit also are expressions of reciprocity and a collective awareness of the costs of smoking and speeding for others. Reciprocity is often expressed in gifts of philanthropy and statements of donors who say they want to give back to society and that which they received from others in the past.

All of the concepts associated with exchange and choice theories – costs, rewards, satisfaction, expectations, comparison levels and comparison level alternatives, profitability, reciprocity – can be used as conceptual tools for assessing family well-being from the perspective of these frameworks. The most obvious application of these concepts is that they can be used to assess the relative rewards and costs associated with a specific family policy or program for those most affected by it. The greater the rewards the program is perceived to provide and the lower its perceived costs – for families – the more it meets the family well-being criterion. The concept of comparison level alternatives can be used to compare the relative costs and rewards of alternative family policies and programs for families, such as foster care reimbursement payments and payments to families under the Temporary Assistance to Needy Families (TANF) program and for different groups of families. Profitability also can be used to assess family well-being as it indeed is used when critics assert that unemployment benefits contribute to high unemployment rates because a job is not "profitable" for laid off workers who critics say come to rely on such benefits rather than gainful employment for their income. And finally, reciprocity, which implies mutuality and interdependence, conveying the idea that people should help, not hurt, others can be used to assess the implications of different policies and programs for families and their well-being – whether they help rather than hurt families – and which ones.

Family Stress Theory

The original family stress model was called a crisis model. It was developed by Reuben Hill (1949, 1958) and called the ABCX model whereby:

- A is the stressor event that places demands on individual families.
- B is the family's resources for meeting the demands arising out of the stressor event.
- C is the family's definition of the situation.
- X is the crisis.

The basic assumption of the model is simple: depending on the resources available to meet the demands of their situation and how they perceive and define it, families may or may not experience a crisis.

The Stressor Event

The stressor event is central to the framework. It is the A factor, the factor that represents the demands, families are required to meet. It may be normative, that is, an expectable taken-for-granted event in the life cycle of the family, such as marriage, the birth of a child, the entry of the child into kindergarten, and so forth. Such events create the need for families to change the ways they function in a variety of ways.

Given declining rates of marriage, some may question the normative status of marriage today. Boss' work (1987) on boundary ambiguity as a source of family stress is relevant here. Boundary ambiguity refers to uncertainty as to who is and is not a member of the family. She measured the concept based on the physical presence but psychological absence of family members, as in the case of families who live together but whose members are preoccupied with their own individual issues or problems, such as joblessness. She also measured it by the psychological presence but physical absence of family members, as in the case of mothers or fathers in the military.

Nonnormative stressors are unexpected and unanticipated life events, such as car accidents, tornadoes, carjackings, earthquakes, winning the lottery, and so forth, that similarly create demands that have the potential of upsetting the balance that families require to function effectively. Such imbalance for families about to become homeless is in part what prompted the Obama administration to create the Homelessness Prevention and Rapid Re-Housing program within its $787 billion economic stimulus package. The program is based on the assumption that once people become homeless, the odds that they may not be able to regain their balance escalates sharply.

Family Resources

Family resources, the B factor, are those material and nonmaterial assets upon which families can draw to meet the demands of their situation. Such resources include (1) family cohesion which develops out of common interests, shared values, mutual affection, and financial interdependence; (2) family adaptability which refers to the ability of families to overcome difficulties and change direction (Olson et al. 1979); (3) satisfactions members derive from meeting the needs of one another and move toward collective goals (Koos 1946); (4) the psychological and physical health of family members; (5) a structure that is organized to meet the needs of family members; (6) time, energy, and money; (7) knowledge and information; and (8) friends and community. Other resources include policies and programs that meet specific demands and needs, such as health insurance to meet demands arising from the illness or failing health of a family member, or child care to meet demands arising from parents' employment or child's developmental needs. Whatever the resource, it must be relevant to the situation and have the potential for maintaining the demand-resource balance of individual families.

Definition of the Situation

Families' subjective definitions and perceptions of the situation, the C factor, is integral to family stress theory, just as it is integral to other family theories, such as exchange and choice theories and symbolic interaction. Families' definitions and perceptions of the situation are based on the meanings they assign to the stressor event, the demands of their situation, and the resources they have available for meeting such demands. How families define their situation also depends on their values and previous experience in dealing with stressful events.

The Crisis

The crisis or X factor refers to the inability of families to function as a result of a stressor event, the absence of resources for meeting the demands of their situation, and their definitions and perceptions of the stressor event. If families have the resources necessary for meeting situational demands and do not perceive or define the situation as a crisis, they may never experience a stressor event in crisis terms, despite the operational or structural changes it may impose on them. This is what is meant by the model: A, the demands arising from a stressor event interacting with B, the family's resources for meeting such demands interacting with C, the family's definition of the situation, and X, the crisis that may or may not occur as a result of the interactions between A, B, and C.

Thus, stressor events create demands that some families are less able to meet than others, threatening the demand-resource balance needed to enable them to function and overwhelming their adaptive capacities. The infusion of government resources such as housing and low interest government loans during periods of natural disasters, such as floods and earthquakes, often help to provide the demand-resource balance families need to avoid a crisis. This was not the case for a family of an 8-year-old boy born with extensive disabilities who required a variety of technological devices in order to live. In a letter to the editor, the mother wrote that because the family's insurance would no longer cover the costs of home health care for children with chronic conditions, it threatened to destroy her family, saying she and her husband would not be able to care for their other two children and provide 24-h medical care for their son at the same time (Westendorp 1994).

The Double ABCX Model

McCubbin and Patterson (1981) elaborate on Hill's original ABCX model by extending it over time to bring longitudinal and process perspectives into the framework. According to McCubbin and Patterson, four additional factors seem to play a role in influencing the course of family adaptation to a stressor event. These include:

- Additional stressors that impinge on the situation, the AA factor, called stress pileup, such where family experiences both normative and nonnormative family events at the same time as when a father of a newborn baby is called into military service.

- Family efforts to generate new or additional resources to bring to bear on the situation, the BB factor.
- Modifications in families' perceptions and views of their situation, the CC factor.
- Family coping strategies that facilitate family adjustments and adaptations to their situation.

Here, it should be noted that different coping strategies could be viewed as the BB factor or AA factor in different situations. For example, alcohol abuse as a coping strategy may increase family strains and tensions for homeless families, thus, acting as an additional demand or stressor for them. Other coping strategies such as going into therapy or volunteering or pursuing additional education might act to alleviate such strains and tensions, thus, acting as additional resources for affected families.

- Family efforts to generate new or additional resources to bring to bear on the situation, the CC factor.
- Modifications in families' perceptions and views of their situation, the CC factor.

It is useful to note here that critics caution the need for cultural sensitivity when assessing families' definitions and perceptions of their situation as it pertains to different ethnic and racial minority families, given that what may be adaptive strategies for some families may be survival strategies for others (Dilworth-Anderson et al. 1993).

Family Coping Strategies that Facilitate Adjustments and Adaptations to the Situation

In a different formulation, coping strategies might be viewed as the BB factor – or the AA factor – in that particular coping strategies, such as alcohol abuse, may contribute to existing family strains and tensions and thus act as additional stressors. Other coping strategies, such as therapy or volunteer work, may alleviate such tensions, in which case these would be additional resources brought to bear on the situation. The denial that some families evidence during periods of natural disasters until they are able to cope with the reality of their situation could be considered similarly. Coping strategies that rely on scarce or inaccessible community resources can compound the stress families experience, the AA factor. Think of families experiencing the oil spill in the Gulf of Mexico or earthquake in Haiti and, more recently, New Zealand and Japan, or for that matter, in all countries and states suffering serious economic dislocations.

Many stories associated with the increase in the number of multi-generational households in the United States or the "doubling up" phenomenon are illustrative of the Double ABCX framework and successive stressor events and attempts to cope with them. One story in particular is that of grandparents undergoing their own financial struggles when they agreed to having their oldest daughter and her family move in with them after they lost their home to foreclosure in 2008. The grandfather subsequently lost his job in early 2009 (Luo 2010). The daughter and her family moved out just a week before another daughter and her family moved in with the grandparents. The latter daughter was laid off in 2007, taking another job only to lose that job as well. Her partner who worked as a flooring contractor lost his job in 2008. The couple looked into shelters but discovered they would not be able to stay together as a family. The daughter said that asking her parents if she and her family could move in with them was the hardest thing she ever had to do after having lived on her own since she was 18 and putting herself through community college.

Although conceding they had no other option, the young couple sometimes regretted moving in with the grandparents. For one, the garrulousness of the grandparents ran counter to the more reticent personality of the young father. Problems ranged from worrying about getting up at night to use the toilet between the parents' and grandparents' bedrooms to the undermining of parents' child-rearing decisions by the grandparents. The daughter subsequently found a job, leaving her partner and child at home with her parents to argue over child-rearing issues. As a way of coping with their situation, the couple spent most of their time in their bedroom when the daughter came home from work, with their child running in and out of the room.

The sharing of expenses was a sensitive intergenerational household issue. While the daughter's food stamps helped with grocery expenses, the couple seldom helped with other expenses, largely because they were paying off creditors and debts to family and friends. As a result of their situation and household arrangements, the young couple's relationship suffered. They argued more frequently. Their sex life, they said, was virtually nonexistent. When the daughter was promoted, receiving a small raise, the couple began to think they might be able to move into their own place. But the grandfather's unemployment benefits were scheduled to expire, leaving the grandparents with no income and exhausted savings – no financial resources. This predicament left the daughter conflicted. She wanted to leave but she also did not want to abandon her parents and compound the stressors of their situation – which could be used to illustrate not only Family Stress Theory and the Double ABCX model but family systems and exchange and choice theories as well.

Conclusion

Thus, to answer the question with which this discussion began, how can family well-being be conceptualized, it can be conceptualized in many different ways – regardless of country. Although it can be discussed nonconceptually in everyday language, the application of different conceptual frameworks allows for a more holistic and contextual approach to the question and a closer examination of the implications of the policies governments enact that affect families – and almost all they enact do – whether directly or indirectly, implicitly or explicitly, intentionally or not. Given the importance of families – regardless of form – not only for individuals but for society and its future, such an examination could facilitate the enactment of family policies that do in fact enhance the well-being of families.

References

Andrews, F. M., & Withey, S. B. (1976). *Social indicators of well-being: Americans' perceptions of life quality*. New York: Plenum.

Blau, P. (1964). *Exchange and power in social life*. New York: Wiley.

Broderick, C. B. (1993). *Understanding family process*. Newbury Park: Sage Publications.

Campbell, A., Converse, P. E., & Rodgers, W. L. (1976). *The quality of American live: Perceptions, evaluations, and satisfactions*. New York: Russell Sage.

Dilworth-Anderson, P., Burton, L., & Johnson, L. (1993). Reframing theories for understanding race, ethnicity, and families. In P. Boss, W. Doherty, R. LaRossa, W. Schumm, & S. Steinmetz (Eds.), *Sourcebook of family theories and methods: A contextual approach* (pp. 627–646). New York: Plenum.

Ekeh, P. (1974). *Social exchange theory*. Cambridge, MA: Harvard University Press.

Frankel, C. (1976). The impact of changing values on the family. *Social Casework, 57*, 355–365.

Gouldner, A. W. (1960). The norm of reciprocity. *American Sociological Review, 25*, 161–178.

Griffin, J. (1986). *Well-being: Its meaning, measurement and moral importance*. Oxford: Clarendon.

Hall, R. (1972). *Organizations: Structure and process*. Englewood Cliffs: Prentice Hall.

Herzog, A. R., Rodgers, W. L., & Woodworth, J. (1982). *Subjective well-being among different age groups*. Ann Arbor: Mi. University of Michigan, Institute for Social Research.

Hill, R. (1949). *Families under stress*. New York: Harper.

Hill, R. (1958). Generic features of families under stress. *Social Casework, 49*, 139–150.

Hill, R. (1971). Modern systems theory and the family: A confrontation. *Social Science Information, 10*, 7–26.

Inglehart, R. (1990). *Culture shift in advanced society*. Princeton: Princeton University Press.

Kamerman, S., & Kahn, A. (1978). *Family policy: Families and government in fourteen countries*. New York: Columbia University Press.

Kantor, D., & Lahr, W. (1975). *Inside the family*. New York: Harper and Row.

Koos, E. L. (1946). *Families in trouble*. New York: Kings Crown Press.

Levi-Strauss, C. (1966). The bear and the barber. *The Journal of the Royal Anthropological Institute, 93*, 1–11.

Litwak, E. (1985). *Helping the elderly: The complementary roles of informal and formal networks*. New York: Guilford.

Luo, M. (2010, December 29). Doubling up in recession-strained quarters. *New York Times*, p. A1.

McCubbin, H., & Patterson, J. M. (1981). *Systematic assessment of family stress resources and coping: Tools for research, education, and clinical intervention*. St. Paul: University of Minnesota, Family Social Science.

Mydans, S. (1994, June 21). Laotians' arrest in killing bares a generation gap. *New York Times*, p. A8.

Nye, I. (1979). Choice, exchange, and the family. In W. Burr, R. Hill, I. Nye, & I. Reiss (Eds.), *Contemporary theories about the family* (Vol. 2, pp. 1–41). New York: Free Press.

Olson, D., Sprenkle, D., & Russell, C. (1979). Circumplex model of marital and family systems: Cohesion and adaptability dimensions, family types, and clinical application. *Family Process, 18*, 3–27.

Read, K. (2011, February 13). Priceless (but with a cost). *Star Tribune*, p. O p1.

Rettig, K., & Bubolz, M. (1983). Perceptual indicators of family life quality. *Social Indicators Research, 12*(4), 417–438.

Rettig, K., Danes, S., & Bauer, J. (1991). Family life quality: Theory and assessment in economically stressed families. *Social Indicators Research, 24*, 269–299.

Roberts, S. (2010, March 22). Facing a financial pinch, and moving in with mom and dad. *New York Times*, p. A21.

Sabetelli, R., & Shehan, C. (1993). Exchange and resource theories. In P. Boss, W. Doherty, R. LaRossa, W. Schumm, & S. Steinmetz (Eds.), *Sourcebook of family theories and methods* (pp. 385–411). New York: Plenum.
Sen, A. (1980). Description as choice. *Oxford Economic Papers*, p. 32.
Sen, A. (1985). Well-being, agency, and freedom. The Dewey lectures 1984. *Journal of Philosophy, 82*, 169–221.
Terreberry, S. (1972). The evolution of organizational environments. In K. Azumi & J. Hage (Eds.), *Organizational systems* (pp. 75–91). Lexington: D.C. Heath.
Thibaut, J. W., & Kelley, H. H. (1959). *The social psychology of groups*. New York: Wiley.
Wallace, C., & Abbott, P. (2012). Social quality, the quality of life and families in Europe. In A. Moreno (Ed.), *Family well-being: European perspectives*. New York: Springer (In process).
Westendorp, K. (1994, April 30). Aaron needs family, not this cruel policy. *Star Tribune*, p. 21A.
Zimmerman, S. L. (1988). *Understanding family policy: Theoretical approaches*. Thousand Oaks: Sage Publications.
Zimmerman, S. L. (1995). *Understanding family policy: Theories and applications*. Thousand Oaks: Sage Publications.
Zimmerman, S. L. (2001). *Family policy: Constructed solutions to family problems*. Thousand Oaks: Sage Publications.

Chapter 3
Social Quality, the Quality of Life and Parents with Young Children in Europe

Pamela Abbott and Claire Wallace

Introduction

This chapter looks at the social quality of families in Europe by focussing upon parents with young children using the European Quality of Life Survey, 2007. It considers the role of employment and unemployment in modifying the quality of life for fathers and mothers in 27 European countries. The aim of this chapter is to test the applicability of the social quality model to this particular group and to look at the variation in European countries.

The quality of life has been an object of European policies as well as a topic of interest to researchers. It is seen as a way of measuring the progress of society which goes beyond economic indicators such as GDP and has been used not just by the EU and the OECD but also by the British and French governments as an indicator of progress (Stiglitz et al. 2009). It is clear that as societies grow more affluent, factors other than economic circumstances start to become more important.

Variations in the quality of life across Europe can be accounted for by social policies and by social institutions that ensure well-being (Bohnke 2006; Watson et al. 2009). Quality of life can be measured using subjective or objective measures, but is usually measured by life satisfaction or subjective well-being (how individuals feel about their lives) on the one hand or happiness, incorporating a more affective dimension, on the other (Diener and Suh 1997). Alternatively, malaise and anomie can be seen as indicators of the lack of quality of life (Watson et al. 2009).

The problem with this approach is that it depends upon a single psychologically derived indicator of well-being and it is therefore concerned with individual satisfaction rather than the situation of the society as a whole. It tends to result in an

P. Abbott (✉) • C. Wallace
School of Social Science, University of Aberdeen, Scotland, UK
e-mail: p.abbott@abdn.ac.uk; claire.wallace@abdn.ac.uk

A. Moreno Mínguez (ed.), *Family Well-Being: European Perspectives*, Social Indicators Research Series 49, DOI 10.1007/978-94-007-4354-0_3,

indefinite list of indicators, which are not theoretically derived. By developing the social quality model, we aim to construct a more sociologically informed and theoretically founded concept of well-being that can better inform us about the quality of life in comparison. We have developed this model elsewhere for Europe as a whole and have demonstrated that it is stable across time and space (Abbott and Wallace 2010; Abbott and Wallace 2011). Here we focus upon how this relates to the experiences of fathers and mothers both at work and at home.

In this chapter, we consider the role of social quality for parents. We look at life satisfaction and then societal quality generally in European societies and then go on to compute a *Model of Societal Quality* for parents of young children in order to understand how different policy frameworks impact upon them using an *Index of Societal Quality*. In this way, we can address the issue of how different aspects of society influence the well-being of parents specifically and how this differs between mothers and fathers. Is employment important for the well-being of mothers? How does it differ across Europe according to cultural norms and policy frameworks? Or are mothers happier staying at home under some circumstances?

The social quality approach arose from an initiative launched under the Dutch presidency of the European Union in 1997 by a network of social scientists. The aim was to counteract the neo-liberal and economistic tendencies within European integration and to put forward an alternative vision of a social Europe based on the EU goals of enhancing social cohesion and combating social exclusion. The aim of the social quality initiative was to develop a theoretically consistent model which could provide a basis for policies and which could be empirically grounded (Beck et al. 1997).

Social quality is defined by the authors of this initiative as 'the extent to which citizens are able to participate in the social and economic life of their communities under conditions which enhance their well-being and individual potential' (Beck et al. 2001: 6–7). Its advocates were concerned to challenge what they saw as the narrowly economistic focus of European social policy with its emphasis on employment as the key to social inclusion, economic growth and competitiveness and argue for a social policy that sustained a liveable society for all (Beck et al. 2001).

In the EU 27, there are marked differences between countries in subjective well-being with a North–South divide in the EU 15 and a marked East–West divide between the EU 15 and the former communist states that are now members. However, in all EU countries, the impact of economic factors is mediated by other factors, notably social support, health and trust (Fahey and Smyth 2004; Bohnke 2006; Watson 2009).

Social quality assumes that well-being is fundamentally concerned with the welfare of societies as well as individuals. The former provides the context in which individuals are able to flourish and grow – the capability structure. Therefore, we need to consider the opportunities that society provides for individuals to build their capabilities and the resources that are available for them to utilise in securing their welfare. We might assume that the higher the quality of a society, the more options

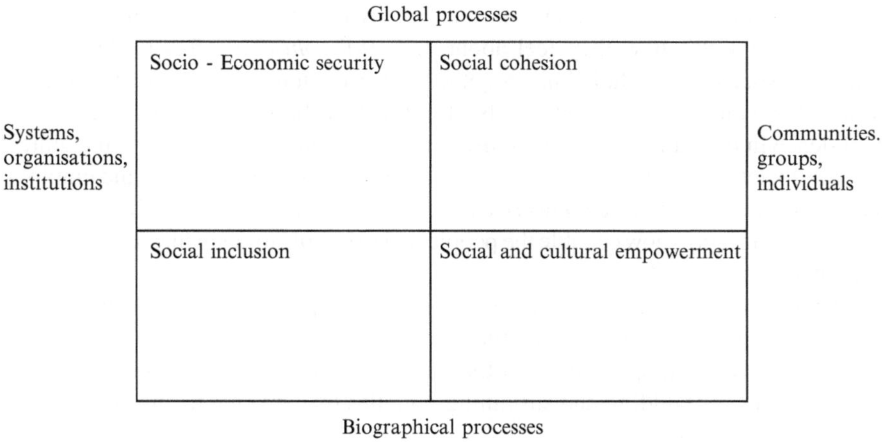

Fig. 3.1 The social quality model

people have to arrange their lives and therefore the more satisfied they will be. However, there are also differences within societies: individuals' perception of the quality of their society is also influenced by their own social status and living conditions (Bohnke 2006). Therefore, agency and the ability to build capabilities are dependent on social and geographical location as well as individuals' perceptions of the opportunities available to them.

The social quality approach does focus on the individual, but as an active subject in a social context. It is concerned with the dialectical and recursive relationship between agency and structure and provides a vision for the future about how the social quality of a society can and should be improved. It provides the essential link between context, action and policies. The social quality approach combines economic and social development by measuring the extent to which the quality of daily life provides for an acceptable standard of living, taking account of the structural features of societies and their institutions as assessed by reference to their impact on citizens. Hence, it incorporates a mixture of structural and individual-level factors, of economic and social dimensions.

Social quality identifies four domains or areas: economic security, social cohesion, social inclusion and social empowerment. They can be illustrated in the diagram below (Fig. 3.1). These are expressed as four quadrants which are the product of the relationship between global processes and biographical processes on the one hand and that between systems and institutions and between communities (Gesellschaft and Gemeinschaft) on the other. The up–down axis of the quadrant represents the relationship between the micro and the macro, the individual and the structural. The left–right axis of the social quality quadrant represents the relationship between system and community, between 'system integration' and 'social integration' in the words of David Lockwood (1992).

Economic security refers not only to income but to how the individual perceives their economic security overall and their release from the day-to-day anxiety of poverty.

Hence, variables need to take into account the living standard of the individual or household and also how they feel about it. *Social cohesion* refers to the way in which the society as a whole knits together at a structural level. Variables for measuring this would include trust, levels of conflict in the society and the extent of confidence in institutions. *Social inclusion* refers to how the individual is integrated into the society through social networks, membership of organisations and employment. *Social and cultural empowerment* is underpinned by good health and education but also refers to how capable the people feel to be able to act in their environment (Nussbaum and Sen 1993).

The social quality model is then concerned to specify the conditions for an inclusive, socially cohesive society that empowers citizens who can enjoy a decent standard of living. It specifies both the conditions for individual well-being and the conditions for building and sustaining societies that are able to ensure the well-being of their members.

Therefore, social quality represents an advance on quality of life approaches because it is more theoretically grounded, because it looks at the social and not just the individual dimensions and because it includes a measure of agency by allowing for social and cultural empowerment. One question might be: which of these quadrants is the most important? In fact, social quality emphasises all parts of the quadrant because it is concerned with the space that this covers. It also enables us to theoretically derive indicators to correlate with subjective life satisfaction by providing a sound basis for selecting indicators. The indicators themselves are measures of the underlying concepts of economic security, social cohesion, social integration and empowerment.

We have already demonstrated that life satisfaction in the contexts as varied as the Commonwealth of Independent States and London is influenced by economic security, social cohesion, social integration and empowerment (Abbott and Sapsford 2006; Abbott 2007; Abbott and Wallace 2011). More recently, we have derived a model from social quality and used it to examine influences on life satisfaction in the EU 27. Using the 2003 and 2007 Living Conditions and Quality of Life Survey, we have demonstrated that our model is stable over time and space. Subjective quality of life is influenced by economic security, social cohesion, social integration and empowerment. For the EU 27, we are able to explain over 40% of the variance in subjective satisfaction.

By constructing an index of societal quality, we can also compare social groups within a given nation as well as comparing societies, and it is to this issue that we now turn.

Societal Quality for Parents

In this chapter, we construct a multidimensional *Index of Societal Quality* using indicators derived from the *European Quality of Life Survey (EQLS)* carried out in all EU countries in 2007. We select indicators for the four domains of the social quality model and then combine the indicators for the four domains to construct a single index of societal quality. This enables us to determine how societal quality varies across the countries of the EU.

Whilst our social quality model (as we have developed it) looks at different dimensions of the quality of society, it can be validated by considering how much it contributes to subjective well-being as a measure of the quality of life at an individual level. We would expect societies with high societal quality to have high levels of life satisfaction. Hence, we would expect people to be dissatisfied if they are not able to enjoy a decent standard of living, do not have confidence in the government and lack general trust, lack social support and feel lonely, and feel unable to take control over their own lives – or though poor health and lack of education lack the capacity to do so. We might expect this to differ between women and men given their differences on these various dimensions.

Family policies vary across Europe, with one of the key differences being the extent to which they support the traditional male breadwinner family or provide support for families where both parents work (Lewis 1992; Daly and Rake 2003; Pfau-Effinger 2005). This distinction is especially critical for parents with very young children. Norms also vary between societies with some reinforcing a traditional gendered division of labour and others being more supportive of both parents having paid employment. We might therefore expect parents to experience the quality of society rather differently from non-parents. We might also expect mothers to experience the social space for action in a society differently from fathers although it is not always clear is the extent to which mothers' (and indeed fathers') expression of preferences is constrained by what is thought to be possible as opposed to being what they would opt for in an ideal world.

The extent to which parents are at home or at work might also affect their social quality. Mothers who stay at home might be expected to suffer greater economic insecurity, to be less integrated into society and to have few possibilities to act on their lives, therefore having lower levels of social and cultural empowerment. Men who stay at home might suffer even more dramatically from this loss of social quality. However, there may be differences across societies as men are encouraged to behave as full-time fathers during parental leave in some countries (notably Sweden) but would find this more difficult in others, where the male breadwinner model has been more the norm (such as Italy). Women from these latter societies might also be more comfortable about leaving the labour market.

Our construction of the *Index of Societal Quality* is constrained by the data that is available, and whilst it is a general model rather than one that includes specific indicators that might additionally structure the social space for parents, it does enable us to identify those societies that seem to provide societal quality for parents and those that do not. It also, of course, gives us a greater understanding of what it is that provides for societal quality beyond economic well-being. It provides the basis for beginning to think about how to construct a society that meets the needs of mothers and fathers and what types of policies will enable them to live satisfying and fulfilling lives whilst they are providing for the economic support and care of their families.

Data

The 2007 European Quality of Life Survey serves as the database for the empirical analysis. In our analysis, we use the data for the 27 member states of the EU a total of 30,626 respondents. The data and a number of publications describing the findings from the survey can be found on the web site of the European Foundation for the Improvement of Living and Working Conditions (http://www.eurofound.europe.eu/). More information on methods and the variables we use can also be found in these publications.[1]

Methods

We consider the extent to which the elements that make up societal quality vary between the countries in general, and for parents with dependent children in particular, by constructing an *Index of Societal Quality*. To do this, we construct a societal quality model which we 'validate' by regressing against subjective satisfaction as the ultimate outcome indicator of individual well-being (Land et al. 2006; Richardson et al. 2008) (we have previously tested the model for stability using the 2003 and 2007 European Quality of Life data set, Abbott and Wallace 2012). We then create a standardised index using the selected indicators. The stages of our analysis are to:

1. Look at the influences on subjective satisfaction by running a series of OLS regression with subjective satisfaction as the dependent variable with the initially selected indicators for each quadrant of the model. This enables us to determine which variables make a significant contribution to explaining variance in satisfaction, i.e. what makes people more or less satisfied with their lives.
2. Run an OLS regression using the enter method (i.e. putting all the variables in at the same time) using all the variables that were significant in the regressions for each quadrant controlling for age and gender.
3. Re-run the regression analysis used at stage 2 controlling for parents and then controlling for country to enable us to see if our model held for parents and if it held for each country, i.e. was it a general model or did it only hold for some groups in society and or some countries.
4. Construct the *Index of Societal Quality* using the variables that contributed significantly to the regression at stage 2. To do this, we recoded all the variables so that they went from poor to high quality, then normalised the variables using the Z statistic and then computed the index using the Z statistic.

[1] We have not provided detailed tables showing the values for all the variables we use for each country. The interested reader can find details in the publications on the foundation's web site.

5. Use analysis of variance to consider how societal quality varies across Europe controlling for country, for men and women, parents and non-parents, for those in employment and not and for different age groups.

In constructing the model, we have selected as indicators variables from a rich data set as indicative of the underlying constructs we are measuring. We were also using data that had not been specifically collected for our purpose, and there were no good indicators of bridging capital, something which is an important indicator of social integration. We tested the model for multicollinearity and found it to be satisfactory as the tolerance of no variable was below 0.4. The levels of single-order correlations between the dependent and independent variable were also tested and found to be acceptable. Scales were computed using principal components analysis with varimax rotation and Cronbach's alpha calculated for each scale. The CAs were all adequate for the number of variables in each scale as no CA was below 0.75.

We computed four scales to use in our analysis, conflict, deprivation and mental health (based upon the one used by the World Health Organization) and housing (the scales were recoded after being computed so that the lowest value was one on the mental health and conflict scales and zero on the deprivation scale to make interpretation easier):

- The conflict scale was computed from the answers to whether or not tension exists between poor and rich, management and workers, men and women and different racial and ethnic groups (CA 0.75). The mean on the conflict scale for the EU 27 was 5.79 on an 11-point scale with 1 being high social conflict and 11 being low (Table 3.1). The society with the highest levels of perceived conflict was Hungary (mean 2.14) and that with the lowest Denmark (mean 7.21). There was no clear pattern in terms of high and low conflict societies in terms of Eastern and Western Europe, Northern and Southern Europe or welfare regimes.
- The deprivation scale was computed from whether or not the following items could be afforded: keeping the home adequately warm; paying for a week's holiday away from home; replacing worn-out furniture; a meal with meat, chicken or fish every second day; buying new cloths and having friends or family for a drink or meal at least once a month (CA 0.827). The scale went from nought (can afford none of the items) to six (can afford all). The EU mean on the deprivation scale was 4.81 and ranged from Bulgaria with a mean of 2.9 to Sweden with a mean of 5.73 (Table 3.2). There was a clear pattern with all the Northern European countries and Italy, Spain and Slovenia being above the mean and the other Southern European countries and the Central European ones being below the mean. There was also a tendency for the SDs to be larger in the Southern and Central European countries than in the Western ones.
- The mental health scale was computed from the experience of the following symptoms over the past two weeks: all the time, most of the time, more than half the time, less than half the time, some of the time or at no time – 'felt cheerful and in good spirit', 'felt calm and relaxed, felt active and vigorous', 'wake up feeling fresh and rested' and 'daily life filled with things of interest' (0.875). The scale went from 1 poor mental health to 26 excellent mental health (Table 3.2).

Table 3.1 Descriptive statistics of scales and key variables

Country										
Means	Mental health scale		Conflict scale		Deprivation scale		Trust in government		Trust in people in general	
Range	1–26 poor to good		1–11 high to low		0–6 afford none to afford all		1–10 low to high		1–10 low to high	
	Mean	SD	Mean	SD	Mean	SD	Mean	SD	Mean	SD
Austria	16.01	4.72	5.88	2.14	5.4	1.29	5.69	2.2	4.8	2.39
Belgium	17.37	4.78	5.59	2.02	5.33	1.28	5.01	2.26	5.57	2.22
Bulgaria	14.62	5.63	6.86	2.18	2.9	2.03	3.31	2.3	4.04	2.13
Cyprus	14.78	5.95	6.88	2.06	4.42	1.63	5.69	2.79	2.51	2.05
Czech Republic	16.16	4.63	5.45	2.20	4.76	1.65	3.62	2.39	4.51	2.4
Denmark	18.00	4.65	7.21	1.91	5.66	0.93	6.62	2.22	7.0	2.31
Estonia	15.16	4.92	5.87	1.89	4.52	1.65	5.61	2.53	5.23	2.39
Finland	17.22	3.84	6.18	1.77	5.6	0,89	6.56	2.09	7.0	1.9
France	16.49	4.91	4.96	2.02	5.34	1.67	5.12	2.26	5.49	1.9
Germany	17.75	4.53	5.35	2.16	5.16	1.44	4.81	2.44	4.82	2.42
UK	16.1	5.3	5.75	2.09	5.36	1.28	4.29	2.41	5.29	2.36
Greece	15.66	5.51	5.63	2.54	4.30	1.88	4.79	2.77	4.15	2.37
Hungary	16.41	4.96	4.13	2.14	3.58	1.88	3.41	2.44	4.63	2.28
Ireland	17.67	4.79	6.45	2.29	5.48	1.94	4.79	2.56	5.77	2.39
Italy	15.58	4.78	5.27	2.27	5.27	1.36	3.84	2.16	4.95	1.93

Latvia	14.6	5.32	6.63	2.2	3.86	1.89	3.26	2.34	4.13	2.45
Lithuania	14.88	5.32	5.64	2.21	3.64	1.94	3.91	2.49	4.31	2.46
Luxembourg	16.98	5.17	5.3	2.4	5.7	0.79	6.09	2.32	5.84	2.02
Malta	14.18	5.22	6.61	2.39	4.35	1.67	5.5	2.78	4.91	2.4
The Netherlands	17.77	4.27	5.6	1.58	5.69	0.9	5.88	1.83	6.53	1.91
Poland	15.43	5.72	5.85	2.1	4.01	1.93	3.53	2.26	4.77	2.24
Romania	14.09	5.97	5.65	2.75	3.34	2.08	4.32	2.49	5.54	2.1
Slovakia	15.28	5.11	6.12	2.22	3.96	1.96	4.91	2.49	4.98	2.35
Slovenia	15.74	4.88	5.14	2.0	5.11	1.45	4.14	2.43	5.18	2.47
Spain	17.17	4.87	5.66	2.61	5.33	1.18	5.39	2.15	5.74	2.16
Sweden	17.76	4.62	6.02	1.67	5.73	0.82	5.72	2.43	6.78	2.30
Portugal	15.61	6.11	6.34	2.53	4.69	1.61	4.27	2.14	4.25	2.09
Mean EU 27	16.14	5.19	5.79	3.8	4.81	1.7	4.78	2.56	5.12	2.43
CA computed scales	0.875		0.745		0.827					

Total number of respondents 30,626

Table 3.2 Descriptive statistics

Country							
	Good/very good health	Finances manage fairly easily/easily/ very easily	Employed	Parent of child under 16 years	Married	Help available Ill	Help available borrow money
Percentage	%	%	%	%	%	%	%
Austria	68.6	72.7	57.6	28.8	61.0	98.2	88.5
Belgium	64.7	66.3	47.5	29.0	65.7	97.9	83.2
Bulgaria	41.7	16.0	46.0	23.0	66.4	95.7	76.3
Cyprus	65.2	43.4	46.9	24.2	74.3	98.5	89.0
Czech Republic	60.2	51.0	55.4	21.8	65.0	98.5	85.8
Denmark	66.3	85.9	48.9	22.1	59.5	98.8	84.7
Estonia	39.2	49.2	47.1	17.1	49.5	96.3	76.2
Finland	61.7	79.5	46.5	24.2	64.8	99.2	90.6
France	70.3	62.8	47.9	29	65.5	98.1	83.1
Germany	65.1	72.5	46.4	22.0	62.4	97.5	82.4
UK	64.5	77.8	45.3	22.9	56.3	97.2	81.1
Greece	72.2	33.4	44.1	21.7	58.0	97.9	94.3
Hungary	47.6	25.2	38.9	21.4	54.9	97.7	68.9
Ireland	80.7	76.4	50.0	27.7	53.3	98.0	87.7
Italy	73.8	57.3	54.6	26.0	58.6	97.4	87.7

Latvia	39.4	36.7	61.4	23.4	50.0	95.9	77.0
Lithuania	35.0	36.3	45.5	19.2	52.2	97.5	86.2
Luxembourg	64.5	84.6	46.0	27.2	68.9	98.0	87.5
Malta	58.7	63.9	44.5	25.2	63.5	99.0	88.2
The Netherlands	66.1	86.7	59.7	30.2	67.8	97.9	81.4
Poland	53.8	46.7	39.9	25.3	63.3	97.4	79.3
Romania	50.9	28.4	44.4	19.9	64.6	98.0	77.3
Slovakia	55.6	50.0	50.8	19.3	59.5	99.3	83.9
Slovenia	55.3	58.9	39.9	14.6	57.9	99.1	93.7
Spain	72.8	58.6	44.6	19.8	62.7	97.4	84.5
Sweden	65.7	86.0	62.4	29.6	70.3	99.2	92.9
Portugal	53.5	65.4	51.3	20.3	59.4	95.4	68.6
EU 27	60.9	58.6	48.2	23.4	61.3	97.8	83.6

Total number of respondents 30,626

The EU 27 mean was 16.14 varying from 14.09 in Romania to 18 in Denmark. Although the pattern is not as clear as for the deprivation scale on the whole, the Northern European countries have the best mental health and the Central European ones the poorest.

- The housing scale was computed from the answers to the following: 'do you lack an indoor flushing toilet' and 'do you lack a bath or shower', coded yes/no (CA 0.847).

The descriptive statistics regarding scales can be found in Tables 3.1 and 3.2.

The Dependent Variable

The dependent variable in the regression analysis was the satisfaction scale – 'All things considered how satisfied would you say you are with your life these days?' – coded 1 (least satisfied) to 10 (most satisfied).

Levels of satisfaction with life vary widely across Europe (Table 3.3) with a North–South and West–East slope. The highest levels of satisfaction are found in Northern Europe with the highest of all in Scandinavia and the lowest levels in East and Central Europe with Bulgaria having noticeable the lowest. Portugal, Greece and Italy have much lower levels of satisfaction than the other EU 15 countries, amongst the lowest in Europe (although Italy's level is somewhat lower than might be expected from other surveys, as is Austria's). Slovenia at rank 12 (mean 7.15) has a level of general satisfaction that places it with the Northwestern European countries, but it is the exception amongst the post-communist countries. Slovenia as we saw above is also comparable to the Northwestern European countries in terms of deprivation. It has an extensive welfare state and has exceptionally good provision for parents of young children in the form of affordable childcare, approaching that of Sweden (Wallace 2003) (see www.hwf.at). Parents are generally slightly more satisfied, even after controlling for age, with the notable exception of those in Denmark, UK, Ireland and Portugal where they are generally less satisfied. However, the differences are relatively small.

Modelling the Quality of Society

We first did a regression for each quadrant of the societal quality model.

Economic Security

As indicators of economic security, we used the following variables:

- The deprivation scale – a computed scale from 0 able to afford none to 6 can afford all items
- The housing scale – a computed scale from 0 neither to 3 both

Table 3.3 Satisfaction European Union 2007

	Satisfaction								
	All			<65 + no kids			<65 + kids <16 years		
Country	Mean	SD	Rank	Mean	SD	Rank	Mean	SD	Rank
Austria	6.84	2.162	15	6.78	2.155	15	7.05	2.171	16
Belgium	7.51	1.739	8	7.49	1.71	7	7.55	1.810	7
Bulgaria	4.90	2.013	27	4.74	2.00	27	5.45	1.962	26
Cyprus	7.05	2.217	14	6.96	2.229	14	7.32	2.162	11
Czech Republic	6.52	2.121	18	6.48	2.12	18	6.68	2.121	=21
Denmark	8.47	1.715	1	8.53	1.72	1	8.26	1.684	3
Estonia	6.65	1.950	17	6.60	1.986	17	6.89	1.753	17
Finland	8.17	1.359	3	8.12	1.393	3	8.33	1.235	2
France	7.25	1.717	10	7.20	1.730	10	7.37	1.680	10
Germany	7.09	2.287	13	7.04	2.297	13	7.24	2.245	13
UK	7.27	2.039	9	7.31	2.037	9	7.16	2.046	14
Greece	6.51	2.069	21	6.42	2.078	22	6.82	2.010	18
Hungary	5.51	2.250	26	5.48	2.239	26	5.61	2.294	25
Ireland	7.59	1.892	6	7.63	1.095	6	7.49	1.856	8
Italy	6.48	1.823	21	6.44	1.824	20	6.60	1.816	23
Latvia	6.03	2.154	24	5.97	2.156	25	6.24	2.138	24
Lithuania	6.20	2.124	23	6.08	2.154	23	6.68	1.963	=21
Luxembourg	7.96	1.819	4	7.94	1.856	4	8.0	1.717	4
Malta	7.54	1.972	7	7.48	2.035	8	7.70	1.764	6
The Netherlands	7.87	1.235	5	7.82	1.264	5	7.98	1.160	5
Poland	6.79	2.079	16	6.69	2.133	16	7.10	1.881	15
Romania	6.46	2.058	22	6.40	2.059	21	6.70	2.039	20
Slovakia	6.56	2.041	18	6.50	2.057	19	6.81	1.958	19

(continued)

Table 3.3 (continued)

	Satisfaction								
	All			<65 + no kids			<65 + kids <16 years		
Country	Mean	SD	Rank	Mean	SD	Rank	Mean	SD	Rank
Slovenia	7.15	1.952	12	7.12	1.966	12	7.29	1.864	12
Spain	7.23	1.760	11	7.18	1.739	11	7.42	1.834	9
Sweden	8.35	1.630	2	8.28	1.706	2	8.53	1.422	1
Portugal	6.12	1.998	25	6.00	1.844	24	5.0	2.001	27
Mean EU 27	7.36	6.386		6.92	2.134		7.20	2.008	

Total number of respondents 30,626

Table 3.4 Regression economic security

	B	Beta	SE
Constant	2.034		.134
HH income	3.278E-5	.041**	.000
Deprivation scale	.288	.236**	.010
Make ends meet	.455	.284**	.013
Food	.320	.047**	.046
Housing	.162	.063**	.017
R2.282			

Total number of respondents 30,626
**$P<0.001$

- The answers to the question *Is your household able to make ends meet*, coded on a 6-point scale from very easily to with great difficulty
- If the household had run out of money to pay for food during last 12 months, coded yes/no
- Household income in euros PPP

The economic security indicators explained just over 28% of the variance with all the variables being significant at the 99.9% level (Table 3.4). The largest contribution to the variance explained was made by the inability to make ends meet followed by the deprivation scale, inability to afford food and poor housing made modest but significant contributions to the variance explained. Income made a significant but weak contribution. This suggests, in line with other research findings (e.g. Bohnke 2008), that satisfaction does not increase in a linear relationship with income but rather that there is a point beyond which increases in income do not lead to increases in general satisfaction. What seems to be important for satisfaction is having an adequate income for an acceptable standard of living.

Societal Cohesion

To measure societal cohesion, we used the following variables:

- The answer to a question on the extent to which people can be trusted – a 10-point scale from low to high
- The answer to a question on trust in government – a 10-point scale from low to high
- The conflict scale – an 11-point computed scale from high to low conflict

All three of the societal cohesion variables made a significant contribution together explaining just over 14% of the variance. General trust in people and trust in government contributed equally and strongly. The conflict scale made a modest but significant contribution (Table 3.5).

Table 3.5 Regression societal cohesion

	B	Beta	SE
Constant	4.793		.041
General trust	.189	.220**	.005
Trust in government	.180	.220**	.005
Conflict scale	.066	.072**	.005
R2.143			

Total number of respondents 30,626
**P<0.001

Social Integration

To measure social integration, we used the following variables:

- Attended a meeting of a trade union/political party/political action group in last year
- Voted in last national election, coded did not vote/voted
- Feel left out of society, coded on a five-point scale coded from strongly agree to strongly disagree
- Marital status, coded not married/married
- Face-to-face contact with children, parents and friends/neighbours living outside household, coded less than once a week/at least once a week
- Non-face-to-face contact with children, parents and friends/neighbours living outside household, coded less than once a week/at least once a week
- Support and advise when ill, depressed and need money urgently, coded no/yes
- Employed, coded no/yes

The social integration indicators together explained 18.3% of the variance (Table 3.6). In terms of social integration, feeling left out made by far the greatest contribution with being able to borrow money and being married making noticeable contributions. Support when ill, being in contact with children and parents, voting and attending meetings of trade unions/political parties were all significant at the 99.9% level but made very modest contributions to the variance explained.

Conditions for Empowerment

To measure conditions for empowerment, we used the following variables:

- The mental health scale – a computed scale coded from 1 to 26 with 1 being the poorest mental health and 26 the best
- The answer to a question on how complicated life is coded on a five-point scale coded from strongly agree 'life is so complicated you cannot find the way' to strongly disagree
- Subjective health coded on a five-point scale from very good to very bad
- Highest level of education (lower secondary or less, upper secondary, post-secondary non-higher, higher education)

Table 3.6 Regression social integration

	B	Beta	SE
Constant	2.437		.175
Support when ill	.614	.042**	.081
Support advice	.157	.013*	.067
Help depressed	.094	.010	.054
Support money	.578	.101**	.032
Married	.403	.093**	.024
Contact parents	−.096	−.021**	.030
Contact children	−.137	−.032**	.030
Contact friends	.077	.014*	.029
Communication parent	.183	.042**	.030
Communication kids	.104	.025**	.030
Communication friends	.102	.004	.133
Feel left out	.730	.345**	.011
Vote	.282	.055**	.027
Going to meetings, TU etc.	−.183	−.027**	.036
Employed	.032	.008	.024
R2.183			

Total number of respondents 30,626
*P<0.01; **P<0.001

Table 3.7 Regression conditions for empowerment

	B	Beta	SE
Constant	2.015		.057
Mental health	.115	.282**	.002
Life complicated	.545	.302**	.010
Health	.230	.104**	.012
Education	.136	.037**	.019
R^2 .281			

Total number of respondents 30,626
**P<0.001

The four indicators for conditions for empowerment together explained 28% of the variance, the same as the economic indicators (Table 3.7). Mental health and life being too complicated made the largest contribution with subjective health making a smaller but noticeable one. Education was significant at the 99.9% level but only made a very modest contribution to the variance explained.

We then carried out a regression including all the variables that were significant for each quadrant. We also controlled for age and gender (Table 3.8). The total variance explained was 44.3% which suggests that we have a model with strong explanatory powers. Age was not significant at the 99.9% level and although gender was, the Beta was very low. The significant variables at the 99.9% level (the cut-off point we set for inclusion in the Index of Societal Quality) were the following: the deprivation scale, not being able to make ends meet, housing deprivation, trust in other people, trust in government, the conflict scale, support when ill, able to borrow money, married, feeling included, the mental health scale, life being too complicated

Table 3.8 Subjective satisfaction (OLS regression) 2007

	Model			Controlling for parent			Controlling for country		
Variables	B	Beta	SE	B	Beta	SE	B	Beta	SE
Constant	5.878		.343	5.870		.342	16.931		1.893
Age	.002	.016	.001	.003	.024*	.001	.003	.021	.015
Gender	.152	.036**	.026	.138	.033**	.026	.139	.033**	.025
Economic									
HH income	.000	–.003	.000	.000	–.002	.000	.000	–.008	.000
Deprivation scale	–.152	–.122**	.010	–.153	–.123**	.010	–.125	–.101**	.010
Make ends meet	–.244	–.153**	.013	–.248	–.156**	.013	–.210	–.132**	.013
Food	.139	.020*	.045	.142	.020*	.045	.246	.035**	.045
Housing	.091	–.34**	.017	.092	.035**	.017	.098	.037**	.017
Societal cohesion									
General trust	.078	.91**	.006	.078	.090**	.006	.064	.074**	.006
Trust in government	.096	.116**	.005	.095	.115*	.005	.076	.092**	.005
Conflict scale	.021	.022**	.006	.021	.023**	.006	.009	.010	..006
Social integration									
Support ill	.059	.032**	.105	.520	.032**	.105	.461	.028**	.103
Support advice	.059	.005	.080	.059	.005	.080	.101	.008	.079
Support money	.191	.031**	.039	.191	.031**	.039	.160	.026**	.038
Married	.307	.071**	.027	.259	.060**	.028	.253	.058**	.027
Contact parents	–.021	–.005	.034	–.028	–.006	.034	–.006	–.001	.034
Contact children	.010	.002	.034	.003	.001	.034	.049	.011	.034
Contact friends	.023	.004	.033	–.028	–.006	.033	.082	.015	.032
Communication parent	.001	.000	.034	–.010	–.002	.034	–.007	–.002	.034
Communication kids	.071	.017	.036	.092	.022*	.036	.065	.015	.036
Feel left out	.224	.107**	.015	.223	.107**	.015	.240	.115**	.015
Vote	.113	.021*	.034	.114	.021*	.034	.068	.013	.033
Meeting TU, etc.	.009	.001	.039	.007	.001	.039	.008	.001	.039

Empowerment									
Mental health	–.081	–.194**	.003	–.081	–.195**	.003	–.086	–.207**	.003
Life complicated	.226	.126**	.013	.225	.125**	.013	.227	.126**	.013
Health	–.151	–069**	.016	–.056	–.015	.024	–.130	–.059**	.016
Education	–.050	–.014	.024	–.146	–.067**	.016	–.088	–.024**	.025
Parent				187	.039**	.033	.0122	.025**	.032
Countries									
Belgium							–122	.025	.032
Denmark							–.117	–.012	.069
Germany							.762	.097**	.058
Greece							.728	.069**	.071
Spain							.680	.050**	.085
France							.301	.034**	.062
Ireland							.184	.012	.095
Italy							.577	.044**	.084
Luxembourg							.156	.012	.088
The Netherlands							.302	.030**	.069
Austria							.707	.057**	.079
Portugal							1.114	.074**	.094
Finland							–.035	–.013	.069
Great Britain							.205	.020	.070
Cyprus							.066	.006	.091
Czech Republic							.496	.048**	.085
Estonia							.533	.048**	.087
Hungary							1.0103	.119**	.076
Latvia							.580	.046**	.096
Lithuania							.452	.039**	.090
Malta							–.073	–.005	.096
Poland							–.016	–.001	.086

(continued)

Table 3.8 (continued)

	Model			Controlling for parent			Controlling for country		
Variables	B	Beta	SE	B	Beta	SE	B	Beta	SE
Slovakia							.475	.044**	.086
Slovenia							.195	.017	.087
Bulgaria							1.182	.089**	.102
Romania							.185	.016	.092
R^2 adjusted	.433			.434			.459		

Sweden = reference country
**$P<0.001$; *$P<0.01$
Total number of respondents 30,626

and health (see above). The conditions for empowerment variables made the largest contribution, followed by the economic variables, followed by the societal cohesion variables with the inclusion variables making the smallest contribution. Not being able to afford to buy food and voting made significant contributions at the 99.9% level, but the Betas were very low.

We then carried out the regression putting in parent as a dummy variable. The variance explained did not change indicating that the model applies to parents as well as non-parents equally. Finally, we entered the countries as dummy variables with Sweden as the reference country. The variance explained increased significantly to just under than 46%, and whilst some of the countries made a significant contribution, the Betas were very modest although slightly stronger for Hungary and Bulgaria where general satisfaction would seem to be somewhat lower than would be predicted by the model. We, therefore, concluded that our model was a general one.

Index of Societal Quality

As the final stage of analysis, we computed the *Index of Societal Quality*. The variables that we used to compute the *Index* were those that were significant at the 99.9% level when the regression analysis was carried out for the whole model: These were for:

- Economic security, deprivation scale and housing scale
- Societal cohesion, most people can be trusted; trust in the government; and conflict scale
- Societal integration: feel left out of society, marital status, support when ill and support when needing money urgently, coded no/yes
- Conditions for empowerment, mental health scale; life is so complicated you cannot find way and self-reported health status

Variations in Societal Quality in Europe

The *Index for Societal Quality* across the EU showed the Nordic countries have the highest societal quality and the Eastern and Central European countries the lowest. In those countries that are above average, men have higher societal quality than women, but in those below average, women have higher societal quality than men. The order of the countries remains the same for parents. However, we can see differences between mothers and fathers on the *Index of Societal Quality* (Fig. 3.2). We can see that in the Nordic countries plus the Netherlands and Luxembourg, all parents, mothers and fathers, employed and unemployed have an above EU average for the *Index of Societal Quality*. In all countries except Luxembourg, employed fathers have the highest *Index*, and in all of these countries with the exception for four Central European countries, Poland, Lithuania, Hungary and Bulgaria, the

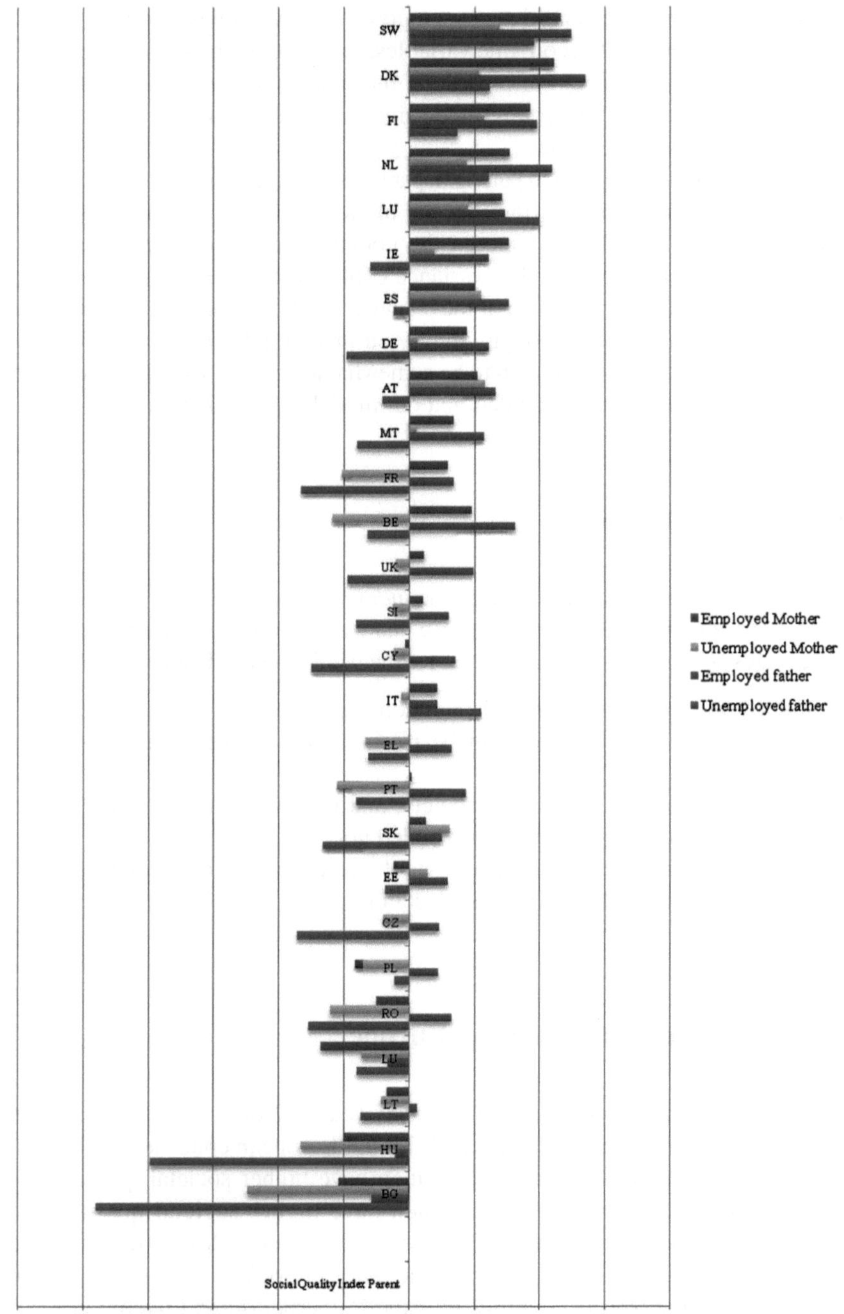

Fig. 3.2 Index of social quality for parents in EU 27, 2007

score is above the EU mean for all parents. Unemployed fathers have a lower score than employed fathers in all countries except Luxembourg and a lower score than employed mothers except in Malta and Lithuania. In all the countries except Austria, Spain, Estonia, Romania, Hungary and Bulgaria, mothers in paid employment have a higher score than mothers who are not employed.

Discussion

Considering the analysis of the *Index of Societal Quality*, we can conclude that country differences are important, although the country differences are similar to those we found in looking at life satisfaction. Therefore, the quality of society, as measured by the *Index of Societal Quality*, helps to produce satisfied people. However, we are now in a position to understand more clearly *why* they are satisfied.

A second important finding is that there were differences for men and for women, with men on the whole having higher societal quality than women. We could hypothesise that fathers' levels of economic security, inclusion and – most importantly – their empowerment are greater.

A third important finding was that the employment status of men and women made an important difference to their social quality. In general, employed fathers scored more highly than non-employed fathers in all countries. Employment was clearly essential for the social quality of fathers, which means that stay-at-home fathers would find it very difficult to manage if they were the ones looking after children. Employed fathers generally scored higher than employed mothers, which suggests that whilst employment is important for mothers, it was still more important for fathers.

For mothers, there was a much more mixed picture. Non-employed mothers generally scored higher than non-employed fathers, indicating that for them staying at home to care for children was not as negative for their social quality as it was for men. The gap between scores for employed and non-employed fathers was much higher than for employed and non-employed mothers, which indicates that for women employment whilst being a mother was not enormously different caring full time for children.

However, in some countries, non-employed mothers scored higher than employed ones so that entering the labour force does not uniformly improve the conditions and satisfaction of mothers with small children.

When we turn to country differences, we find that societal quality was highest for employed fathers in Nordic countries and lowest for unemployed men in Central and Eastern Europe. Unemployment therefore hits fathers differently depending upon where they live. The lack of social security and the low level of benefits in Central and Eastern Europe as well as an ideological commitment to a 'male breadwinner role' whilst children were young are important in this respect.

The countries where non-employed mothers scored more highly than employed mothers (or not much lower) were the ones where family policy encourages women to take on a full-time caring role and have intermittent attachment to the labour market. Countries where family policy encourages women to have paid employment are ones where employed mothers score more highly than unemployed mothers and the gap is relatively large.

Conclusions

The analysis has shown that societal quality is a good predictor of life satisfaction for both parents and non-parents alike, although societal quality was a little higher amongst parents than amongst non-parents. The societal quality of employed and non-employed mothers and fathers did vary according to the work-care regime of the country. In all countries, employed fathers had the highest societal quality, whilst for employed mothers, this varied according to whether the norm was for them to return fairly soon to full-time work or whether they lived in a country where extended periods of leave for childcare were more usual. Therefore, societal quality is shaped by the policy environment.

Combining, as we have the social quality approach with measuring what is important in determining individual life satisfaction, we can consider what social policy needs to encompass if it is both to meet individual needs and underpin the development of competitive, dynamic societies. Social quality provides the basis for a meta-theory for developing public policy and for its implementation – for the practice of public policy. In this respect, labour market as well as income maintenance policies are important for fostering economic security and social integration of individuals into the society. Economic policy is concerned with allowing independence, labour market policy with opening ways for participation and social policy with securing dignity and fostering solidarity. The policy context shapes societal quality by providing socio-economic security or social inclusion or by providing the basis for social and cultural empowerment.

Our analysis indicates that a society delivers societal quality when citizens have sufficient income to enjoy a decent standard of living, can place trust in people generally and in government, feel that they are integrated into society, have good physical and mental health and feel empowered to take control over their lives. From the point of view of parents, it is important that policies allow them to integrate work and care, but this is more important in some societies than in others and impacts differently upon mothers and fathers. The analysis shows that it is important to take into account not just individual but also societal aspects of well-being, which can be analysed using the social quality model.

References

Abbott, P. (2007). Social quality, quality of life and happiness in London. In *Global metropolitan forum, assessing happiness and competitiveness in major world metropolises*. Seoul.

Abbott, P., & Sapsford, R. (2006). Happiness and general satisfaction in post-soviet Russia and Ukraine. *Journal of Communist Studies and Transition Politics, 23*, 181–2002.

Abbott, P., & Wallace, C. (2010). Explaining economic and social transformations in post-Soviet Russia, Ukraine and Belarus. *European Societies, 12*, 653–674.

Abbott, P., & Wallace, C. (2012). Social quality: A way to measure the quality of society. *Social Indicators Research.* (forthcoming).

Beck, W., Maesen, V., & Walker, A. (1997). *The social quality of Europe*. The Hague: Kluwer Law International.

Beck, W., Van der Maesen, L., Fleur, Th, & Walker, A. (2001). *Social quality: A vision for Europe*. The Hague: Kluwer Law International.

Bohnke, P. (2006). *First European quality of life survey: Life satisfaction, happiness and sense of belonging*. Dublin: European Foundation for the Improvement of Living and Working Conditions.

Bohnke, P. (2008). Does society matter? Life satisfaction in and Enlarged Europe. *Social Indicators Research, 87*, 189–210.

Daly, M., & Rake, K. (2003). *Gender and the welfare state*. Cambridge: Polity Press.

Diener, E., & Suh, E. (1997). Measuring quality of life: Economic, social and subjective indicators. *Social Indicators Research, 40*, 189–216.

Fahey, T., & Smyth, E. (2004). Do subjective indicators measure welfare? Evidence from 33 societies. *European Societies, 6*(1), 5–27.

Land, K., & Lamb, V. et al. (2006). Measuing trends in child well-being. An evidence-based approach. *Social Indicators Research, 80*, 105–132

Lewis, J. (1992). Gender and the development of welfare regimes. *European Journal of Social Policy, 2*, 159–173.

Lockwood, D. (1992). *Solidarity and Schism: 'The problem of disorder' in Durkheimian and Marxist sociology*. Oxford/New York: Oxford University Press.

Nussbaum, M., & Sen, A. (Eds.). (1993). *The quality of life*. Oxford: Clarendon.

Pfau-Effinger, B. (2005). Welfare state policies and the development of care arrangements. *European Societies, 7*, 321–348.

Richardson, D., & Hoelscher, P. et al. (2008). Child well-being in central and easern European countries and the Commonwealth of independent states. *Child Indicators Research, 1*, 211–250

Stiglitz, J., Sen, A., & Fitoussi, J. P. (2009). *Commission on the measurement of economic performance and social progress*. Paris: The Commission.

Wallace, C. (Ed.). (2003). *Country contextual reports*. Vienna: Institute for Advanced Studies, HWF Project.

Watson, D., Pichler, F., & Wallace, C. (2009). *Subjective well-being in Europe*. Dublin: European Foundation for the Improvement of Living and Working Conditions.

Part II
Family, Child Poverty and Well-Being

Chapter 4
Child Poverty and Child Well-Being in Italy in a Comparative Framework

Daniela Del Boca and Anna Laura Mancini

Introduction

Several international reports show that child poverty rates have increased over recent years in European countries. The ECHP (European Community Household Panel) data show that in the second half of the 1990s, the risk of poverty among children remained relatively stable at around 20% in the EU-15 while it tended to decline slightly, from 17% to 15%, among the population as a whole. In the southern European countries, including Italy, the risk of poverty rates among children remained at around 25%.[1] The OECD also recently combined data from national sources in order to estimate trends in poverty rates since the early 1990s.[2] These show that in a number of countries, including in Italy, the gap between child poverty and overall[3] poverty rates widened in the late 1990s and early 2000s.

[1] This comparison unfortunately cannot take into account that underground economy is much higher in southern European countries especially Italy and Spain.

[2] The OECD uses a different definition of relative income poverty based on 50% of the median disposable income, and on a different equivalence scale, which implies that levels and trends in poverty based on this definition might differ to some extent from levels and trends calculated using the ECHP and EU-SILC data.

[3] A major difficulty in performing poverty analysis at the individual level arises from the assessment of intra-household distribution. While not the focus of this report, it is important to account for the role of joint consumption, externalities and lack of information about the assignment of goods in the household in generating "a veil of ignorance" over the intra-household distribution of welfare (Ravaillon 1996; Peluso and Trannoy 2007).

D. Del Boca (✉)
CHILD, Collegio Carlo Alberto, Department of Economics, University of Turin, Turin, Italy
e-mail: dani.delboca@unito.it

A.L. Mancini
Bank of Italy, Turin, Italy
e-mail: annalaura.mancinicancel_at_@gmail.com

A. Moreno Mínguez (ed.), *Family Well-Being: European Perspectives*,
Social Indicators Research Series 49, DOI 10.1007/978-94-007-4354-0_4,

The purpose of this chapter is to examine several dimensions of relative and absolute poverty among children, with a special focus on the Italian case, and to explore its underlying factors, mainly related to the nature of the labour market and the structure of the welfare state. Given that child poverty outcomes result from complex interactions between joblessness, in-work poverty and the impact of transfers, the countries achieving the best outcomes are those that are performing well on all fronts, notably by combining strategies aimed at facilitating access to employment and enabling services (childcare, etc.) with income support (social transfers other than pensions).

The next two sections describe the main characteristics of children at risk of poverty in the Europe Union and in Italy using the most recent available data. Section "Social Transfers to Families and Children" analyses the recent public intervention in support of families and children directed to reduce poverty rates. Section "Childcare Opportunities: The Impact on Children Well-Being" reports recent data on childcare opportunities and empirical results on the impact of childcare on children well-being. Section "The Dynamics of Child Poverty" considers the dynamics of child poverty across Italian regions. Section "Other Aspects of Child Poverty: Early School Leaving and Underage Working" examines another dimension of children poverty which is related to the human capital of children. Section "Conclusions" concludes.

Child Poverty in the European Union

The problem of child poverty and the main underlying factors vary consistently in scale and in nature across the EU. The report on "Child poverty and child well-being in the European Union" presented by the European Commission in 2010 compares the level, the persistence and the causes of child poverty in different member states using the European Union Statistics on Income and Living Conditions (EU-SILC) (EC Commission 2010). The extent (risk of poverty), the severity (poverty gaps) and the duration of child poverty (poverty persistence) are analysed in 11 states together with their determinants and the role played by the public welfare.

The risk of poverty is higher for children (20% in the EU-27) than for the population as a whole (17% in the EU-27), and in most countries, it increases with the age of the child. The patterns and the timing of family formation, family dissolution and the overall family composition affect significantly child's risk of poverty. In particular, in most European countries (Italy being the biggest exception), a child is more likely to be poor if he lives with a lone parent. At the same time, children who live in large families (three or more children) face a lower probability of being poor, but they account for the largest share of children at risk of poverty. At the EU level, 37% of children in single-parent households are at risk poverty, while only 24% of children on large families are at risk of poverty, but they account for more than 25% of poor children.

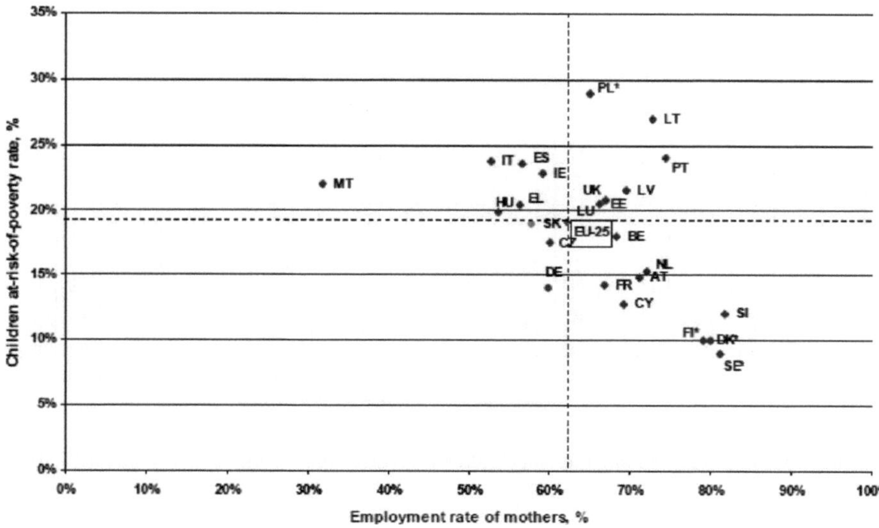

Fig. 4.1 Employment rates of mothers and child poverty (EC Commission 2008) (Source: EU-SILC (2005) – income year 2004 (income year 2005 for IE and UK) and LFS)

Child poverty can be related to two main phenomena: joblessness and working poor. In some countries, joblessness is a key factor in determining child poverty risk. On average, according to EU-SILC data, children in jobless households account for 25% of all children at risk of poverty, this proportion rising to 40% in Belgium, the UK and Ireland. However, most children live in households where on average only one parent works but his salary is not enough to insure the household against the risk of poverty. In the EU as a whole, children in single-earner households are at four times greater risk of poverty, the situation being particularly worst in the southern countries. A strong attachment to the labour market reduces significantly the risk of poverty among children irrespectively to the family structure. For these reasons, the employment of mothers seems to be crucial in significantly reducing the risk of poverty among children (see Fig. 4.1). In most countries identified among the best relative performers with regard to the risk of child poverty, mothers' employment rates are over 65% (Del Boca et al. 2009). Therefore, in-kind and money transfers designed to enhance women labour market participation also have a positive effect in reducing child poverty.

Child poverty is sensitive to the welfare system and in particular to the degree of horizontal (across generations) and vertical (in favour of poor) redistribution. In general, low effectiveness is observed when a low level of transfer is associated with poor targeting (like in southern countries). However, generous transfers might also have an undesirable negative effect on labour market participation, implying a negative long-run effect on poverty.

Countries who successfully limit child poverty are characterized by a combination of three main factors: high labour market participation of parents, low in-work

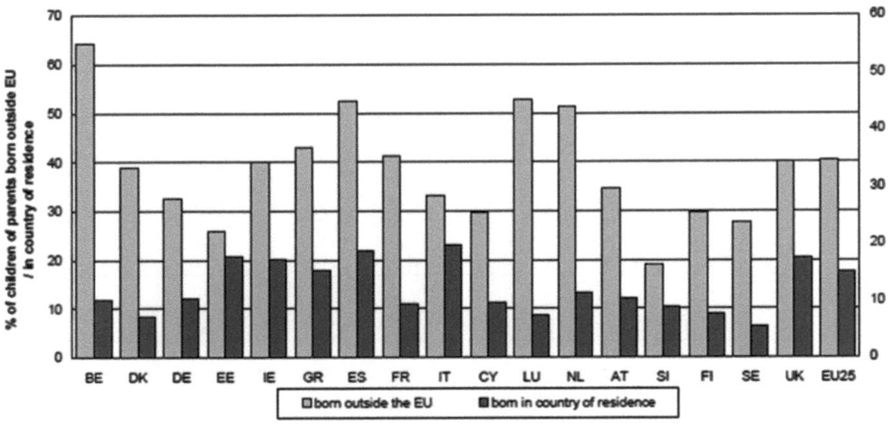

Fig. 4.2 Risk of poverty among migrant children (%) (EC Commission 2008) (Source: EU-SILC 2005)

poverty and effective income support (both in-kind and monetary policies). At the opposite end, countries with a high risk of poverty among children (like southern countries) are characterized by single-earner households, high levels of in-work poverty and ineffective income support policies. Moreover, often these countries also lack of efficient in-kind services to support both children development and parents' work.

Among the group of most vulnerable children, all European countries share the difficult situation of migrant children, in particular of non-EU migrant children. In the overall majority of European countries, there is a substantial poverty gap between migrant children and native children (see Fig. 4.2). Part of this gap can be explained by the fact that migrant children sum up some of the main reason underlying child poverty: they are more likely to live in big families (with three or more siblings), in jobless or single-earner families and with parents with low level of education and therefore also low earning capacity.

Characteristics of Children at Risk of Poverty in Italy

According to Italian National Institute for Statistics (ISTAT) latest statistics, overall poverty from 1997 to 2009 remained relatively stable in Italy (11% of households and 13% of individuals), but its composition changed significantly. In relative terms, poverty among elderly reduced while poverty among young children increased. In 2009, 17% of children were poor in relative terms and 6.2% were poor in absolute terms. Looking at EU-SILC data, in Italy, 25.4% of children are at risk of poverty according to the latest data. This proportion is higher than among the population as a whole (19.8%) and much higher than the average proportion of children at risk

Table 4.1 At risk of poverty rate of children (%) by household characteristics

	Italy	EU-25
All	25.4	19.8
Single-parent household	34.4	35.5
Two adult 3+ children	42.0	24.5
Couple: both work full-time	3.4	5.0
Couple: one works full-time, one jobless	33.5	22.3
Both jobless	63.4	61.0
Mother <30	38.7	37.0
Mother low education	37.6	35.5

Source: EU-SILC 2007

of poverty in the EU-25 (19.1%). Moreover, the difference between the risk of poverty for children and for the overall population is wider in Italy than in the EU as a whole.

As Table 4.1 shows, there are two main groups of households at risk of poverty: lone parents[4] and large families with three or more children. Though the risk of poverty among the first is slightly below the EU average, the risk among large families is much higher than the EU average. While, therefore, 15% of children live in households with more than three children, the risk of poverty for them is over 50% higher than for other children. For children of lone parents, the risk of poverty is also much higher than for others, but these account for only around 8% of children, lower than the EU average. Relative to children with no siblings, children with one sibling show a 20% greater risk of experiencing poverty; the risk rises to 33% among children with two or more siblings (Billari and Zuanna 2008).

The EU-SILC data also indicate that the risk of poverty increases with the age of children in Italy (older children are more likely to have siblings, and the number of children accordingly increases their risk of poverty). The risk of poverty of children is also related to the age of the parent: just above 40% of children whose mother or father is below 30 are at risk of poverty, again 50% higher than for children on average, reflecting the relationship between a parent's age and their earnings.

The presence of other adults in the household increases the risk of poverty in a different way depending on the type of household (36% for single parent living with another adult and 28% for couples with two children), perhaps reflecting the fact that the adult in question might be either a young person or an elderly parent being supported from the household's income.[5]

[4] The risk of poverty of children living with lone parents is higher in families where the lone parent is the mother. Living with a single mother indeed increases the risk to 37% (in line with the EU average) compared to only 20% for those living with a lone father (this latter share however needs to be interpreted with caution in all member states because of the small sample size).

[5] Brandolini and Saraceno (2007) show that the share of young lone mothers is low in Italy, noting that the figure might be underestimated, since in most cases young unmarried mothers tend to live with their parents.

In the EU as a whole, the employment rate of women with children is lower than those who do not have children (62%, against 70%); but in Italy, it is much lower (53% against 60% and 34% with 3 or more children). In order to understand better the extent to which parental employment is the key to raise the income of households to adequate levels, we need to examine the extent to which people of working age are employed and whether, if so, they work part-time or full-time, throughout the year or only for a part of the year. A work intensity index can be calculated for households defined in relation to the employment situation of all working-age members (who are not students) over the income reference period (12 months). A work intensity of 1 refers to households in which all working-age adults are working full-time over the whole year, and a work intensity of 0 corresponds to a "jobless" household where no one is working. Values in between indicate the extent to which those in the household are working part-time or only for part of the year.

In practice, in households where work intensity is between 0 and 0.5, almost 60% of the children are at risk of poverty; when work intensity is between 0.5 and 1, the proportion is reduced by half (29.5%). Both figures are much higher than the EU-25 averages (respectively 47.5% and 19.9%). The risk of poverty is especially high (around 79%) for children living in jobless households. While the risk is lower for those with parents working part-time, it is still much higher than in the EU average. It should also be noted that having at least one parent in a job with a temporary contract implies a risk of poverty of 25%, much higher than for children where this is not the case.

The picture doesn't change much when we look at absolute poverty instead of relative poverty. The estimate of absolute poverty is calculated on the basis of a poverty threshold which corresponds to "the minimum monthly expenditure necessary to purchase a basket of goods and services considered essential for an acceptable standard of living for a given family".[6] This threshold varies (by construction) according to family size, age composition, geographic area and city size. The basket includes three macro-components: food, housing and residual consumption (other items such as education, health and transportation).

According to ISTAT (see Table 4.2), the rate of absolute poverty in Italy in 2009 is 4.7%, and it varies significantly across regions and among different family types. The rate in the south (7.7%) is much higher than in the north (3.6%) and the centre of Italy (2.7%).

Looking at family types, the highest level of absolute poverty is concentrated among large families (with three or more children) and in particular in families with young children. The poverty rate of households with five members (9.2%) is more than twice as high as for households with two (3.8%) and three (4.2%) members. Moreover, for households with three children under 18, the proportion increases to 9.1%.

From 2005 to 2009, the incidence of poverty on average slightly increased, but it increased markedly for families with three or more children (from 8.0% in 2005 to

[6] "Rapporto sulla povertà assoluta in Italia nel 2007", ISTAT, Rome.

Table 4.2 Incidence of absolute poverty in 2005 and 2009 by regions

	2005				2009			
	North	Centre	South	Italy	North	Centre	South	Italy
Incidence of poverty (%)								
Family	2.7	2.7	6.8	4.0	3.6	2.7	7.7	4.7
Individual	2.5	2.4	7.0	4.1	3.7	2.7	8.5	5.3

Source: "Rapporto sulla povertà assoluta in Italia nel 2007", ISTAT

9.1% in 2009). One of the reason beyond this increase is that very little has been done in this decade for families and young children either in monetary transfers or services. In the next two sections, we focus on recent interventions concerning monetary transfers and childcare opportunities.

Social Transfers to Families and Children

In Italy, the composition of social transfer shows that the pension component accounts for the most important share (80%) while very little is directed to families and children.[7]

There are basically no, or very limited, measures targeted directly at poor children, and most of the welfare transfers and benefits are targeted to families in which at least one parent works on a regular basis. Moreover, the level and effectiveness of social spending are among the lowest in the EU. The impact of government transfers has been explored in several research papers using EUROMOD, the findings of which have been summarised by the Social Situation Observatory (see EC Report Children Poverty in the EU 2008). In this report, transfers are estimated to reduce the risk of poverty by only 21% in Italy, in contrast to 42% in the EU.

Between 2007 and 2010, three policy measures for poor families have been introduced. The first consisted of a transfer for families with a large number of children (assegno di sostegno), the second (Bonus famiglia[8]) was a tax deduction for the year 2009 in favour of poor families, while the third (Social Card[9]) were

[7] In fact, the proportion of transfers going to pensions is larger than in any other EU country, which is only to a small extent explained by the larger number of people in retirement.

[8] The Bonus famiglia was directed to Italian low-income families in 2009. Its amount varied from EUR 200 to EUR 1,000 depending on the number of members (including children) and on family income. People living alone were eligible only if they received a pension (i.e. it is an income support policy for elderly people in this case).

[9] The Social Card is a cash transfer to support household expenditure (electric/gas bill or shopping) of poor families. Households with at least 1 child younger than 3 as well as individuals older than 65 with an equivalent annual income below EUR 6,000 are eligible. Given these criteria, it is mainly targeted to poor elderly more than low-income families with children. Moreover, the amount involved is very limited (EUR 40 per month). See Monti (2008) for more details.

again monetary transfers targeted at poor households. All the three measures were quite limited in their amount, and they benefited elderly people much more than households with young children.

The impact of these policies was analysed by Baldini and Pellegrino (2008) in a micro-simulation model based on the Bank of Italy data. They show that the Social Card increased the income of recipients in the bottom decile of the income distribution by 8%, while the Bonus famiglia by only 5%. Given its poor performance, in 2010, the Social Card was reformed and an evaluation procedure is planned for 2011 before extending the new rules to the whole population. Also in 2010, the third national action plan for child poverty was approved by the *"Osservatorio nazionale per l' Infanzia"* (National Council for Childhood), closing finally a gap that lasted for almost 6 years (the second action plan was approved in 2002). This action plan refers to the fight against child poverty and social exclusion as a primary goal of welfare policies; however, the plan does not entail any concrete policy suggestion nor the rules to set up the monitoring of the plan implementation.

As already mentioned in the previous section, there is negative correlation between mother working and children poverty. An indirect way, then, to prevent children poverty is to support the employment of mothers.

In Italy, besides the lower participation rates of mothers, a large proportion of women leave the labour market after the first child and never return afterwards (Bratti et al. 2005). In spite of the poor starting point and of empirical evidence of the positive effect of mothers work on children poverty, no intervention was done to provide incentive to women work. In contrast, the School Reform (2009) appears to go in the opposite direction by both shrinking directly female employment (substantial cuts in the number of teachers in primary and secondary school, 81% of which are women) and reducing the services to support female labour (reduction of the full-time schedule in preschool and primary education). Given the lack of other services (such as after-school programmes), the full-time schedule in preschool and primary school is one of the most important ways to support households in reconciling work and family.

Unfortunately, the most recent strategic document on family policies published by the Ministry of Labor (Italy 2020) also points in this "no intervention" direction. According to this document, in fact, the most effective way to sustain women's work remains the help that other family members (adult children, grandparents and so on) can give in taking care of children[10] with no particular need to increase the public intervention in this field.

Childcare Opportunities: The Impact on Children Well-Being

Childcare services are an important way to support women in reconciling family and work (Del Boca 2002; Del Boca et al. 2005, 2009).

[10] Page 17 of the "Programma di azioni per l'inclusione delle donne nel mercato del lavoro".

In Italy, the childcare options for working parents remain more limited than in other EU countries. In the northern European countries, parents can decide whether to use a combination of part-time and childcare or to use parental leave (in some countries both parents can take a part-time leave) (De Henau et al. 2008a). Moreover, they can choose among private, public or informal services.

The available options for Italian parents are more limited, given less private and public childcare options as well as less part-time opportunities and shorter and less paid parental leave. Indeed, it's only since 2000 that fathers are encouraged to take parental leave in Italy.[11] In spite of the reputation for high quality,[12] childcare opportunities are limited and a large proportion use informal care or take care directly for their children.

The EU-SILC data shows that about 20% of children use childcare in Italy. While 27% of parents with income above the poverty line use formal childcare for children 0–2, only 17.5% of the families below the poverty line do. It is a question of availability as well as costs. In terms of availability, while childcare for children 3–5 is very widespread in Italy, childcare for children 0–2 is still quite limited. Moreover, facilities are less available in areas where poverty risk is higher.[13]

A mismatch between the features of public childcare and mothers' labour supply is evident in Italy. Since the public childcare system offers very limited hours of operation, only nonworking mothers or those employed in part-time jobs find it useful (Del Boca and Vuri 2007). In other countries, such as the UK and the Netherlands, childcare availability is also poor and the opening hours limited, but a large number of part-time jobs make it easier for mothers to reconcile work and motherhood. In countries like Denmark and Sweden, instead, opening hours are 11 h a day. Such a degree of availability is of great help to parents with very young children who need to combine their family and professional responsibilities.

Bratti et al. (2005) show that in-kind transfers, such as childcare opportunities, have been an important way to encourage women to remain in the labour market after childbearing. As shown by Fig. 4.3, women who live in areas where childcare is widely available have a lower probability of leaving the labour market after childbirth.

The proportion of children in public childcare in Italy varies across regions. In the northern regions, it is around 20–25%, while in most southern regions, it is less than 5% (as a percentage of the number of children 0–3 living in those areas). It is

[11] Father taking 3 months is entitled to one additional month of parental leave (it implies that he can leave for 4 months). The leave is an individual entitlement, but the total amount of the parental leave taken by two parents cannot exceed 10 months or 11 if the father takes at least 3 months.

[12] De Henau et al. (2008b) compare public childcare provision.

[13] The results obtained with the EU-SILC are higher than those reported by the Multiscope Survey of ISTAT 2007 (17.2%). This is mainly due to a difference in the definitions used. EU-SILC includes more childcare opportunities than Multiscope. In addition, given the different timing of the two surveys during the year, the number of the children 0–1 is different in the two surveys. Freguja and Cutillo (2009) showed that once two surveys are corrected for the different definitions, the discrepancy between the two data sources is not statistically significant.

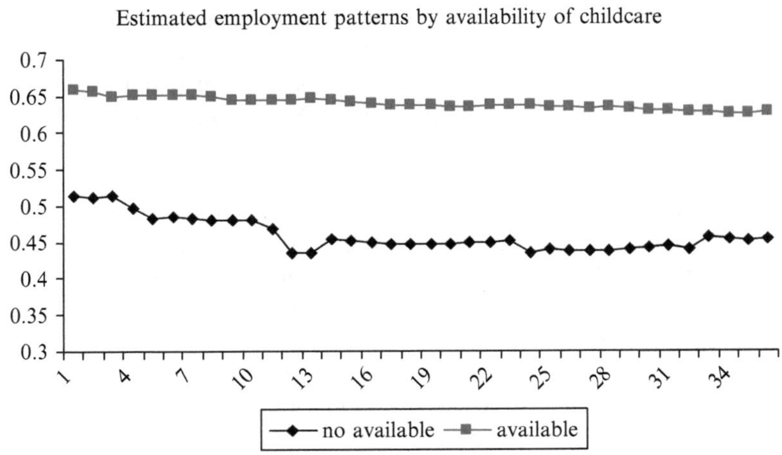

Fig. 4.3 Estimated employment patterns by availability of childcare

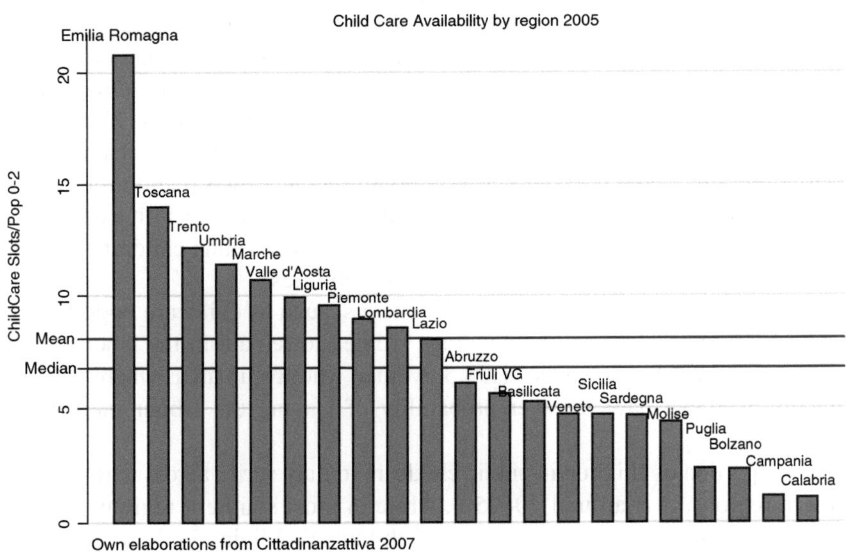

Fig. 4.4 Childcare availability by region (2005)

not a coincidence that the southern regions are also the ones with lowest female participation rates (less than 25% against 60% in the north) and with fewer children (1.30 children for woman against 1.5 in the north) (Del Boca and Rosina 2009; Zollino 2008) (Fig. 4.4).

Different accessibility rates created a situation of severe rationing of public childcare in some areas of the country, especially in the south. In these regions, women have difficulties to find a job in the formal labour market and are unemployed or work in the underground economy.

In a situation of lack of childcare and income support for children, grandparents and family ties are of key importance. Indeed, they provide flexible help at zero cost. However, the support of grandparents may be reduced in the future because of the postponement of the pensionable age of women as well as their greater mobility which is likely to mean that fewer of them live nearby.

Public childcare in Italy is also more expensive than in other countries. Public subsidy accounts for about 80% of the total cost in Italy, while in Spain and France, it is between 90% and 100%. Private childcare is also more expensive, about 30% more than public childcare (Del Boca et al. 2005). Hourly childcare costs are higher in the private sector than in the public sector both for children under 3 years of age (8.25 vs. 7.67) and between 3 and 5 years of age (4.16 vs. 2.61).

However, the low proportion of young children using childcare does not depend only on the lack of availability or the relatively high costs but depends also on "cultural resistance" of Italian families to delegate the care of the young children. According to an ISTAT survey (2005), almost two thirds of families with children 0–2 prefer to take care directly of their children, while 19% report to prefer the use of childcare facilities and are able to use them, and 23% of them report to be rationed (the most important reasons are lack of availability in the area, high costs and inconvenient hours of service). In a recent work, Del Boca and Vuri (2007) analyse the impacts of a costs reduction and an increased supply of childcare. Their results show that a reduction in childcare costs would have an impact on mother's labour supply only in the north, where childcare is more widespread and well established and therefore well known and "trusted" by mothers.

An increase in the availability of childcare affects positively the likelihood of participating in the labour market, especially of those women with low education (Del Boca et al. 2009). On another hand, the availability of childcare impacts also child cognitive outcomes at a later stages. In area where public childcare is more widespread, children test scores in elementary school are significantly higher (Brilli et al. 2011).

Therefore, it appears that more relevant policies should be aimed to increase the supply of publicly provided childcare places rather than policies aimed to reduce the costs. An understanding of the importance of these factors is relevant in the evaluation of childcare policies following the Barcelona recommendation.[14] This is also particularly important in Italy, where the majority of families with children have also only one child and children would benefit not only from the educational aspects but also from the socialization aspects of the childcare system.

[14] "Member states should remove disincentive to female labour force participation and strive, taking into account the demand for childcare facilities and in line with national patterns of provision, to provide childcare by 2010 to at least 90% of children between 3 years old and the mandatory school age and at least 33% of children under 3 years of age" Conclusioni della Presidenza, Barcellona, 15–16 marzo 2002.

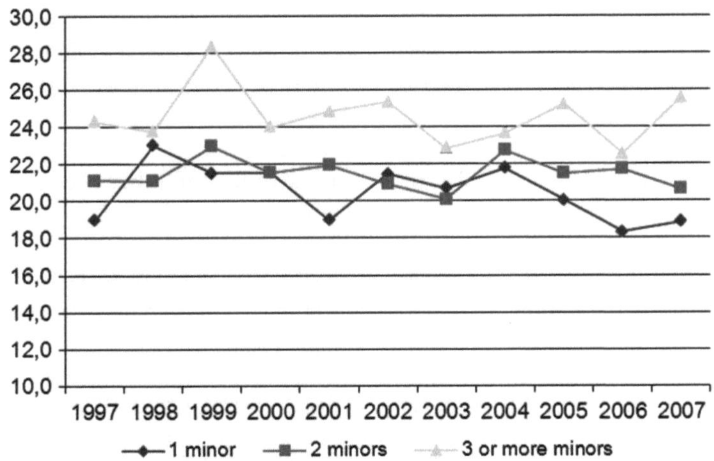

Fig. 4.5 Relative poverty risk over time among families with minor by number of children

The Dynamics of Child Poverty

The way the risk of poverty has changed over time is also important. According to data from ISTAT, poverty among families with children seems to have been relatively stable during the period 1997–2007. It has, however, increased among families with three children or more[15] (from 24.3% in 1997 to 26.8% in 2007). Figure 4.5 shows the relatively poverty risk among families with minor children.

However, one of the most significant dimensions is still the territorial one. If we compare families with at least one minor child across regions, we see that the risk of poverty is much higher in the southern regions (around 22%) than in the north (around 17%) (Fig. 4.6).

It is also important to look at the duration, or persistence, of poverty among children. The "static" approach measuring the spread and intensity of poverty at a given moment in time should be supplemented by a longitudinal analysis of individual experiences to indicate how long children remain in poverty since the policy significance is very different if children remain for only a limited time with income below the poverty threshold than if this is a permanent, or almost permanent, state of affairs. However, very little is currently known on the duration and persistence of poverty for those living in Italy, owing to the limited availability of panel data with repeated measurements on individuals' well-being over relatively long time periods.

The EU-SILC longitudinal data can be used to throw light on this issue. According to the data from 2004 to 2006, just over 13% of children aged 0–15 in 2004 were living below the poverty line in that year but also in the two following years.

[15] Probably because of a lack of effective support to large families.

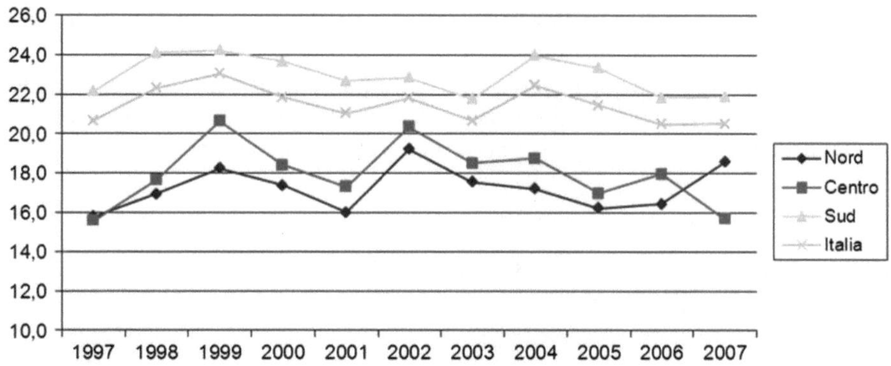

Fig. 4.6 Relative poverty risk in Italy among families with at least one minor over time and regions

Brandolini (2005) used data from the Bank of Italy's Survey on Household Income and Wealth (SHIW). However, the SHIW has a number of limitations for the study of the duration of poverty at the individual level. First, its panel component is very small and, second, its biannual release makes it impossible to detect poverty spells that last less than 2 years (which, as we will see, are numerous).

More recently, Devicienti and Gualtieri (2007) exploited the panel aspect of the ECHP to study in parallel the dynamics of a number of alternative definitions of poverty.[16] Income poverty is defined here in terms of equivalent household income, subjective poverty is defined according to an individual's own assessment of ability to make ends meet given available financial resources, and the index of "lifestyle deprivation" is obtained by combining the survey's information on the lack of possession of a number of items deemed as "essential" in contemporary western life. For each poverty definition, the transitions in and out of poverty and the poverty persistence are estimated and compared.

The results show that despite frequent re-entry into income poverty, exits are relatively rapid, making most spells of low income of short duration. The results of the multivariate models show that people at risk of poverty broadly share the same characteristics. People living in households with many children and with low levels of education are, therefore, those with higher risk of persistent poverty compared to the rest of the population. The situation may be even worse for those living with a nonworking head of household (unemployed, out of the labour force) or working an insufficient number of hours, although these variables were not always statistically significant. The household's area of residence and mother's employment are also crucial factors. This is not surprising for a country like Italy, characterized by a long-standing territorial dualism, with an underdeveloped and slowly growing south and a poorly performing labour market, characterized by high rates of long-term

[16] Income poverty, subjective poverty and a multidimensional index of lifestyle.

unemployment and youth unemployment rate and one of the lowest female participation rates in Europe.

The probability of leaving poverty was lowest for families with children. Among them, families with nonworking mother and parents with low levels of education and living in the south have the lowest probability of leaving poverty.

Other Aspects of Child Poverty: Early School Leaving and Underage Working

Child poverty is also strongly related to human capital investment. Individuals with a low level of education are at strong disadvantage in the labour market and are at greater risk of poverty.

The Ministry of Education published a report on dropouts and early school leavers for lower and higher secondary schools in Italy to check progress towards the Lisbon targets in education and training (to reduce the number of early school leavers by 50% by 2010).[17] In what follows, dropouts are students who leave school in a particular year before completing their studies, while early school leavers refers to those aged 18–24 with at most lower secondary education (Licenza Media) no longer studying. For the academic year 2006–2007, the number of dropouts was equal to 0.2% of the total number of students attending lower secondary school and 1.6% of those attending upper secondary school. In 2006, early school leavers in Italy amounted to 20.8% of those aged 18–24 (as against an EU average of 15.3%). The high rate of early school leaving is evident not only in the southern regions but also in some regions of the north where the labour market for low-skilled workers is relatively attractive.

Since 2009, data for child cognitive achievements are provided by INVALSI assessment gathered by the National Evaluation Service (*Servizio Nazionale di Valutazione*, in Italian). These data show that cognitive outcomes are correlated with families' socioeconomic status (Campofiori et al. 2010). Both Italian and math scores are higher among children in higher educated and higher income households.

The regional differences in the results of the Pisa-OECD (2007) tests show worse results for children in the south. In particular, the score for mathematical competence is 448 for southern students against 515 for northern students. This large territorial difference in student performance is quite surprising, given the highly centralized nature of the Italian educational system. Bratti et al. (2007) show that the most significant factors are the school infrastructures and the state of the local labour market, in terms of both employment probability and extension of the irregular and illegal economies.

The phenomenon of early school leaving and low scores is likely to be linked to child labour. In Italy, school is compulsory until 16 years old, and child work is not

[17] Ministro dell Istruzione "La dispersione scolastica 2007" Roma 2008.

allowed until 14 years old. According to a CGIL report[18] (2005), 400,000 children aged <18 are working (Paone and Teselli 2000; CGIL 2005). From a geographical point of view, underage labour is more widespread in southern Italy (60% of the total), although it is relatively common in the north of the country as well (40%).

According to this study, child labour is caused by not only economic but also "cultural" poverty. Besides economic aspects, therefore, the cultural attitudes of the underage workers' families and their immediate social environment are also important. For example, in many cases, the family tends to dismiss the value of education compared with work, with the latter seen as a factor which enables individual fulfilment. Consequently, numerous minors view work as a means to satisfy their needs through obtaining money. Moreover, small family-run firms tend to view child labour as a resource which facilitates their operations.

ISTAT (2002) finds that 0.5% of children aged 7–10 work, 3.7% of those 11–13 and 11.6% of those older than 14. According to ISTAT, 80% of working children aged 7–10 live in a family at risk of poverty (ISTAT 2002). School dropout, early school leaving and underage working therefore seem to be more likely among children at risk of poverty.

A large recent literature developed mainly in the USA and UK has raised the issue of the importance of early intervention. Since children cognitive and non-cognitive skills are more "malleable" at the early stage, it is crucial to invest earlier than later in life (Carneiro and Heckman 2003). The family plays a powerful role in shaping these abilities, contributing both genetic endowments and pre- and postnatal environments, which interact to determine the abilities, behaviour and talents of children. Some families do this task poorly, with detrimental consequences for their children. From a variety of intervention studies, it emerges that it is possible to partially compensate for exposure to adverse environments if high-quality interventions are made sufficiently early in children's lives. The remediation efforts that appear to be most effective are those that supplement family resources for young children from disadvantaged environments. Since the family is the fundamental source of inequality in all societies, programmes that target children from disadvantaged families can have substantial economic and social returns.

The recent OECD's publication on child well-being (OECD 2009) shows that Italian government spending on children is close to the OECD average overall, but Italy spends only 80% of the OECD average for younger children and half what is spent in later years. Despite this average overall spending, in many areas, Italian children do less well than their peers in other countries. Even given historically low Italian fertility rates, just under one in two Italian children live in overcrowded conditions (48%) compared to fewer than one in three in the OECD overall (30%). Equally, one in three children lives in poor local environmental conditions compared

[18] A qualitative survey was conducted which covered a total of 16 territorial units (large cities, medium-to-small towns and provinces) deemed particularly significant in terms of the extent of child labour. In each of these units, minors were contacted in meeting places like coffee shops, amusement arcades, youth clubs and schools. A total of 600 interviews were conducted.

to one in four children on average across the OECD. Italian children do very poorly at school. Italy has the 4th worst average educational performance, and the second largest gap between good and poor performers, after Mexico. The number of Italian youth not in employment, education or training reflects the poor schooling outcomes, again being the third worst in the OECD after Mexico and Turkey.

In many OECD countries, there is a particular concern about outcomes of the children of immigrants. There is little in the way of internationally comparable data on outcomes for these children. However, the PISA survey records the student's birthplace, allowing an exploration of experiences of non-native relative to native-born children for educational deprivation. The data show that non-native students are more educationally deprived than native children in 17 out of 26 OECD countries. Migrant educational deprivation is particularly marked among the Nordic and continental European member countries (with the Netherlands and Sweden as exceptions) and is less strong among the Anglophone countries (the United States, Australia, the United Kingdom, New Zealand and Canada).

Immigrant children not only face a persistently higher risk of poverty, but they also are disadvantaged in terms of schooling outcomes. In fact, INVALSI data shows that cognitive outcomes are lower for immigrant children. The gap between foreigners and native-born Italians in advancement from one grade to the next has widened steadily from elementary school through secondary school (see INVALSI 2008–2010). In elementary school in the 2006–2007 school year, for example, the rate of advancement was 96.4% among foreign students compared with 99.9% among native-born Italians. In middle school, the share fell to 90.5% compared with 97.3% among the native born, and it fell to 72% in secondary school compared with 86.4% among the native born.

Conclusions

All data sources measuring children poverty rates show similar results. The two main groups of households at risk of poverty are households with minor children and large families with three or more children, in particular when they live in the south.

In this chapter, we report the differences between children poverty rates among European countries and discuss the various factors determining the high poverty rates among children in Italy.

The high poverty rate among children in Italy is determined by the combination of rigidities and limitations of labour market opportunities for mothers, the limited in-kind services and the low monetary support for households with children.

The recent policy proposals do not seem to address properly the issue of child poverty, being more focus on elderly needs. In fact, they still neglect the issue of child poverty as well as strategies to encourage the participation of women in the workforce. Policies which would appear particularly appropriate to the Italian case include the extension of childcare schools and other fundamental social services, the promotion of part-time and other work arrangements suitable to the needs of women during childcare years.

The EU recommendation to raise women's employment to 60% is at this point an unreachable target (the female participation rate being only 47%). In order to reach this target, the EU has recommended an increase in public childcare availability (33% of children) and the creation of more part-time jobs (as part of the overall Employment Strategy).

All the results indicate that women with lower education (and income) are more sensitive to changes in income and prices—a finding that is consistent with economic theory as well as previous empirical results. Recent policy measures unfortunately do not seem so far to go in this direction with potential negative implications for child poverty rates.

Acknowledgements We thank Chiara Noè and Silvia Pasqua (CHILD-Collegio Carlo Alberto) for useful suggestions. The research was partially financed within the project "Parental and Public Investments and Child Outcomes" by the Collegio Carlo Alberto which is gratefully acknowledged.

References

Baldini, M., & Pellegrino, S. (2008). Si fa presto a dire Bonus, lavoce.info. December 10, 2008

Billari, F., & Zuanna, D. (2008). *La rivoluzione nella culla. Il declino che non c'e*. Milano: EGEA.

Brandolini, A. (2005). *Income inequality and poverty in Italy*. Rome: Bank of Italy.

Brandolini, A., & e Saraceno, C. (2007). *Poverta' e benessere*. Rome: Il Mulino.

Bratti, M., Del Bono, E., & Vuri, D. (2005). New Mothers' labour force participation in Italy: The role of job characteristics. *Labour, 19*(1), 79–121.

Bratti, M., Checchi, D., & Filippin, A. (2007, February). *Territorial differences in Italian students' mathematical competencies: Evidence from Pisa 2003* Iza Discussion Paper No. 2603.

Brilli, Y., Del Boca, D., & Pronzato, C. (2011). Exploring the roles of child care, *Collegio Carlo Alberto Notebooks 214* .

Campofiori, E., Figura, E., Papini, M., & Ricci, R. (2010). Un indicatore di status socio economico culturale degli allievi della quinta primaria in Italia, *INVALSI Wp 27/2010*.

Carneiro, P., & Heckman, J. J. (2003). Human Capital Policy. In J. J. Heckman, A. B. Krueger, & B. M. Friedman (Eds.), *Inequality in America: What role for human capital policies?* (pp. 77–239). Cambridge, MA: MIT Press.

CGIL. (2005). *Mai piu lavoro minorile*. Rome: CGIL.

De Henau, J., Meulders, D., & O'Dorchai, S. (2008a). Parents' care and career. Comparing parental leave policies. In D. Del Boca & C. Wetzels (Eds.), *Social policies, labour markets and motherhood: A comparative analysis of European countries*. Cambridge: Cambridge University Press.

De Henau, J., Meulders, D., & O'Dorchai, S. (2008b). Making time for working parents: Comparing public childcare provision. In D. Del Boca & C. Wetzels (Eds.), *Social policies, labour markets and motherhood: A comparative analysis of European countries*. Cambridge: Cambridge University Press.

Del Boca, D. (2002). The effect of child care on participation and fertility. *Journal of Population Economics, 15*(3).

Del Boca, D., & Rosina, A. (2009). *Famiglie Sole*. Bologna: Il Mulino.

Del Boca, D., & Vuri, D. (2007). The mismatch between employment and child care. *Journal of Population Economics, 20*(4), 805–832.

Del Boca, D., Pasqua, S., & Pronzato, C. (2005). Employment and fertility in Italy, France and the UK. *Labour, 4*, 2005.

Del Boca, D., Locatelli, M., & Vuri, D. (2005). Child care choices of Italian households. *Review of Economics of the Household, 3*, 453–477.

Del Boca, D., Pasqua, S., & Pronzato, C. (2009). Motherhood and employment in institutional contexts: An European perspective. *Oxford Economic Papers, 61*(Suppl 1), i147–i171.

Devicienti, F., & Gualtieri, V. (2007, August). *The dynamics and persistence of poverty in Italy Labor Collegio Carlo Alberto.*

EC Commission. (2008). *Child poverty and well being in the EU.* Current status and way forward.

EC Commission. (2010). *Child poverty and child well being in the European Union.*

Freguja, C., & Cutillo, C. (2009). *Child care report.* Unpublished manuscript Rome 2009 available at request.

ISTAT. (2002). *Bambini, lavori, e lavoretti: Verso un sistema informativo sul Lavoro Minorile.* Rome: ISTAT.

Monti, P. (2008). *L'età rende iniqua la Card* www.lavoce.info. December 10, 2008.

OECD. (2007). *PISA 2006 science competencies for tomorrow's world.* Paris: OECD.

OECD. (2009). *Doing better for children.* Paris: OECD.

Paone, G., & Teselli, A. (2000). *Lavoro e lavori minorili.* Rome: Ediesse.

Peluso, E., & Trannoy, A. (2007). Does less inequality among households mean less inequality among individuals? *Journal of Economic Theory, 133*(1), 568–578.

Ravaillon, M. (1996). Issue in measuring and modelling poverty. *The Economic Journal, 108*, 1328–1343.

Zollino, P. (2008). *Il difficile accesso ai servizi di istruzione per la prima infanzia in Italia: i fattori di offerta e di domanda.* Banca d'Italia.

Chapter 5
Child Well-Being and Lone Parenthood Across the OECD

Simon Chapple

Introduction

What is the causal impact of being in a lone parent family on child well-being? This chapter uses a simple meta-analysis to address this primary question. The question breaks down into two secondary ones. The first question is whether there is a casual effect on well-being of being bought up in a lone parent family. The second is how large is the effect. The chapter focuses on the impact of lone parent family structure either on account of having never partnered or, alternatively, having separated or divorced. This review takes a strongly cross-country, cross-OECD perspective. The aim is to develop a piece of work which is accessible to and speaks to the interests of policymakers, while sacrificing the minimum of analytical rigour.

In considering the impact of family structure on child well-being, a very wide variety of dimensions of family structure have been researched. However, most of the research focus has been on lone parents (or divorce or separation) or stepfamilies, on one hand, compared to intact cohabiting and legally married families on the other. Since it has been the primary policy concern in the OECD countries where it has been a social policy issue, this survey focuses primarily on whether being raised in a lone parent family has an impact on child well-being, compared to being bought up with two biological parents in an intact family.

Issues of lone parent family structure have also been on the political and policy agenda in some OECD countries. However, in order to consider these broader public policy issues in a well-rounded fashion and to consider possible policy responses, further research questions in addition to those posed by this chapter need investigation. The survey will not consider the efficacy of policies to change family structure, nor will it consider social policy measures to compensate for any negative causal effects

---

S. Chapple (✉)
Social Policy Division, OECD, Paris, France
e-mail: simon.chapple@oecd.org

A. Moreno Mínguez (ed.), *Family Well-Being: European Perspectives*,
Social Indicators Research Series 49, DOI 10.1007/978-94-007-4354-0_5,

of different family structures. Such additional information is necessary to make evidence-based policy in the area. These policy issues will be returned to briefly in the conclusion.

Child well-being, the outcome of focus in this review, has different dimensions. In the absence of a single, over-arching and generally accepted measure of well-being, child well-being is viewed here as multidimensional across a variety of outcome domains (Pollard and Lee 2003). Most typically, the measures available are measures of well-being deficits for children. The approach here will be to use whatever measures of well-being are employed by researchers. Child well-being, as interpreted here, also has a strong inter-temporal or life-cycle dimension. In considering the possible impacts of family structure, this review considers the well-being of children now, their future well-being as children and as independent adults.

Some researchers have remarked on the dominance of Anglophone research on the impact of family structure on child well-being and questioned its generalisability to other OECD countries (Bukodi and Dronkers 2003, p. 3). The point is well taken. It is a motivation here to explore research from as many OECD countries as possible. That said, however, it remains true that research is dominated by researchers and data from the Anglophone OECD countries. There are a variety of possible reasons for this dominance, including the dominance of English language scientific publications, the greater perception of lone parenthood as a policy problem in Anglophone countries, and the stronger history of longitudinal data sets in those countries, data sets which are better suited to answering causal questions about the impacts of lone parenthood as well as measuring exposure over the child life cycle to such family structures.

There is a considerable amount of high-quality primary United States research on the issue, as well as good literature syntheses and meta-analyses, Amato and Keith (1991b) and Amato (2000a) being canonical examples of the latter. More recently, the United States journal *The Future of Children* published a special issue on "Marriage and Child Well-being". This special issue covers a significant amount of the ground traversed by this chapter. Thus, a consideration of its conclusions and its strengths and weaknesses forms a very convenient jump-off point for a study on the wider OECD research. All papers in the issue are by United States academics and all focus on United States research literature and implications. A United States focus is unsurprising, since United States research is likely to be most directly relevant to inform to United States policy. Additionally, as already remarked, much of what is known about the impact of family structure on child well-being comes from the United States, although the relative preponderance of United States research does appear to be declining (Ermisch and Francesconi 2001a, p. 251).

The *Future of Children* issue nicely contextualises recent United States debates about family, family structure and its effects on children. Frequently, the perception of those outside the United States is that the pro-marriage line is driven by conservative religious forces. The reality is rather more complex. According to the special issue at least, a broad spectrum of American society appears supportive of marriage – a particular form of two-parent family structure – to support child well-being (Nock 2005). The editors of the special issue make it clear that they believe the United States research evidence supports a broad consensus view that "children benefit [on a variety of dimensions of well-being] from growing up with two married biological parents" (p. 8). The United States consensus, at least according to the *Future of Children*, is that certain family structures – in particular lone parent families – can have negative effects on child well-being. However, the editors also point out that there is considerable disagreement about appropriate policy responses within the broad consensus spectrum to the identified problem.

There are two papers in this collection of particular interest to this review. The first, by Thomas and Sawhill, considers the impact of family structure, in terms of legally married, cohabiting and lone parent households, on the economic well-being of children. The second, by Amato, considers the impact of family structure on cognitive, social and emotional functioning of children.

In terms of economic well-being (equivalised after tax income), Thomas and Sawhill (2005) conclude that children in married households fare better in terms of income than children in cohabiting couples who in turn fare better than children in lone parent households, at least in the United States. While acknowledging that the relationship between family structure and child economic well-being may not be causal, Thomas and Sawhill conclude that a significant amount of it is caused by lone parenthood. Thomas and Sawhill also argue that "[t]he availability of child support for single-parent families and the marriage penalties in the tax and transfer system reduce but rarely completely offset the economic benefits of marriage" (p. 57). These results are not automatically generalisable across the OECD, as other OECD countries have very different approaches to tax-benefit policies relating to families and child support systems (see Skinner et al. 2007), publicly provided child care, and so forth, which may change these patterns. Observation suggests that lone parent supports are frequently more generous or stronger outside the United States.[1]

Amato (2005) concludes that children growing up with two continuously married parents are less likely to experience a wide range of cognitive, emotional and social problems, both during childhood and also into adulthood. Amato is confident that this conclusion can be taken as a true treatment effect of family structure. Nevertheless, he also makes the point that the effect sizes on child outcomes from different family structures are fairly small.

The United States consensus proclaimed in 2005 in the special edition of the *Future of Children* may however be premature. In a strongly contrasting United States view from about the same time, Ginther and Pollak (2003, p. 9) observe that "[t]he lack of a consensus about the effect of family structure on children's outcomes is striking". And in a further recent United States review, Liu (2007, p. 2) suggests that "evidence on whether divorce itself has a causal impact on children is

[1] This study does not consider the issue of whether lone parenthood impacts adversely on the household income to which children are exposed. There is a literature on child poverty statics and dynamics across the OECD which usually look at tabulations of family structure (amongst other things), including lone parent family structure, against income poverty transitions. There is also a smaller literature on lone parent family structure and material living standards. For reasons of space, this literature is not further considered.

far from conclusive", while it is also disputed by Hoekstra (2006) and Stevenson and Wolfers (2008).

Rather than simply repeat the existing recent United States surveys and shorter, select surveys which typically accompany all of the new published empirical contributions to the literature, something that adds more policy value is undertaken here. This chapter focuses attention on research on child well-being outcomes and lone parent family structure in non-United States OECD countries and examines the extent to which it supports United States research. At the same time, it is important to note that the United States and non-United States literatures are not independent of one another. Non-United States researchers draw on United States research methods and conclusions, attend conferences with their United States counterparts, publish in the same journals, and may have attended the same universities for their educations. In addition, while it is sometimes seen as simply summarising United States research, Amato's (2000a) meta-analysis, used here to provide the comparative United States meta-analysis, actually draws on research in at least several other OECD countries, including the United Kingdom, Canada, the Netherlands and New Zealand.[2]

The focus here will be on research published in the 1990s or later. Narrowing the temporal focus renders the task more manageable by concentrating on the most recent and therefore the most informative research. It also focuses on the higher quality end of the research spectrum as research techniques improve over time. Linguistic limitations mean, however, that the research base will be English language dominated. This is not quite the problem it may seem at first blush, since English is increasingly the international language of social sciences in much of the non-English-speaking OECD.

Why Lone Family Structure Might Matter for Family Well-Being

This section provides a tour of the impacts that lone parent family structure, arising either out of being born into a lone parent family or parental divorce or separation, may have on children's well-being and development (see Amato 2000a, b, pp. 1270–1273; Amato 2005, pp. 82–84; Hill et al. 2001 for brief summaries).[3]

Children living in lone parent families are less likely to have as much income as children living in intact families. Often separation means the direct loss of a family

---

[2] This conclusion has been deduced from the reference list in Amato (2000a), where five out of the 67 studies are definitely from outside the United States. Some of the remaining 62 studies may also rely on non-United States data, though this is difficult to establish without a detailed article-by-article examination. Unfortunately, no separate data or detail is presented in the article to allow examination of variation of effect sizes between different countries included in the sample.

[3] Hill et al. (2001, pp. 273–276) provide a well-referenced summary which divides the theories in three broad streams – "stress theory", "social control theory" and "economic hardship theory".

earner but may also increase the difficulty and cost of the custodial parent effectively supplying labour and generating an income themselves. There is also the loss of parental assets like houses if these are shared equally between parents (although a family house may stay in possession of the custodial parent following separation, providing a flow of imputed income to the custodial parent and child which is often not accounted for in many studies). Causal linkages in terms of material resources available for parental investment in children, or in terms of higher levels of parental stress, may then connect poorer material outcomes with other adverse child well-being outcomes. The lower leisure available to lone parents, because of increases in paid and unpaid work, may also contribute to stress.

Parental separation or geographic absence also often means a loss of or reduction in contact with the noncustodial parent. With this loss, children lose the time, networks and skills of that parent. There may also be loss of extended family networks and resources on the side of the noncustodial parent's family as well.

Parental separation can result in a wide variety of changes in children's living situations. Schools, child care and residence may all change. Relationships with friends and extended family members may also suddenly change. Change, especially sudden change across numerous dimensions of life, can be stressful for children. Additionally, separation may leave the custodial parent with considerable mental health problems, including depression, as well as causing high levels of stress for reasons which may be material and emotional. The resulting parental stress and depression can impact on the child's well-being and development.

Post-separation, children may be exposed to considerable open parental conflict and antipathy, for example, through custody disputes, both informal and legal, which may have negative impacts on their well-being and development.

Children of lone parent families may be exposed to a variety of social stigmas in environments as varied as the wider family, peer groups, schools, the media and welfare officers. This stigma may be internalised by the child and lead to poorer current and long-term outcomes for these children.

There may also be positives in growing up in a lone parent family compared to the counterfactual of two biological parents. If the absent parent would have contributed to creating an environment which involved high amount of parental conflict in the home, had problems of mental health or alcohol or drug abuse, was likely to abuse or demean the child or the other parent, lacked an income and stable employment, or was prone to criminal behaviour, it is quite plausible the child would be better off growing up without that parent (Amato 2000a).

A Cross-OECD Meta-Analysis

A straightforward meta-analysis of effect sizes, with results presented as a percentage of a standard deviation of the dependent outcome variable, was undertaken. The method broadly follows Amato (2000a). Studies were located through a comparatively unstructured search of strings of keywords (like "parental divorce", "lone parents", "child well-being", and so on) through several online databases including PubMed and RePEc (including published working papers and, in a few cases, online conference papers) during the middle months of 2007, and then through a secondary analysis of bibliographies of these articles. The approach to determining the data set to be considered was as follows. Only literature published after 1990 was considered, the arbitrary early cut-off date designed partly to avid consideration of material which is too old and partly to constrain the size of the analysis. Only English language literature was considered. English is the predominant international language of social science. Therefore, most researchers seek to publish their quality material to access the widest intellectual audience possible. Thus, in all probability, little has been missed and that which is missed is likely to be of poorer quality. The meta-analysis is based on articles published from 1990s. The cut-off date for publications was July 2007.

To be included, studies had to contain a sample of children living with only one parent. Sometimes these studies did not distinguish the reasons for lone parenthood (in other words, some children were being bought up as lone parents because of the death of a parent and some because of parental divorce or separation). Such studies are included here, unlike in Amato, to increase the number of available studies and increase countries' representation. In any case, given life expectancy across the OECD, numbers of children in lone parent families because of parental death will usually be small. Finally, in the sense that parental death represents a "natural experiment" which may not suffer from the same selection on unobservable variables as parental divorce or separation (see above), it may be of value to include child of widows and widowers in a sample of lone parents in any case.

The focus was a comparison of lone parent structures to two-parent intact families. For example, in some cases, distinctions were used between intact versus non-intact families, or lone versus two parents, where lone parents may be due to either death or parental separation, and where two parents' structures may be a consequence of remarriage. Typically, the effect size in terms of a comparison of lone mother versus to a biological and intact family, or the closest on offer to this, was selected.

The standard method of estimating an effect size is to subtract the outcome variable for children living in a single-parent family from that for children in an intact family and divide it by the polled group standard deviation. Where a pooled standard deviation was not available or could not be readily constructed, the standard deviation for the largest subgroup – typically that for children from intact families – was used. Where the publication did not provide the information, a variety of methods were used to convert results into effect sizes.[4]

This chapter also broadly follows the taxonomic approach to effects of Amato (2000a), with some added categories (e.g. Amato does not consider adult outcomes

[4] See Chinn (2000) for some useful examples for calculating effect sizes from odds ratios and logit and probit estimation.

of children who experience a lone parent family structure). Outcomes were classified into the following categories:

- Academic achievement
- Conduct/behaviour/delinquency/ADHD
- Depression/anxiety/happiness
- Self-concept/esteem
- Social relations
- Physical health (additional)
- Employment/income (additional)
- Other (a catch-all category, additional)

Outcomes within each category – with the exception of the catch-all "other" category – are clearly more intuitively comparable than between categories.

Again following Amato, effect sizes are calculated for each independent sample in the study. Typically, independent samples were provided where differential results were produced by sex. If there were several results provided by an independent sample within each outcome category, then a simple within-category average effect was calculated.

Outcomes were also classified by age, again largely following Amato. Seven age categories were used based on school ages. These age categories were preschool, primary school, secondary school, mixed primary and secondary school, college/university, adults and other. Where outcomes were for groups of children of different ages but falling within the eight age ranges, they were averaged to give a figure for the age category.

Mostly classification into one of the eight outcome categories was straightforward. However, from time to time, some more considered decisions needed to be made to fit outcomes into these eight categories. A degree of judgement was required. For example, smoking, drinking and drug taking were classified as conduct/behaviour/delinquency – forms of externalising behaviour – if these were teenage outcomes, and as physical health, as risk factors, if these were adult outcomes. Additionally, physical reasons for hospitalisation (including suicide attempts) were coded as physical health, while adult hospitalisation due to alcohol, drugs and psychiatric disease was coded as "other". Truancy was considered as a form of externalising behaviour, as were violence and criminal outcomes for those who were not adults. Suicidal ideation or suicide attempts were classified as depression/anxiety/happiness, while actual suicide was classified as physical health.

The method distinguishes three different types of effect sizes:

1. Effect sizes for mean differences, controlling for pre-divorce variables
2. Effect sizes based on simple mean differences
3. Effect sizes for mean differences, controlling for post-divorce variables

The preferred method was analysing child outcomes, post- to pre-separation, controlling for child and family observables prior to the split. Failing such an approach, raw differences, post- to pre-separation, were used if available.

Analyses that adjusted only for age and sex and other family forms were considered to be examples using simple mean differences. If such simple mean differences were not available, coefficient estimates post- to pre-separation including adjustments for post-divorce factors were used. Where there was any uncertainty about whether controls were pre- or post-divorce, they were coded as post-divorce. Studies which used a mixture of pre- and post-divorcee variables were coded as post-divorce.

Amato (2000a) provides United States results used as a point of comparison. However, the studies for his work are not uniquely from the United States. There are United Kingdom, Canadian, Dutch and New Zealand studies included in his meta-analysis as well. Amato does not acknowledge the possibility of systematic differences in effect sizes between these different country estimates in his sample due to differences in society, economy or social welfare policies. No United States studies were included in this meta-analysis.

Averaged effect sizes considered here are likely to be biased upwards because the majority are raw unadjusted differences, which do not allow for selection bias. In addition, the numbers here are likely to be biased upwards because of a number of recent studies using sibling-fixed effects techniques, which found few significant effects, which could not be included. Effect sizes could not be calculated and included for these studies because insufficient information was provided.

Finally, there is no doubt that more work could yield more effect sizes. The cut-off date for the search was end of July 2007.

The total number of studies used is 122. The number of effect sizes collected is 893. These were summarised down into 367 average effect sizes by domain. While the aggregate number of 367 effect sizes is impressive, the number of effect sizes by OECD country varies widely. The large numbers of United Kingdom, Canadian and Finnish studies stick out, in part probably because those countries have good longitudinal surveys which have addressed these questions, and a sufficient number of lone parents to ensure meaningful cell sizes. A number of countries had very few, or no (in the case of Japan), studies. Little in the way of special effort was made to bolster the numbers for under-represented countries.

The average unweighted effect size from the 367 effect sizes for all the 122 studies included here is −0.230 which compares to the figure of −0.288 reported by Amato (2000a), taken from 67 largely United States studies published in 1990s with 177 effect sizes. Amato's overall conclusion is that this figure of −0.29 fits into the generally accepted "small" definition of effect size. Thus, if anything, the rest of the OECD in total is towards the smaller end of small. The minimum effect size and the maximum effect size found were both similar to the Amato study. In 345 cases of cases, the effect of being bought up in a lone parent was negative (94%, compared to 88% for Amato), and in 22 cases, the effect was positive.

To the extent that the comparison is valid, effect sizes also differ substantially on average between non-United States OECD countries. Effect sizes for the Anglophone

Table 5.1 Effect sizes by country

	N	%	Average	SD
Australia	7	2	−0.297	0.338
Austria	4	1	−0.098	0.162
Belgium	7	2	−0.200	0.160
Canada	26	7	−0.186	0.122
Czech Republic	1	0	−0.101	N/A
Denmark	21	6	−0.248	0.277
Finland	54	15	−0.314	0.170
France	12	3	−0.205	0.190
Germany	18	5	−0.173	0.208
Greece	4	1	−0.328	0.257
Hungary	10	3	−0.250	0.111
Iceland	9	2	−0.254	0.163
Ireland	3	1	−0.251	0.087
Italy	7	2	−0.231	0.086
Japan	0	0	N/A	N/A
Korea	1	0	−0.128	N/A
Luxembourg	1	0	−0.225	N/A
Mexico	1	0	−0.083	N/A
Netherlands	23	6	−0.173	0.134
New Zealand	5	1	−0.181	0.134
Norway	24	7	−0.236	0.218
Poland	1	0	−0.135	N/A
Portugal	3	1	−0.060	0.060
Slovak Republic	6	2	−0.132	0.078
Spain	7	2	−0.161	0.191
Sweden	29	8	−0.268	0.154
Switzerland	2	1	−0.130	0.054
Turkey	5	1	−0.649	0.469
United Kingdom	76	21	−0.187	0.159
Anglophone	116	32	−0.195	0.164
Nordic	135	37	−0.281	0.281
Continental W. European	107	29	−0.185	0.185
Total	367	100	−0.230	0.198

and Continental Western European countries are very similar, with those in the Nordic countries being, perhaps surprisingly, somewhat higher (Table 5.1).[5]

Turning now to estimation method, the data reveal that the majority of studies – nearly three in every four – were methodologically naïve raw mean differences between outcomes for child of lone parents and a control. Only a minority of studies

[5] Two Norwegian researchers, Breivik and Olweus (2006, p. 61), observe "[a] fairly common view holds that children's risks of negative outcomes associated with family dissolution are generally small or nonexistent in Scandinavia and clearly smaller than what is usually found in the United States".

Table 5.2 Effect sizes by estimation method

	N	%	Average	SD
Pre-divorce controls	49	13	−0.171	0.187
Raw mean differences	273	74	−0.256	0.200
Post-divorce controls	45	12	−0.136	0.153

Table 5.3 Effect sizes by type of data set

	N	%	Average	SD
Clinical	70	19	−0.313	0.292
Random samples or population data	297	81	−0.210	0.162

controlled for pre-divorce variables and a similar number presented effect sizes after controlling for post-divorce variables (recall the latter were only employed when no raw mean difference effect sizes could be calculated. They may over-control for selection). As expected, post-divorce controls gave the lowest average effect size, followed by pre-divorce controls. Mean raw differences, as expected, which provide no controls for selection, show the highest effect size. Even for mean raw differences, it is worth noting the effect size is still in the range customarily considered small. Given the predominance of raw mean differences in the effect size sample, it is likely that the true mean estimated effect size of −0.230 is upwardly biased (Table 5.2).[6]

About one in every five effect sizes was from a clinical sample. Clinical samples, as one might anticipate, showed a substantially larger mean effect size than random samples (which also include population-based data sets). Furthermore, outcomes measured from multiple item questionnaires were associated with a smaller effect size than single item questions. But the difference was reasonably small, being −0.222 for multiple items compared to −0.242 for single items. Overall, the pattern of coefficients between studies was as expected, following Amato and Keith (1991b) and Amato (2000a), with methodologically more sophisticated studies generating lower effect sizes (Table 5.3).

The most common domain examined for consideration of an impact of lone parenthood was academic attainment, with over a quarter of studies addressing some form of educational outcome. Externalising and internalising mental health problems and physical health problems all had a similar degree of prominence. This meta-analysis was much more heavily weighted towards educational outcomes than Amato (41% of the first five outcome domains compared to 22% for Amato) but much the same on conduct and depression (24% in both cases here compared to

[6] Amato (2005) also calculates mean weight effect sizes, which weights the individual effect size by its sample size. This method provides a better estimate of the effect size in the population. This weighting was not done here because of the significant number of studies which did not report the population sizes of the treatment and control groups. However, it is noteworthy that in Amato's study, this reduced effect sizes by domain by between one third and one half. There is no reason to believe that a similar reduction would not occur if the non-United States OECD data were re-weighted, again suggesting further upward bias in the effect sizes reported here.

Table 5.4 Effect sizes by outcome domain – a comparison with Amato (2000a)

	Mean unweighted effect size – Amato	Mean unweighted effect size – this study	Difference
Academic achievement	–0.26	–0.19	0.07
Conduct/behaviour/ delinquency/ADHD	–0.33	–0.29	0.04
Depression/anxiety/ happiness	–0.31	–0.20	0.11
Self-concept/esteem	–0.24	–0.13	0.11
Social relations	–0.28	–0.20	0.08
Total – five domains above	–0.29	–0.22	0.07

Table 5.5 Effect sizes by outcome domain

	N	%	Average	SD
Academic achievement	100	27	–0.192	0.150
Conduct/behaviour/ delinquency/ADHD	59	16	–0.288	0.206
Depression/anxiety/happiness	58	16	–0.203	0.163
Self-concept/esteem	8	2	–0.130	0.126
Social relations	18	5	–0.198	0.123
Physical health	67	18	–0.207	0.187
Employment/income	12	3	–0.214	0.202
Other (a catch-all category)	45	12	–0.339	0.298
Total	367	100	–0.230	0.198

23% in both cases for Amato). Self-concept and social relations were markedly under-represented (3% and 7%, respectively, compared to 16% in both cases for Amato). A major reason for this difference in shares by outcome domain is the use of OECD PISA data on differences for educational outcomes of children in lone parent families in this study.

What about effect sizes by domain? There are five domains where this study and Amato's overlap. Where the five domains are shared in common between the two studies, this study generates an average effect size of –0.216 (recall Amato's directly comparable figure of –0.288). By domain, this study finds a much lower impact on all outcomes (where comparable), with the exception of conduct, than Amato. It is the inclusion of domains which are not considered by Amato which boosts the average effect size found here (Table 5.4).

Lone parenthood effect sizes found for the non-United States OECD were larger for externalising than for internalising problems, not a result emerging to the same extent out of Amato's meta-analysis. This larger effect size for externalising compared to internalising behaviour found in the non-United States OECD may reflect any or all of (a) a true effect (b) the poor performance of instruments for internalising behaviour, something inherently harder to measure than externalising behaviour or (c) selection effects being stronger for externalising behaviour (Table 5.5).

Table 5.6 Effect sizes by age range

	N	%	Average	SD
Preschool	13	4	−0.178	0.209
Primary school	39	11	−0.262	0.266
Secondary school	165	45	−0.218	0.169
Mixed primary and secondary	34	9	−0.255	0.156
College	3	1	−0.042	0.138
Adults	66	18	−0.281	0.247
Other	47	13	−0.180	0.153

Table 5.7 Effect sizes by sex

	N	%	Average	SD
Male	80	22	−0.236	0.235
Female	78	21	−0.211	0.151
Both	209	57	−0.234	0.198

The number of effect sizes by age group reveals a distinct bias towards observing effects on secondary school age children, with approaching half of effect sizes being for this group (again partly reflecting the inclusion of PISA data for secondary school pupils). The next most popular age group for study was outcomes for children who had experienced a lone parent family structure as adults. The number of effect sizes for preschoolers was small, probably because the range of child outcomes collected in the early years is low and also because fewer children are in a lone parent family at this life-cycle stage.

> Of interest here is that moderate effect sizes were found into adulthood.[7] In fact, adult effect sizes were found to be the largest of any age group. This finding indicates that cause or selection into being a child of a lone parent is a marker which lasts well into adulthood (Table 5.6).

The majority of effect sizes mix males and females, but about a fifth respectively are for males and females separately. There is some very minor tendency for mean effect sizes to be larger for males. The absolute value of the size differences is almost certainly unimportant for policy purposes. On the other hand, Amato (2000a, p. 361) finds "modest support for the notion that divorce has stronger effects on boys than girls, at least in some domains" (see also Amato 2000b, pp. 1283–1284) (Table 5.7).

Effect sizes may differ between countries due to the different composition of the sample of effect sizes. To account for compositional differences, a simple multivariate regression as run, including outcome domains, whether differences were

[7] Recall Amato (2000a) does not consider adult outcomes. Young adult outcomes are however considered in relationship to lone parenthood in Amato (1999).

raw or controlled before and after divorce, stage of life cycle of the affected child, whether the sample was random or convenience, and country dummies. In terms of significant coefficients at a 5% level, the existence of pre- and post-divorce controls reduced effect sizes, with post-divorce controls having a larger effect, as anticipated. Random samples had significantly lower effect sizes than convenience samples. In terms of country effect sizes, Australia, Finland and Turkey had significantly higher effect sizes than the default (the United Kingdom), while Germany was significantly lower.

Overall, one might consider the small effect sizes found above to be an upper limit. For a number of reasons, it is likely that there are some upward biases imparted by the methods employed here to summarise the data and by the fact that so many of the studies do not control for any form of selection into lone parenthood.

General Policy Conclusions

Despite limited data for comparison of both levels and trends in lone parenthood across the OECD, it is clear that many countries have experienced substantial rises in numbers of lone parents over the last generation. These rises have been pronounced in some Anglophone countries. It is also clear that in most OECD countries, a significant minority of children will experience a lone parent family at some point in their life cycle. These changes have placed lone parent family structures on the policy agenda in some OECD countries. What is not clear is whether the trend to increased shares of lone parents will continue in countries with high rates of lone parenthood, or whether saturation has now been reached.[8] What is also not clear is whether countries currently with low rates of lone parenthood will converge to those with higher rates. In fact, the causes which have given rise to differential changes in rates of lone parenthood across the OECD have not been well investigated (in part because of the weaknesses in the data).

For policymakers, the first point to note is that, in comparison say to some policy-related literatures like the impact of education on earnings or even the employment effects of minimum wages, the empirical literature on the impact of family structure on child outcomes is at an immature stage. The immaturity is signalled by the lack of a consensus regarding the existence of a causal effect of lone parent family structure. To draw stronger conclusions means the application of particularly strong priors to the existing body of evidence. The quotation below illustrates the cautious recent approach taken by some researchers to the question:

> Our findings are that there is currently no unambiguous proof that growing up in a lone-parent family has adverse effects for later-life outcomes (with the exception of the effect

[8] There is some evidence of stabilisation and even recent decline in proportions of lone parents, for example, in New Zealand.

> on smoking). To reiterate, this does not mean that there is no effect. It means that the size and direction of the effect is not known for sure (for important statistical reasons). Indeed, our results are consistent with the effects being adverse (Francesconi et al. 2005, p. 48).

However, despite the ambiguity, researchers are also holding out some hope that a more precise conclusion may be able to be drawn in the (indefinite) future:

> Identification of a causal impact [of family structure on child well-being] must, however, await data which contain sufficiently convincing instruments that allow family structure to be modelled as an endogenous variable (Ermisch and Francesconi 2001a, p. 263).

In their position of caution, the researchers cited above are also reflecting a more general shift towards scepticism, within the economics profession at least, of using results from traditional multivariate analysis to determine causality. Moffitt (2005, p. 91) puts it this way: "[w]ithin economics, thinking about causal estimation has shifted dramatically in the past decade towards a more pessimistic reading of what is possible and a retreat in the ambitiousness of claims to causal determination". It is fair add to this that, in addition, economists as a profession tend to be both more technically focussed on conditions required for causal identification and perhaps hence more sceptical about identifying cause and effect that many in other disciplines – such a psychology, sociology and demography – who have contributed to the literature on lone parenthood and child well-being.

What policy conclusions are possible? Putting aside the causal question, something more definitive can be said on size of any effect. The meta-analysis, undertaken here, and in conjunction with Amato's similar study of (mostly) United States research, suggests that at a maximum that the likely causal effect sizes of being bought up in a lone parent family are at best small. In addition, the meta-analysis undertaken here, due to the dominance of raw mean effect sizes and use of unweighted estimates, delivers estimates of the average size of the lone parent effect on children which are almost certainly still too high. Additionally, it seems likely that the average effect for non-United States OECD countries is somewhat smaller than for the United States. The finding here that the non-United States OECD generates on average lower effect sizes than the United States may be seen to offer some support for a more sceptical view of the lone parent literature outside the United States. However, there is one important caveat to this scepticism – the Nordics generate quite similar effect sizes to the United States.

The largest effect sizes found in the meta-analysis in a well-defined category were for externalising behaviour. Externalising behaviour has clear social costs to third parties, as well as to the individual who has those issues. Again, the temptation to regard this finding as causal is strong, but there are obvious selection mechanisms whereby people who are unable to successfully sustain a relationship are more likely to have children who have behavioural problems without there being a causal link from the resulting family structure into externalising child behaviour.

Small effect sizes of being bought up as a child in a lone parent family structure were found into adulthood. In fact, adult effect sizes were found were the largest of any age group. A further interesting, if somewhat negative, finding was little evidence that males in the non-United States OECD are more affected by lone parenthood than females. This finding would suggest that recent deteriorating relative performance, especially in education, by boys in several OECD countries is unlikely to be able to be readily attributed to rising numbers of children being bought up by lone parents.

The extent to which different welfare regimes across the OECD influence the transmission of causal effects of lone parenthood is extremely difficult to judge, since the causal effects of lone parenthood are so difficult to define. However, it is the case that there are some differences between OECD countries in terms of the impact of lone parenthood. The extent to which these differences can be put down to policy choices regarding welfare regimes is unclear. There are other differences between countries, not simply welfare regime variation, which may account for inter-country differences in between children of lone parents and children in intact families. For example, parental selection into lone parenthood may differ across countries, due to factors like cross-country differences in divorce laws or the social stigma of divorce. Sociocultural differences across the OECD are obvious in relation to family issues, and these differences may be responsible for observed cross-country differences. And for policymakers, even if it was known conclusively that differences in causal effects of lone parenthood on child outcomes were due to the differences in the operation of welfare states, this would not positively identify which dimension of policy difference across a wide range of benefits and services in kind (including education and housing policies), singularly or interactively, were responsible for the outcome difference. It is noteworthy that the few studies found here which explicitly discussed such questions were either extremely reluctant to attribute differences to policy or found that their results contradicted their priors.

A surprising conclusion of the meta-analysis was the higher than average effect sizes found in the Nordic countries, with an overall average which was very similar to the mean United States effect size found by Amato (2000a). It was anticipated, prior to commencing this work, that the re-distributional nature of these states towards lone parents would overcome other environmental or selection factors leading to worse results for children in such families. Consequently, children of lone parents in the United States would be considerably worse off in terms of well-being measures than Nordic children. The results presented here suggest that there are other things going on. The unexpected result of the meta-analysis in this regard actually broadly concurred with other very recent evidence found in the literature review, for example, the recent comparative studies of Breivik and Olweus (2006), Bjorklund et al. (2007a) and PISA. Nevertheless, the consensus on this matter is not unanimous, at least for Norway (see Phipps 1998).

The meta-analysis reveals that the average size effects are small, but this does not, however, mean the effects are necessarily unimportant as a policy issue. Most effect sizes in almost all multivariate regression studies of social phenomena are small. Effects can also found across a wide range of outcomes, across much of the child and young adult life cycle, and, in addition, may affect a considerable group of children. Of course, given the considerable apparent variation in exposure to lone parenthood across different OECD countries, this means that lone parenthood will be a greater policy concern in countries with higher rates of lone parenthood, all other things being equal.

The effect sizes considered in the meta-analysis are average effects. Again, only on the basis of strong assumptions are these effect sizes those most relevant to policy. For any particular policy being contemplated, the relevant effects are the effects of reducing separation for the currently intact families which are marginal to the policy change. Different sorts of families are likely to be marginal to different policy changes.

Policymakers need to additionally keep in mind that average effects conceal an enormous amount of variation. Many children bought out with lone parents do well on all counts. Many children bought up in stable two-parent families do poorly. This is because many other factors – some well understood and others less so – influence the social outcomes of interest for children (Amato 2005). This additionally means that crudely targeting resources towards lone parents, in addition to possibly reinforcing social stigma which may undermine well-being of children from lone parent families, is likely to lead to high false positives (providing a service to children of lone parent families who have no need of it) and high false negatives (not providing a service to many children of two-parent families have need of it).

The meta-analysis also shows that the methodologically more sophisticated studies, in terms of several indicators of sophistication, tend to yield smaller effect sizes. The most robust conclusion is that higher quality research designs typically show a smaller and less statistically significant effect on lone parent family structure on child well-being than more traditional bivariate or multivariate methods. However, the results depend on the method, the sample and the country. Given the comparatively few studies using higher quality designs, it is not possible to say definitively which one of these three possible dimensions is driving the results. It should be also recalled that these designs are better for answering causal questions, but they still rely on some important maintained hypotheses for identification of causal effects.

Policy levers to change children's experience of lone parent family structure or change the impact on children of a lone parent family structure are not a core part of this review. But if there is a casual effect of lone parenthood on children's outcomes, a further issue becomes the relative efficacy and cost of a very broad range of policies to (a) encourage people who are unlikely to form a stable family unit to more carefully consider decisions to have children, (b) to encourage parents who may be at risk of separating to consider staying together and (c) to compensate children who find themselves in a lone parent family structure from any adverse causal consequences of their family structure. The costs of the various policies to influence child well-being via influencing family structure will then have to be compared against the social benefits of so doing. Information on relative policy efficacy in this area is, at best, patchy and – probably for most member states of the OECD – non-existent.

In conclusion, policymakers should be aware that the current immature state of the literature does not allow strong conclusions to be drawn regarding the impact of lone parenthood on child well-being in the absence of additional strong priors.

There is certainly enough in the literature to suggest policymakers should be concerned about the implications of family structure for child well-being and should keep a close eye on social trends in terms of changes in family structure as well as on the developing social scientific literature on the impact of family structure on child well-being. However, there does not seem to be enough in the literature, in the absence of application of extra-scientific priors in terms of identification, to advocate radical policy change, especially if levers to change family form are at all costly to undertake or uncertain in effect. What should be clear from this review is that this is an area of social science which is rapidly expanding, in terms of new estimation techniques, in terms of growth of useful longitudinal data sets and in terms of countries where the impact of lone parenthood is being researched. It may well be that in another decade research will cast a more precise and certain light on the questions addressed above in this chapter.

Acknowledgements I am very grateful to Professor Maria Bacikova-Sleskova for undertaking a special run of her Slovak data set for this study on request (Sleskova et al. 2006). I also thank my colleagues Mark Pearson and Willem Adema for their useful comments. The usual disclaimers apply.

References

Agerbo, E., Nordentoft, M., & Mortensen, P. B. (2002). Familial, psychiatric, and socioeconomic risk factors for suicide in young people: Nested case–control study. *British Medical Journal, 325*, 74–79.

Albert, C. (2000). Higher education demand in Spain: The influence of labour market signals and family background. *Higher Education, 40*, 147–162.

Albertini, M., & Dronkers, J. (2003). *Intergenerational effects of divorce in a mediterranean society* (EUI Working Paper SPS 2003/11). European University Institute, Florence Badia Fiesolana: Department of Political and Social Sciences.

Alcon, M., & Pedersen, J. (2001). Family as a child development context and smoking behaviour among school children in Greenland. *International Journal of Circumpolar Health, 60*(1), 52–63.

Almqvist, F., Kumpulainen, K., Ikäheimo, K., Linna, S.-L., Henttonen, I., Huikko, E., Tuompo-Johansson, E., Aronen, E., Puura, K., Piha, J., Tamminen, T., Räsänen, E., & Moilanen, I. (1999). Behavioural and emotional symptoms in 8–9-year-old children. *European Child & Adolescent Psychiatry, 8*(Supplement 4), IV/7–IV/16.

Amato, P. (1991). Parental absence during childhood and adult depression. *The Sociological Quarterly, 32*, 543–546.

Amato, P. (1999). Children of divorced parents as young adults. In E. M. Hetherington (Ed.), *Coping with divorce, single parenting, a remarriage: A risk and resilience perspective.* Mahwah: Erlbaum.

Amato, P. (2000a). Children of divorce in the 1990s: An update of the Amato and Keith (1991) Meta-analysis. *Journal of Family Psychology, 15*, 355–370.

Amato, P. (2000b). Consequences of divorce for adults and children. *Journal of Marriage and the Family, 62*, 1269–1287.

Amato, P. (2002). Good enough marriages: Parental discord, Divorce, and children's well-being. *Virginia Journal of Social Policy & the Law, 9*, 71–94.

Amato, P. (2005). The impact of family formation change on the cognitive. Social and emotional well-being of the next generation. *The Future of Children, 15*(2), 75–96.

Amato, P., & Booth, A. (2001). The legacy of marital discord: Consequences for children's marital quality. *Journal of Personality and Social Psychology, 81*, 627–638.
Amato, P. R., & Cheadle, J. (2005). The long reach of divorce: Tracking marital dissolution and child well-being across three generations. *Journal of Marriage and the Family, 67*, 191–206.
Amato, P. R., & DeBoer, D. (2001). The transmission of divorce across generations: Relationship skills or commitment to marriage? *Journal of Marriage and the Family, 63*, 1038–1051.
Amato, P., & Gilbreth, J. G. (1999). Nonresident fathers and children's well-being: A meta-analysis. *Journal of Marriage and the Family, 61*(3), 557–573.
Amato, P., & Keith, B. (1991a). Separation from a parent during childhood and adult socio-economic attainment. *Social Forces, 70*, 187–206.
Amato, P., & Keith, P. (1991b). Parental divorce and the well-being of children: A meta-analysis. *Psychological Bulletin, 110*, 26–46.
Amato, P., & Sobolewski, J. M. (2001). The effects of divorce and marital discord on adult children's psychological well-being. *American Sociological Review, 66*, 900–921.
Anders, B., Ginther, D., & Marianne, S. (2007). Family structure and child outcomes in the United States and Sweden. *Journal of Population Economics, 20*, 183–201.
Andersson, G. (2002). Children's experience of family disruption and family formation: Evidence from 16 FFS countries. *Demographic Research 7*(7). Available at http://www.demographic-research.org
Antecol, H., & Bedard, K. (2007). Does single parenthood increase the probability of teenage promiscuity, substance use, and crime? *Journal of Population Economics, 20*, 55–71.
Antecol, H., Bedard, K., & Helland, E. (2001). *Does single parenthood increase the probability of teenage promiscuity, drug use, and crime? Evidence from divorce law changes* (Claremont Colleges Working Papers 2001–11). Claremont Colleges.
Aral, N., Gursoy, F., & Dizman, H. (2006). A comparison of depression in children with and without mothers. *Psychological Reports, 99*(2), 619–629.
Artis, J. (2007). Maternal cohabitation and child well-being among kindergarten children. *Journal of Marriage and Family, 69*(1), 222–236.
Aseltine, R. (1996). Pathways linking parental divorce with adult depression. *Journal of Health and Social Behaviour, 34*, 133–148.
Barnow, S., Lucht, M., & Freyberger, H. J. (2001). Influence of punishment, emotional rejection, child abuse, and broken home on aggression in adolescence: An examination of aggressive adolescents in Germany. *Psychopathology, 34*(4), 167–173.
Baumer, J. H., Hunt, L. P., & Shield, J. P. (1998). Social disadvantage, family composition, and diabetes mellitus: Prevalence and outcome. *Archives of Disease in Childhood, 79*(5), 427–430.
Baydar, N. (1988). Effects of parental separation and re-entry into union on the emotional well-being of children. *Journal of Marriage and the Family, 50*, 967–981.
Berntsson, L., & Kohler, L. (2001). Long-term illness and psychosomatic complaints. *European Journal of Public Health, 11*(1), 35–42.
Biblarz, T., & Raftery, A. E. (1999). Family structure, educational attainment, and socioeconomic success: Rethinking the 'pathology of matriarchy'. *The American Journal of Sociology, 105*(2), 321–365.
Bjarnason, T., Davidaviciene, A., Miller, P., Nociar, A., Pavlakis, A., & Stergar, E. (2003). Family structure and adolescent cigarette smoking in eleven European countries. *Addiction, 98*, 815–824.
Björklund, A., & Sundström, M. (2006). Parental separation and children's educational attainment: A siblings approach. *Economica, 73*, 605–624.
Björklund, A., Ginther, D., & Sundström, M. (2007a, November). *Does marriage matter for children? Assessing the causal impact of legal marriage* (IZA DP No. 3189).
Björklund, A., Ginther, D., & Marianne, S. (2007b, March 1). *Is cohabitation bad for children? Assessing the causal impact of legal marriage on child outcomes* (Princeton Working Paper).
Blakely, T., Atkinson, J., Kiro, C., Blaiklock, A., & D'Souza, A. (2003). Child mortality, socioeconomic position, and one parent families: Independent associations and variation by age and cause of death. *International Journal of Epidemiology, 32*, 410–418.

Block, J. H., Block, J., & Gjerde, P. F. (1986). The impact of divorce on children. *Journal of Marriage and the Family, 57*, 619–648.

Bockelbrink, A., Heinrich, J., Schäfer, I., Zutavern, A., Borte, M., Herbarth, O., Schaaf, B., Von Berg, A., Schäfer, T., & for the LISA Study Group. (2006). Atopic eczema in children: Another harmful sequel of divorce. *Allergy, 61*, 1397–1402.

Bonell, C., Allen, E., Strange, V., Oakley, A., Copas, A., Johnson, A., & Stephenson, J. (2006). Influence of family type and parenting behaviours on teenage sexual behaviour and conceptions. *Journal of Epidemiology and Community Health, 60*(6), 502–506.

Booth, A., & Amato, P. R. (2001). Parental predivorce relations and offspring postdivorce well-being. *Journal of Marriage and the Family, 63*, 197–212.

Borgers, N., Dronkers, J., & van Praag, B. (1996). Different forms of two- and lone-parent families and the well-being of their children in secondary education. *Social Psychology of Education, 1*, 147–169.

Bosman, R., & Louwnes, W. (1988). School careers of children from one-parent and two parent families. *Netherlands Journal of Sociology, 24*, 98–116.

Bradshaw, J., & Finch, N. (2002). *A comparison of child benefit packages in 22 countries*. United Kingdom, Department of Work and Pensions.

Breivik, K., & Olweus, D. (2006). Children of divorce in a Scandinavian welfare state: Are they less affected than United States children? *Scandinavian Journal of Psychology, 47*, 61–74.

Brodzinksy, D., Hitt, J., & Smith, D. (1993). Impact of parental separation and divorce on adopted and nonadopted children. *The American Journal of Orthopsychiatry, 63*(3), 451–460.

Bukodi, E., & Dronkers, J. (2003, November 13–16). *Family structure and educational attainment in Hungary*. Paper presented at the second conference of The European network for empirical and comparative research on the sociological aspects of divorce, Tilburg, The Netherlands.

Butters, J. E. (2005). Promoting healthy choices: The importance of differentiating between ordinary and high risk cannabis use among high-school students. *Substance Use & Misuse, 40*(6), 845–855.

Capron, C., Thérond, C., & Duyme, M. (2007). Brief report: Effect of menarcheal status and family structure on depressive symptoms and emotional/behavioural problems in young adolescent girls. *Journal of Adolescence, 30*(91), 175–179.

Carbonneau, R., Tremblay, R. E., Vitaro, F., Dobkin, P. L., Saucier, J. F., & Pihl, R. O. (1998). Paternal alcoholism, paternal absence and the development of problem behaviors in boys from age six to twelve years. *Journal of the Study of Alcohol, 59*(4), 387–398.

Case, A., Lin, I.-F., & McLanahan, S. (2001). Educational attainment of siblings in step-families. *Evolution and Human Behaviour, 22*, 269–289.

Casquel, E. (2003, January 16). *The effect of labour market conditions and family background on educational attainment of Spanish youngsters* (ISER Working Paper). http://www.iser.essex.ac.uk/pubs/workpaps/pdf/2003–01.pdf.

Chase-Lansdale, P. L., Cherlin, A. J., & Kiernan, K. E. (1995). The long-term effects of parental divorce on the mental health of young adults: A developmental perspective. *Child Development, 66*(6), 1614–1634.

Cheng, H., Dunn, J., O'Connor, T., Golding, J., & the ALSPAC Study Team. (2006). Factors moderating children's adjustment to parental separation: Findings from a community study in England. *Journal of Abnormal Psychology, 34*(2), 239–250.

Cherlin, A. (2005). American marriage in the early twenty-first century. *The Future of Children, 15*(2), 33–55.

Cherlin, A. J., Furstenberg, F. F., Chase-Lansdale, P. L., Kiernan, K. E., et al. (1991). Longitudinal studies of effects of divorce on children in Great Britain and the United States. *Science, 252*(5011), 1386–1389.

Cherlin, A. J., Furstenburg, P. L., Chase-Lansdale, P. L., & McRae, C. (1998a). Effects of parental divorce on mental health through the life course. *American Sociological Review, 63*, 239–249.

Cherlin, A., Chase-Landsdale, P. L., & McRae, C. (1998b). Effects of parental divorce on mental health through the life cycle. *American Sociological Review, 63*, 239–249.

Chinn, S. (2000). A simple method for converting an odds ratio to an effect size for use in meta-analysis. *Statistics in Medicine, 19*, 3127–3131.

Christoffersen, M. N., & Soothill, K. (2003). The long-term consequences of parental alcohol abuse: A cohort study of children in Denmark. *Journal of Substance Abuse Treatment, 25*(2), 107–116.

Corak, M. (2001). Death and divorce: The long-term consequences of parental loss on adolescents. *Journal of Labour Economics, 19*(3), 682–715.

Crowder, K., & Teachman, J. (2004). Do residential conditions explain the relationship between living arrangements and adolescent behavior? *Journal of Marriage and the Family, 66*, 721–738.

Csorba, J., Rózsa, S., Vetro, A., Gadoros, J., Makra, J., Somogyi, E., Kaczvinszky, E., & Kapornay, K. (2001). Family- and school-related stresses in depressed Hungarian children. *European Psychiatry, 16*, 18–26.

Curtis, L. J., Dooley, M. D., Lipman, E. L., & Feeny, D. H. (2001). The role of permanent income and family structure in the determination of child health in Canada. *Health Economics, 10*(4), 287–302.

D'Onofrio, B., Turkheimer, E., Emery, R., Heath, A., Madden, P., Slutske, W., & Martin, N. (2006). A genetically informed study of the processes underlying the association between parental martial instability and offspring adjustment. *Developmental Psychology, 42*(3), 486–499.

D'Onofrio, B., Turkheimer, E., Emery, R., Harden, P., Slutske, W., Heath, A., Madden, P., & Martin, N. (2007a). A genetically informed study of the intergenerational transmission of marital instability. *Journal of Marriage and the Family, 69*, 793–809.

D'Onofrio, B., Turkheimer, E., Emery, R., Maes, H., Silberg, J., & Eaves, L. (2007b). A children of twins study of parental divorce and offspring psychopathology. *Journal of Marriage and the Family, 69*, 793–809.

de Goede, M., Spruijt, E., Maas, C., & Duindam, V. (2000). Family problems and youth unemployment. *Adolescence, 35*(139), 587–601.

Deding, M., Lausen, M., & Andersen A. R. (2007). *Starting school. The effect of early childhood factors on child well-being. Programme area 4: The effects of welfare policy* (Working Paper 2).

Demers, M., Brodeur, J. M., Mouton, C., Simard, P. L., Trahan, L., & Veilleux, G. (1992). A multivariate model to predict caries increment in Montreal children aged 5 years. *Community Dental Health, 9*(3), 273–281.

Doherty, W., & Needle, R. (1991). Psychological adjustment and substance use among adolescents before and after a parental divorce. *Child Development, 62*(2), 328–337.

Dronkers, J. (1994). The changing effects of lone parent families on the educational attainment of their children in a European welfare state. *Sociology, 28*(1), 171–191.

Dronkers, J. (1999). The effects of parental conflicts and divorce on well-being of pupils in Dutch secondary school. *European Sociological Review, 15*(2), 195–212.

Duncan, G. (with Hill, M., & Yeung, W-J. J.) (1997). Childhood family structure and young adult behavior. *Journal of Population Economics, 14*(2), 271–299.

Elliot, B. J., & Richards, M. P. M. (1991). Children and divorce: Educational performance and behaviour before and after parental separation. *International Journal of Law and the Family, 5*, 258–276.

Ellis, B. J., et al. (2003). Does father absence place daughters at special risk for early sexual activity and teenage pregnancy? *Child Development, 74*, 801–821.

Ellwood, D., & Jencks, C. (2001). *The growing differences in family structure: What do we know?* Unpublished manuscript, Harvard University, Boston.

Ely, M., West, P., Sweeting, H., & Richards, M. (2000). Teenage family life, life chances, lifestyles and health: A comparison of two contemporary cohorts. *International Journal of Law, Policy and the Family, 14*, 1–30.

Erik, L. K., Skrondal, A., Vertio, H., & Helgason, A. (1998). To what extent do parents strive to protect their children from environmental tobacco smoke in the Nordic countries? A population-based study. *Tobacco Control, 7*(1), 56–60.

Ermisch, J., & Francesconi, M. (2001a). Family structure and children's achievements. *Journal of Population Economics, 14*(2), 249–270.

Ermisch, J., & Francesconi, M. (2001b). Family matters: Impacts of family background on educational attainments. *Economica, 68*(270), 137–156.

Esping-Anderson, G. (1990). *The three worlds of welfare capitalism*. Princeton: Princeton University Press.

Evenhouse, E., & Reilly, S. (2004). A sibling study of stepchild well-being. *Journal of Human Resources, 39*(1), 248–276.

Evren, C., Kural, S., & Cakmak, D. (2006). Clinical correlates of childhood abuse and neglect in substance dependents. *Addictive Behaviours, 31*, 475–485.

Eydoux, A., & Letablier, M.-T. (2007). *Les familles monoparentale en France*. Serie rapport de vecherche No.36 centre d'études de l'émploi, Noisy-le-Grand, Juin.

Fergusson, D., Horwood, J., & Lynskey, M. (1994a). Parental separation adolescent psychopathology and problem behaviours. *Journal of the American Academy of Child and Adolescent Psychiatry, 33*(8), 1122–1131.

Fergusson, D., Lynskey, M., & Horwood, J. (1994b). The effects of parental separation. The timing of separation and gender on children's performance on cognitive tests. *Journal of Child Psychology and Psychiatry, 35*(6), 1077–1092.

Fleming, D. M., & Charlton, J. R. H. (1998). Morbidity and healthcare utilisation of children in households with one adult: comparative observational study. *British Medical Journal, 316*(May), 1572–1576.

Fombonne, E., & Vermeersch, S. (1997). Children of the GAZEL Cohort: I--Prevalence of contacts with the medico-educational system for psychological reasons, and associated factors. *Revue Epidemiology et Santé Publique, 45*(1), 29–40 [Article in French].

Forehand, R., Armistead, L., & David, C. (1997). Is adolescent adjustment following parental divorce a function of pre-divorce adjustment? *Journal of Abnormal Child Psychology, 25*, 157–164.

Francesconi, M., Jenkins, S., & Siedler, T. (2005, September). *The impact of family structure during childhood on later-life attainment*. Anglo-German Foundation for the Study of Industrial Society.

Francesconi, M., Jenkins, S., & Siedler, T. (2006, July). *Childhood family structure and schooling outcomes: Evidence for Germany* (Discussion Papers 610). Berlin: DIW Berlin.

Frankel, D. (2006, May 19). *How does family structure affect children's outcomes? Evidence from the civil war* (Staff General Research Papers with number 12819). Ames: Iowa State University. Department of Economics.

Franz, M., Lensche, H., & Schmitz, N. (2003). Psychological distress and socio-economic status in single mothers and their children in a German city. *Social Psychiatry and Epidemiology, 38*, 59–68.

Frisch, M., & Hviid, A. (2006). Childhood family correlates of heterosexual and homosexual marriages: A national cohort study of two million Danes. *Archives of Sexual Behaviour, 35*(5), 533–547.

Fröjd, S., Marttunen, M., Pelkonen, M., von der Pahlen, B., & Kaltiala-Heino, R. (2006). Perceived financial difficulties and maladjustment outcomes in adolescence. *European Journal of Public Health, 16*(5), 542–548.

Fronstin, P., Greenburg, D., & Robins, P. (2001). Parental disruption and the labour market performance of children when they reach adulthood. *Journal of Population Economics, 14*, 137–172.

Gähler, M. (1998). Self-reported mental well-being among adult children of divorce in Sweden. *Acta Sociologica, 41*(3), 209–225.

Garib, G., Garcia, T. M., & Dronkers, J. (2003, November 13–16). *Are the effects of different family forms on children's educational performance related to the demographic characteristics and family policies of modern societies?* Paper presented at the second conference of the European network for empirical and comparative research on the sociological aspects of divorce, Tilburg, The Netherlands.

Garnefski, N., & Diekstra, R. (1997). Adolescents from one parent, stepparent and intact families: Emotional problems and suicide attempts. *Journal of Adolescence, 20*, 201–208.
Gennetian, L. (2005). One or two parents? Half or step siblings? The effect of family composition on young children's achievement. *Journal of Population Economics, 18*(3), 415–436.
Gertler, P., Levine, D., & Ames, M. (2003). *Schooling and parental death* (Working Paper No. C03–128). Berkeley: Centre for International and Development Economics Research.
Ginther, D. K., & Pollak, R. A. (2003, April). *Does family structure affect children's educational outcomes?* NBER Working Paper Series (Working Paper 9628).
Ginther, D. K., & Pollak, R. A. (2004). Family structure and children's educational outcomes: Blended families, stylized facts, and descriptive regressions. *Demography, 41*(4), 671–696.
González, L. (2005). The determinants of the prevalence of single mothers: A cross country analysis, institute for the study of lobour, Discussion paper (IZA DP No. 1677).
González, L., & Vitanen, T. (2006, October). *The effect of divorce laws on divorce rates in Europe* (Working Paper number 2006003). Sheffield: The University of Sheffield. Department of Economics
González, L., & Vitanen, T. (2008). *The long run effects of legalizing divorce on children*. Paper to royal economic society annual conference, Warwick University, March.
Griesbach, D., Amos, A., & Currie, C. (2003). Adolescent smoking and family structure in Europe. *Social Science and Medicine, 56*, 41–52.
Grogger, J., & Ronan, N. (1995, September). *The intergenerational effects of fatherlessness on education attainment and entry level wages*. National Longitudinal Surveys. U.S. Department of Labour. Bureau of Labour Statistics.
Gunther, N., Slavenburg, B., Feron, F., & van Os, J. (2003). Childhood social and early developmental factors associated with mental health service use. *Social Psychiatry and Psychiatric Epidemiology, 38*, 101–108.
Hammer, T., & Vaglum, P. (1990). Initiation, continuation or discontinuation of cannabis use in the general population. *British Journal of Addiction, 85*(7), 899–909.
Hansagi, H., Brandt, L., & Adreasson, S. (2000). Parental divorce: Psychological well-being, mental health and mortality during youth and young adulthood. A longitudinal study of Swedish conscripts. *European Journal of Public Health, 10*(2), 86–92.
Hao, L., & Matsueda, R. (2006). Family dynamics through childhood: A sibling model of behavioural problems. *Social Science Research, 35*, 500–524.
Hao, L., & Xie, G. (2002). The complexity and endogeneity of family structure in explaining children's misbehaviour. *Social Science Research, 31*, 1–28.
Harland, P., Reijneveld, S. A., Brugman, E., Verlove-Vanhorick, S. P., & Verhulst, F. C. (2002). Family factors and life events as risk factors for behavioural and emotional problems in children. *European Child & Adolescent Psychiatry, 11*, 176–184.
Harper, C. C., & McLanahan, S. (1999). *Father absence and youth incarceration. Centre for research and child well-being* (Working Paper Number 99–03).
Hassani, K., Kosunen, E., & Rimpela, A. (2006). The use of oral contraceptives among Finnish teenagers from 1981 to 2003. *Journal of Adolescent Health, 39*, 649–655.
Haveman, R., & Wolfe, B. (1994). *Succeeding generations*. New York: Russell Sage.
Hill, M., & Callister, P. (2003, November 13–14). *Is 'single parent family' a misnomer misdirecting research and policies?* Paper for presentation at Family Demography Conference, Bethesda, MD.
Hill, M., Yeung, W. J. J., & Duncan, G. (2001). Childhood family structure and young adult behaviours. *Journal of Population Economics, 14*(2), 271–299.
Hoekstra, M. (2006, February 9). *Just kidding dear. Using dismissed divorce cases to identify the effect of parental divorce on student performance*. www.econ.pitt.edu/papers/mark_divorce_paper.pdf
Hope, S., Power, C., & Rodgers, B. (1998). The relationship between parental separation in childhood and problem drinking in adulthood. *Addiction, 93*(4), 505–514.
Huurre, T., Junkkari, H., & Aro, H. (2006). Long-term Psycho-social effects of parental divorce. *European Archives of Clinical Neuroscience, 256*, 256–263.

Huurtig, T., Taanila, A., Ebeling, H., Miettunen, J., & Moilanen, I. (2005). Attention and behavioural problems of Finnish adolescents may be related to the family environment. *European Child & Adolescent Psychiatry, 14*, 471–478.

Icks, A., Rosenbauer, J., Strassburger, K., Grabert, M., Giani, G., & Holl, R. W. (2007). Persistent social disparities in the risk of hospital admission of paediatric patients in Germany – prospective data from 1277 diabetic children and adolescents. *Diabetic Medicine, 24*, 440–442.

Isir, A. B., Todemir, M., Kücüker, H., & Dulger, H. E. (2007). Role of family factors in adolescent delinquency in an Elazig/Turkey reformatory. *Forensic Science, 52*(1), 125–127.

Isohanni, M., Oja, H., Moilanen, I., & Koiranen, M. (1994). Teenage alcohol drinking and non-standard family background. *Social Science Medicine, 38*(11), 1565–1574.

Jens, L. (1990). Mentally retarded criminal offenders in Denmark. *The British Journal of Psychiatry, 1990*(156), 726–731.

John, E., Francesconi, M., & Pevalin, D. J. (2004). Parental partnership and joblessness in childhood and their influence on young people's outcomes. *Journal of the Royal Statistical Society A, 167*(1), 69–101.

Johnson, J., & Mazingo, C. (2000). *The economic consequences of unilateral divorce for children*. Champaign: Office of Research. University of Illinois.

Jonathan, G. (2004). Is making divorce easier bad for children? The long run implications of unilateral divorce. *Journal of Labor Economics, 22*(4), 799–834.

Jonsson, J. O., & Gähler, M. (1997). Family dissolution, family reconstitution, and children's educational careers: Recent evidence from Sweden. *Demography, 34*(2), 277–293.

Jonsson, F., Njardvik, U., Olafsdottir, G., & Gretarsson, S. (2000). Parental divorce: Long-term effects on mental health, family relations and adult sexual behaviour. *Scandinavian Journal of Psychology, 41*, 101–105.

Joshi, H., Cooksey, E., Wiggins, R., McCulloch, A., Verropoulou, G., & Clarke, L. (1999). Diverse family living situations and child development: A multi level analysis comparing longitudinal evidence from Britain and the United States. *International Journal of Law, Policy and the Family, 13*(3), 292–314.

Kaltiala-Heino, R., Rimpelä, M., Rantanen, P., & Laippala, P. (2001). Adolescent depression: the role of discontinuities in life course and social support. *Journal of Affective Disorders, 64*, 155–156.

Kapornai, K., Gentzler, A., Tepper, P., Kiss, E., Mayer, L., Tamás, Z., Kovacs, M., & Vetró, Á. (2007). Early developmental characteristics and features of major depressive disorder among child psychiatric patients in Hungary. *Journal of Affective Disorders, 100*(1), 91–101.

Kendler, K. S., Neale, M. C., Prescott, C. A., Kessler, R. C., Heath, A. C., Corey, L. A., & Leaves, L. J. (1996). Childhood parental loss and alcoholism in women: A causal analysis using a twin-family design. *Psychological Medicine, 26*, 79–95.

Kerr, D., & Michalski, J. (2007). Family structure and children's hyperactivity problems: A longitudinal analysis. *The Canadian Journal of Sociology, 32*(1), 85–112.

Kestilä, L., Koskinen, S., Martelin, T., Rahkonen, O., Pensola, T., Aro, H., & Aromaa, A. (2005). The determinants of health in early adulthood: What is the role of parental education, childhood adversities and own education? *European Journal of Public Health, 16*(3), 305–314.

Kestilä, L., Koskinen, S., Martelin, T., Rahkonen, O., Pensola, T., Aro, H., & Aromaa, A. (2006). Influence of parental education, childhood adversities and current living conditions on daily smoking in early adulthood? *European Journal of Public Health, 16*(6), 617–626.

Kotimaa, A. J., Moilanen, I., Taanila, A., Ebeling, H., Smalley, S. L., McGough, J. J., Hartikainen, A. L., & Jarvelin, M. R. (2003). Maternal smoking and hyperactivity in 8-year-old children. *Journal of the American Academy of Child and Adolescent Psychiatry, 42*(7), 826–833.

Krein, S. F. (1986). Growing up in a single parent family: The effect on education and earnings of young men. *Family Relations, 35*, 161–168.

Krein, S. F., & Beller, A. H. (1988). Educational attainment of children from single-parent families: Differences by exposure, gender and race. *Demography, 25*, 221–234.

Kuh, D., & Maclean, M. (1990). Women's childhood experience of parental separation and their subsequent health and socioeconomic status in adulthood. *Journal of Biosocial Science, 22*(1), 121–135.

Kumpulainen, K. (2000). Psychiatric symptoms and deviance in early adolescence predict heavy alcohol use 3 years later. *Addiction, 95*(1), 1847–1857.

Kumpulainen, K., & Räsänen, E. (2002). Symptoms and deviant behaviour among eight-year olds as predictors of referral for psychiatric evaluation by age 12. *Psychiatric Services, 53*(2), 201–206.

Laftman, S. B., & Östberg, V. (2006). The pros and cons of social relations: An analysis of adolescents' health complaints. *Social Science and Medicine, 63*, 611–623.

Lamerz, A., Kuepper-Nybelen, J., Wehle, C., Bruning, N., Trost-Brinkhues, G., Brenner, H., Hebebrand, J., & Herpertz-Dahlmann, B. (2005). Social class, parental education, and obesity prevalence in a study of six-year-old children in Germany. *International Journal of Obesity, 29*, 373–380.

Lang, K., & Zagorsky, J. (2001). Does growing up with a parent absent really hurt? *Journal of Human Resources, 36*(2), 253–273.

Langille, D., Hughes, J., Murphy, G., & Rigby, J. (2005). Socio-economic factors and adolescent sexual activity and behaviour in Nova Scotia. *Canadian Journal of Public Health, 96*(4), 313–318.

Lanz, M., Iafrate, R., Rosnati, R., & Scabini, E. (1999). Parent–child communication and adolescent self-esteem in separated, inter-country adoptive and intact non-adoptive families. *Journal of Adolescence, 22*, 785–794.

Larsson, B., & Sund, A. M. (2007). Emotional/behavioural, social correlates and one-year predictors of frequent pains among early adolescents: Influences of pain characteristics. *European Journal of Pain, 11*, 57–65.

Ledoux, S., Miller, P., Choquet, M., & Plant, M. (2002). Family structure, parent–child relationships and alcohol and other drug use among teenagers in France and United Kingdom. *Alcohol and Alcoholism, 37*(1), 52–60.

Leeners, B., Neumaier-Wagener, P., Kuse, S., Irawan, C., Imthurn, B., & Rath, W. (2006). Family stability during childhood and the risk to develop hypertensive diseases in pregnancy. *Early Human Development, 82*, 441–446.

Li, L., & Power, C. (2004). Influences on childhood height: Comparing two generations in the 1958 British birth cohort. *International Journal of Epidemiology, 33*, 1320–1328.

Li, L., Manor, O., & Power, C. (2004). Early environment and child-to-adult growth trajectories in the 1958 British birth cohort. *American Journal of Clinical Nutrition, 80*, 185–192.

Lintonen, T., Rimpelä, M., Vikat, A., & Rimpelä, A. (2000). The effects of societal changes on drunkenness trends in early adolescence. *Health Education Research, 15*(3), 261–269.

Lissau, I., & Sorensen, T. (1994). Parental neglect during childhood and increased risk of obesity in young adulthood. *The Lancet, 343*, 324–327.

Liu, S. (2007, July 16). *Is my parent's divorce to blame for my failure in life? A joint model of child educational attainments and parental divorce, paper*. Miami: Department of Economics, University of Miami.

Locard, E., Mamelle, N., Billette, A., Miginiac, M., Munoz, F., & Rey, S. (1992). Risk factors of obesity in a five year old population, parental versus environmental factors. *International Journal of Obesity, 16*(10), 721–729.

Lont, A., & Dronkers, J. (2004). Parental divorce and the well-being of adolescent children. Changes between 1984–1999 in the Netherlands. In W. Glatzer, S. von Below, & M. Stoffregen (Eds.), *Challenges for quality of life in the contemporary world. Advances in quality-of-life studies, theory and research* (pp. 249–270). Dordrecht/Boston/London: Kluwer.

Lundberg, S., & Pollak, R. (2007, February). *The American family and family economics*. National Bureau of Economic Research (NBER Working Paper 12908).

Mahler, P., & Winkelmann, R. (2004, November). *Single motherhood and (un)equal educational opportunities: Evidence for Germany* (IZA Discussion Paper No. 1391).

McLanahan, S., & Bumpass, L. (1988). Intergenerational consequences of family disruption. *The American Journal of Sociology, 94*(1), 130–152.

McLanahan, S., & Sandefur, G. (1994). *Growing up with a single parent*. Cambridge: Harvard University Press.

McMunn, A., Nazroo, J., Marmot, M., Boreham, R., & Goodman, R. (2001). Children's emotional and behavioural well-being and the family environment: Findings from the health survey for England. *Social Science & Medicine, 53*, 423–440.

Meezan, W., & Rauch, J. (2005). Gay marriage, same sex parenting, and America's children. *The Future of Children, 15*(2), 97–115.

Miller, P., & Plant, M. (1999). Truancy and perceived school performance: An alcohol and drug study of United Kingdom teenagers. *Alcohol and Alcoholism, 34*(6), 886–893.

Moffitt, R. (2005). Remarks on the analysis of causal relationships in population research. *Demography, 42*(1), 91–108.

Morrison, D. R., & Cherlin, A. J. (1995). The divorce process and young children's well-being: A prospective analysis. *Journal of Marriage and the Family, 57*, 800–812.

Murray, A., & Sandqvist, K. (1990). Father absence and children's achievement from age 13 to 21. *Scandinavian Journal of Educational Research, 34*(1), 3–28.

Noack, P., Krettek, C., & Walper, S. (2001). Peer relations of adolescents from nuclear and separated families. *Journal of Adolescence, 24*, 535–548.

Nock, S. (2005). Marriage as a public issue. *The Future of Children, 15*(2), 13–28.

O'Connor, T., Caspi, A., DeFries, J. C., & Plomin, R. (2000). Are associations between parental divorce and children's adjustment genetically mediated? An adoption study. *Developmental Psychology, 36*(4), 429–437.

Ostberg, A.-L., Lindblad, U., & Halling, A. (2003). Self-perceived oral health in adolescents associated with family characteristics and parental employment status. *Community Dental Health, 20*, 159–164.

Otten, R., Engels, R., van de Ven, M., & Bricker, J. (2007). Parental smoking and adolescent smoking stages: The role of parents' current and former smoking, and family structure. *Journal of Behavioural Medicine, 30*(2), 143–154.

Pagani, L., Tramblay, R. E., Vitaro, F., Kerr, M., & McDuff, P. (1998). The impact of family transition on the development of delinquency in adolescent boys: A 9-year longitudinal study. *Journal of Child Psychology and Psychiatry, 39*(4), 489–499.

Pagani, L., Boulerice, B., Vitaro, F., & Tremblay, R. (1999). *Effects of poverty on academic failure and delinquency in Boys: A change and process model approach.*

Painter, G., & Levine, D. (2000). Family structure and youths' outcomes: Which correlations are causal? *Journal of Human Resources, 35*(3), 524–549.

Parera, N., & Surís, J.-C. (2004). Having a good relationship with their mother: A protective factor against sexual risk behaviour among adolescent families? *Journal of Pediatrics and Adolescent Gynecology, 17*, 267–271.

Park, H. (2007). Single-parenthood and children's reading performance in Asia. *Journal of Marriage and the Family, 69*, 863–877.

Phipps, S. (1998, September). *Outcomes for children in Canada, Norway, and the United States: A microdata comparison*. Halifax: Department of Economics, Dalhousie University.

Phipps, S. (2002). The well-being of young Canadian children in international perspective: A functionings approach. *Review of Income and Wealth, 48*, 493–515.

Piketty, T. (2003, December). *The impact of divorce on school performance: Evidence from France. 1968–2002.* Centre for Economic Policy Research (Discussion Paper No. 4146).

Piko, B. F., & Fitzpatrick, K. M. (2007). Socioeconomic status. Psychosocial health and health behaviours among Hungarian adolescents. *European Journal of Public Health, 17*(4), 353–360.

Pollard, E., & Lee, P. (2003). Child well-being: A systematic review of the literature. *Social Indicators Research, 61*, 59–78.

Pong, S.-L., Dronkers, J., & Hampden-Thompson, G. (2003). Family policies and children's school achievement in single- versus two-parent families. *Journal of Marriage and the Family, 65*, 681–699.

Ponnet, K., Vermeiren, R., Jespers, I., Mussche, B., Ruchkin, V., Schwab-Stone, M., & Deboutte, D. (2005). Suicidal behaviour in adolescents: Associations with parental marital status and perceived parent-adolescent relationship. *Journal of Affective Disorders, 89*, 107–113.

Quinlivan, J., Tan, L., Steele, A., & Black, K. (2003). Impact of demographic factors, early family relationships and depressive symptomatology in teenage pregnancy. *The Australian and New Zealand Journal of Psychiatry, 38*, 197–203.

Rainer, W. (2006). Parental separation and well-being of youths. *Journal of Socio-economics, 35*(2), 197–208.

Ram, B., & Hou, F. (2003). Changes in family structure and child outcomes: Roles of economic and familial resources. *Policy Studies Journal, 31*(3), 309–330.

Reichman, N., Corman, H., & Noonan, K. (2003). *Effects of child health on parents' relationship status*. National Bureau of Economic Research (NBER Working Paper 9610).

Ribar, D. (2004). *What do social scientists know about the benefits of marriage? A review of quantitative methodologies*. Institute for the Study of Labour, Discussion Paper (IZA DP No. 998).

Richards, M., & Wadsworth, M. E. J. (2004). Long term effects of early adversity on cognitive function. *Archives of Disability and Childhood, 89*, 922–927.

Rodgers, B. (1994). Pathways between parental divorce and adult depression. *Journal of Child Psychology and Psychiatry, 35*(7), 1289–1308.

Romelsjo, A., Kaplan, G., Cohen, R., Allenback, P., & Andreasson, S. (1992). Protective factors and social risk factors for hospitalization and mortality among young men. *American Journal of Epidemiology, 135*(6), 649–658.

Ruschena, E., Prior, M., Sanson, A., & Smart, D. (2005). A longitudinal study of adolescent adjustments following family transitions. *Journal of Child Psychology and Psychiatry, 46*(4), 353–363.

Sandefur, G., & Wells, T. (1997). *Using siblings to identify the effects of family structure on educational attainment*. Institute for Research on Poverty (Discussion Paper no. 1144–97).

Sandefur, G., & Wells, T. (1999). Does family structure really influence educational attainment? *Social Science Research, 28*(December), 331–357.

Sanz-de-Galdeano, A., & Vuri, D. (2006). Parental divorce and students' performance: Evidence from longitudinal data. *Oxford Bulletin of Economics and Statistics, 69*(3), 321–328.

Sauvola, A., Koskinen, O., Jokelainen, J., Hakko, H., Jarvelin, M.-R., & Rasanen, P. (2002). Family type and criminal behaviour of male offspring: The northern Finland 1966 birth cohort study. *The International Journal of Social Psychiatry, 48*(2), 115–121.

Shaw, D. S., Emery, R. E., & Tuer, M. D. (1993). Parental functioning and children's adjustment in families of divorce: A prospective study. *Journal of Abnormal Child Psychology, 21*, 119–133.

Sidebotham, P., Golding, J., & the ALSPAC Study Team. (2001). Child maltreatment in the 'children of the nineties'. A longitudinal study of parental risk factors. *Child Abuse & Neglect, 25*, 1177–1200.

Sigle-Rushton, W., Hobcraft, J., & Kiernan, K. (2005). Parental divorce and subsequent disadvantage: A cross-cohort comparison. *Demography, 42*(3), 427–446.

Sjöberg, R., Nilsson, K., & Leppert, J. (2005). Obesity, shame and depression in school-aged children: A population-based study. *Pediatrics, 116*, 389–392.

Skinner, C., Bradshaw, J., & Davidson, J. (2007). *Child support policy: An international perspective* (Department for Work and Pensions Research Report. vol. 405). Corporate Document Services. Leeds.

Sleskova, M., Tuinstra, J., Geckova, A. M., van Dijk, J., Salonna, F., Groothoff, J., & Reijneveld, S. (2006). Influence of parental employment status on Dutch and Slovak adolescents' health. *BMC Public Health, 6*, 250.

Sourander, A., & Helstä, L. (2005). Childhood predictors of externalizing and internalizing problems in adolescence. *European Child & Adolescent Psychiatry, 14*, 415–423.

Sourander, A., Helstelä, L., Ristkari, T., Ikäheimo, K., Helnius, H., & Piha, J. (2001). Child and adolescent mental health service use in Finland. *Social Psychiatry and Psychiatric Epidemiology, 36*, 294–298.

Sourander, A., Aromaa, M., Pihlakoski, L., Haavisto, A., Rautava, P., Helenius, H., & Sillanpää, M. (2006). Early predictors of deliberate self-harm among adolescents. A prospective follow-up study from age 3 to age 15. *Journal of Affective Disorders, 93*, 87–96.

Spence, S., Najman, J., Bor, W., O'Callaghan, M., & Williams, G. (2002). *Maternal anxiety and depression, poverty and marital relationship factors during early childhood as predictors of anxiety and depressive symptoms in adolescence, 43*(4), 457–469.

Spencer, N. (2005). Maternal education, lone parenthood, material hardship, maternal smoking, and longstanding respiratory problems in childhood: Testing a hierarchical conceptual framework. *Journal of Epidemiology and Community Health, 59*, 842–846.

Spruijt, Ed, & DeGoede, M. (1996). Changing family structure and adolescent well-being in the Netherlands. *International Journal of Law Policy and the Family, 10*, 1–16.

Spruijt, Ed, DeGoede, M., & Vandervalk, I. (2001). The well-being of youngsters coming from six different family types. *Parent Education and Counselling, 45*, 285–294.

Stevenson, B., & Wolfers, J. (2008, January 27). Divorce and children: What do we know? *Cato Unbound.*

Strohscheim, L. (2005). Parental divorce and child mental health trajectories. *Journal of Marriage and the Family, 67*, 1286–1300.

Sun, Y. (2001). Family environment and adolescents' well-being before and after parents' marital disruption: A longitudinal analysis. *Journal of Marriage and the Family, 63*(3), 697–713.

Suris, J.-C., & Parera, N. (2005). Being old-for-grade and drug use: Not such a clear connection. *Act Paediatrica, 94*, 1807–1814.

Sweeting, H., West, P., & Richards, M. (1998). Teenage family life, lifestyles, and life chances: Associations with family structure, Conflict with parents and joint family activity. *International Journal of Law, Policy and the Family, 12*, 15–46.

Taanila, A., Ebeling, H., Kotimaa, A., Moilanen, I., & Jarvelin, M.-R. (2004). Is a large family a protective factor against behavioural and emotional problems at the age of 8 years? *Acta Paediatrica, 93*, 508–517.

Theodorakis, Y. A., Papaioannou, A., & Karastogianidou, K. (2004). Relations between family structure and students' health-related attitudes and behaviours. *Psychological Reports, 95*(3 Pt 1), 851–858.

Thomas, A., & Sawhill, I. (2005). For love and money? The impact of family structure on family income. *The Future of Children, 15*(2), 57–74.

Thomsen, Ph. (1994). Children and adolescents with obsessive compulsive disorder: An analysis of socio-demographic background. *Psychopathology, 27*, 303–311.

Thrane, N., Sondergaard, C., Schonheyder, H. C., & Sorensen, H. T. (2005). Socioeconomic factors and risk of hospitalization with infectious diseases in 0- to 2-year-old Danish children. *European Journal of Epidemiology, 20*, 467–474.

Timothy, B., & Gottainer, G. (2000). Family structure and children's success: A comparison of widowed and divorced single-mother families. *Journal of Marriage and the Family, 62*(2), 533–548.

Ulusoy, D., & Demir, N. O. (2006). Situational runaway adolescents. A study on risk factors from a Turkish sample. *International Journal of Adolescent Medical Health, 18*(2), 271–280.

Undheim, A. M., & Sund, A. M. (2005). School factors and the emergence of depressive symptoms among young Norwegian adolescents. *European Child & Adolescent Psychiatry, 14*, 446–453.

Valle, A.-K., Torgersen, L., Roysamb, E., Klepp, K.-I., & Thelle, D. (2005). Social class, gender and psychosocial predictors for early sexual debut among 16 year olds in Oslo. *European Journal of Public Health, 15*(2), 185–192.

VanderValk, I., Spruijt, Ed, de Goede, M., Meeus, W., & Maas, C. (2004). Marital status, marital process and parental resources in predicting adolescents emotional adjustment: A multilevel analysis. *Journal of Family Issues, 25*, 291–317.

VanderValk, I., Spruijt, Ed, de Goede, M., Maas, C., & Meeus, W. (2005). Family structure and problem behavior of adolescents and young adults: A growth-curve study. *Journal of Youth and Adolescence, 34*, 533–546.

Vatten, L. J., & Skjaerven, R. (2003). Effects on pregnancy outcome of changing partner between first two births: Prospective population study. *British Medical Journal, 327*(7424), 1138–1141.

Vikat, A., Rimpelä, A., Kousnen, E., & Rimpelä, M. (2002). Sociodemographic differences in the occurrence of teenage pregnancies in Finland in 1987–1998: A follow-up study. *Journal of Epidemiology and Community Health, 56*, 659–668.

Vingilis, E., Wade, T., & Adlaf, E. (1998). What factors predict self-rated physical health? *Journal of Adolescence, 21*, 83–97.

von Kries, R., Toschke, A., Koletzko, B., & Slikker, W. (2002). Maternal smoking during pregnancy and childhood obesity. *American Journal of Epidemiology, 156*(10), 954–961.

Wadsworth, M., Hardy, R. J., Paul, A. A., Marshall, S. F., & Tate, T. J. (2002). Leg and trunk length at 43 years in relation to childhood health, diet and family circumstances; evidence from the 1946 national birth cohort. *International Journal of Epidemiology, 31*, 383–390.

Weitoft, G. R., et al. (2003a). Mortality, severe morbidity, and injury in children living with single parents in Sweden: A population-based study. *The Lancet, 361*(9354), 289–295.

Weitoft, G. R., Hjern, A., Haglund, B., & Rosén, M. (2003b). Mortality, severe morbidity, and injury in children living with single parents in Sweden: A population based study. *The Lancet, 361*, 289–295.

Wicks, S., Hjern, A., Gunnell, D., Lewis, G., & Dalman, C. (2005). Social adversity in childhood and the risk of developing psychosis: A national cohort study. *Amercian Journal of Psychiatry, 162*(9), 1652–1657.

Wilson, C. M., & Oswald, A. J. (2005). *How does marriage affect physical and psychological health? A survey of the longitudinal evidence*. Institute for the Study of Labour Discussion Paper (IZA Discussion Paper No. 1619).

Woessman, L. (2004, September). *How equal are educational opportunities? Family background and student achievement in Europe and the United States*. Institute for the Study of Labour Discussion Paper (IZA DP No. 1284).

Wojtkiewicz, R. A. (1993). Simplicity and complexity in the effects of parental structure on high school graduation. *Demography, 30*(4), 701–717.

Zafiriadis, K., Livaditis, M., Xenitidas, K., Diamanti, M., Tsatalmpasidou, E., Sigalas, I., & Polemikos, N. (2005). Social and psychological characteristics of Greek secondary school students with learning difficulties. *Journal of Adolescence, 28*, 741–752.

Part III
Work Family Balance and Gender

Chapter 6
Parental Leave Policies, Gender Equity and Family Well-Being in Europe: A Comparative Perspective

Karin Wall and Anna Escobedo

Introduction

Leave policies and the protection of working parents' rights have changed significantly in Europe during the last few decades. While policies introduced immediately after World War II were largely based on a male-breadwinner model, the post-1970s policies have recognised the increase in maternal employment, the growing diversity of work/family arrangements and working parents' needs for state support in caring for young children. Paid maternity leave and paid or unpaid parental leave are now available throughout Europe – Western, Central and Eastern – and policy developments have encouraged more gender-neutral leaves and longer periods of paid leave (Deven and Moss 2005).

Two questions may be raised regarding the changing nature of leave policies. The first is whether these changes have shifted policy away from the male-breadwinner model, thereby reinforcing gender equity both in employment and in care work. Welfare state literature and feminist literature aiming to incorporate gender into the former reveal complex and often contradictory consequences of leave policies. Paid leave schemes and childcare services are generally seen to strengthen women's ties to paid work (Ruhm 1998; Glass and Riley 1998) by raising female employment rates, reducing new mothers' labour-market exits, and decreasing their job turnover.

K. Wall (✉)
Institute of Social Sciences, University of Lisbon, Lisbon, Portugal
e-mail: karin.wall@ics.ul.pt

A. Escobedo
Department of Sociology and Organisational Analysis, University of Barcelona, Barcelona, Spain
e-mail: anna.escobedo@ub.edu

A. Moreno Mínguez (ed.), *Family Well-Being: European Perspectives*, Social Indicators Research Series 49, DOI 10.1007/978-94-007-4354-0_6,

On the other hand, leave provisions, in particular, of longer duration, are also shown to have negative effects on women's employment by eroding their human capital and making them less attractive to employers, when compared to the male workforce (Morgan and Zippel 2003; Bergman 2009). The debate on what constitutes a gender-friendly state also reveals different approaches, with some scholars emphasising the extent to which states support women's economic independence (Sainsbury 1999) while others underline the role of the state in granting women entitlements to 'time for care' and recognising women's preferences (Knijn and Kremer 1997). 'Employment' and 'care' perspectives do not necessarily clash. As some literature has pointed out, the impact of longer and more generously paid periods of leave does not always have clear-cut effects. Moreover, recent analysis of changes in leave policies in Europe shows that the trend towards more generosity in leave does not necessarily increase gender equality (Wall 2007a; Ray et al. 2010; Thévenon 2011). In fact, generosity and gender egalitarianism emerge as different dimensions and have to be analysed separately.

The second question is whether these changes have resulted in cross-national convergence or divergence and also, in the case of dispersion, if the clustering of countries is linked to the typology of welfare regimes proposed by welfare studies (Esping-Andersen 1990). Comparative analysis on the convergence of leave policies in industrialised countries has shown that, in spite of some common trends and some long-standing broad geographical patterns, these changes have had different levels of magnitude across countries and have consequently maintained or even increased divergence (Gauthier 2002; Thévenon 2011). Moreover, the fourfold typology of welfare regimes, in spite of its usefulness in highlighting differences across policy regimes, is not clearly visible. More importantly, it does not help us to fully understand the processes of variation within and across groups of countries.

These two questions imply a third challenge which is taken up in this chapter. If the nature of leave policy is changing and traditional welfare state analysis does not adequately account for variation, then it is important to understand what else is shaping the maintenance of diversity. The approach developed in this chapter suggests that there are different *leave policy models* underpinning developments in leave in European societies. Drawing on some fundamental dimensions of the work-care-leave-gender conundrum, both at the level of policies and of changing expectations and practices, we will seek to identify this diversity. Two issues are of particular significance. First, what processes of change in cultural norms and social practices, related to motherhood, fatherhood and work-family balance after the birth of a child, may be identified in European policies and societies? Secondly, how does gender equity in employment and care interact with leave policy generosity in these processes?

In the next section, we discuss the methodological framework. In the third section, we describe the models. In the last section, we look at the usefulness of such an approach to understand major trends and cross-national differences in leave policies in Europe.

Methodology and Data

An explorative analysis of contemporary 'leave policy models' will be carried out on the basis of an interpretative approach which seeks to identify a diversity of empirically based ideal types by looking at some fundamental dimensions of work-leave-gender policies, culture and practices. Selection of three main analytical dimensions took into account the literature addressing the complex interplay between leave systems and work-family, gender and welfare regimes.

Leave Systems

Many comparative studies have tackled the task of describing leave systems across countries. Analyses have focused on one main indicator, the generosity of leave, by examining the duration and the type of job-protected leave. Recent studies have gone beyond this approach by examining payment (level of compensation or full-time equivalent) and the degree of gender equity. In this chapter, we will draw on four interrelated indicators (Tables 6.1, 6.2, 6.3, 6.4, 6.5, 6.6, and 6.7). First, since unpaid leave is known to have extremely low take-up rates, we will look at total *post-natal paid* leave[1] as well as *well-paid* leave within the former. Two other indicators concern the *degree of individualisation* (individual and non-transferable versus family entitlement to leave) and *gender equity*. Father's specific entitlements (through paternity leave, the father's quota or the bonus in the duration of leave when shared by the two parents) and flexibility regarding who may use leave will be examined as measures of gender equity; outcomes (e.g. father's take-up rates) will be examined when available. Finally, it is important to consider whether gender equity is a major objective of leave policy and to understand this in the context of each country's *specific pathway* regarding gender equality and the leave system.

Gender and Work/Family Models

To understand the meanings of 'leave', it is important to analyse interconnections between leave systems and other areas of family life and policy such as the articulation between work and care. Expectations and policies related to gender roles and work-family balance may be more or less supportive of working parents and usually emphasise different perspectives on how children should be cared for during the leave period.

[1] Including the compulsory paid weeks of post-natal leave for mothers and the paid weeks which may be taken after that.

At least two important variables may be seen to underpin the social construction of gender roles in work/family articulation.[2] The first is related to the *conjugal division of work* (who should work outside the home, who should care for young children, who actually does so and whether paid work is full time or part time). For example, strong agreement with the ideal of the husband as provider and the wife as secondary provider (part-time work) makes it difficult for the mother not to assume her conventionally assigned role of main childcarer (Crompton 1999). The second concerns the *social construction of motherhood* and how it is seen to relate to fatherhood (Leira 1992; McMahon 1995; Pfau-Effinger 1999). Motherhood may be interpreted as a long phase of life in which the special tasks of caring totally absorb women's capacity for work, thereby excluding employment altogether or reducing it for some years, or as a life stage which does not absorb women's capacity for work so that maternal employment does not have a negative impact on children and should be managed alongside childcare responsibilities which are shared with the father.

There is substantial literature on changing work-family models during the last few decades in European societies. Some of this literature suggests a more or less linear move from the male-breadwinner model towards a dual-earner/dual-carer model, while other identifies a shift towards an 'adaptive' model where women's preferences go towards part time or no employment while children are young (Treas and Widmer 2000; Hakim 2003). In contrast with these perspectives, other approaches have highlighted a diversity of models. Viewing Western European development over the last few decades, Pfau-Effinger (1999) identifies five gendered cultural models, two more traditional and three modern. Cross-national analysis of attitudes and practices related to the gendered division of paid and unpaid work has also highlighted a plurality of models (Wall 2007b; Aboim 2010).

In order to capture diversity in work-family models, it is important to consider a variety of data since female employment rates may be biased by including or excluding women who are on parental or childcare leave according to national regulations (e.g. in Finland, women on parental leave are considered as employed but inactive when they are on childcare leave while receiving a home-care-related allowance). Besides female employment rates and part-time work, it is essential to look at cultural expectations and recent policy debates, as well as differences in the activity rates of women with and without children and the gendered divisions of work in couples with children below 3.

[2] The concept of 'work/family articulation' refers to the processes and practices whereby individuals and families develop specific strategies to manage paid and unpaid work. The latter may include cutting back on working hours, taking leave, adapting parents' work schedules or delegating care for young children to professional or informal carers. 'Reconciliation' and 'balancing' are terms currently used to analyse this process. But they can imply that some form of conciliation or equilibrium between the two spheres is always achieved, and this represents an analytical drawback. We therefore prefer the more neutral concept of 'articulation' between work and family life.

Welfare Regimes and the Leave-Services Connection

A third dimension is the social construction of *the relationship between working parents and the Welfare State*. In European society, there are different ideological frameworks regarding this relationship. From one point of view, care for children may be regarded primarily as a responsibility of the state. The underlying ideal is that children are future citizens; therefore, public institutions are seen as competent in fulfilling the task of care and early education. Caring for children, however, may alternatively be considered as primarily the task of families – the underlying attitude being that children are seen as needing special care (by parents or especially by the mother) to become competent individuals. This ideological framework is strong in Central and Eastern Europe but may also be found in other countries and is part of an on-going policy debate on family well-being in all European countries (Esping-Andersen 2003). One of the main consequences of this debate for policies is the stronger or weaker emphasis on state responsibility in supporting working parents through day care services (adapted to parents' working hours). The linkages established between the leave system and access to services (e.g. ensuring that day care is available when leave ends) are therefore of particular importance. Consideration of this dimension will be based on data concerning the intensity (average opening hours) and prevalence (coverage rates) of ECEC (early childhood education and care services), as well as developments in the coordination between the end of leave and services.

For the 22 countries under discussion,[3] we examined the comparative evidence describing variations in leave systems and their connections to the other dimensions. The models must be seen as exploratory. Research has shown that typologies have to be systematically reviewed since all models, rooted as they are in specific cultural and historical paths, are dynamic and may shift or even deviate substantially over time. In fact, trying to find some pattern in these variations, we previously identified five leave policy models which, seen in the light of recent changes, needed to be revised (Wall 2007a). As a result, we have added two other models. This does not mean that the number of models must be continually multiplied; new models may appear, but some models may also merge over time due to convergence. However, the 'non-fits' that only represent one or two countries are essential to understanding how new pathways and realities are emerging, within a larger context of both convergence and divergence. Given that the main reason for this typology is its usefulness in understanding diversity, the two models describe countries (Germany, Austria, Portugal) where recent changes have made them into interesting case types.

[3]Sweden, Denmark, Iceland, Norway, Finland, Slovenia, France, Belgium, Germany, Austria, Poland, Estonia, Hungary, Czech Republic, Netherlands, UK, Ireland, Switzerland, Portugal, Spain, Italy, Greece.

Data for the 22 countries on leave systems, ECEC services, maternal employment and couples' employment patterns were taken from the reviews and statistical data collected by the International Network on Leave Policy and Research, in particular, the Annual Reviews of the last 6 years (Moss and O'Brien 2006; Moss and Wall 2007; Moss and Korintus 2008; Moss and Fusulier 2009; Moss and Kocourkovà 2010; Moss 2011). Eurostat data was used for female employment rates and part-time work. Since the data is available on-line,[4] we only include the tables on leave systems which were drawn up for this chapter on the basis of the 2011 review.

Leave Policy Models in Europe

The 'One-Year-Leave' Gender-Equality-Orientated Model

The 'one-year-leave' model is associated with leave arrangements that provide approximately *one year of paid leave* (9–13 months) *with full or very high compensation of previous earnings* (Table 6.1). In the four countries (Sweden, Iceland, Denmark and Slovenia) that fit this model most closely, there is an initial short maternity leave followed by a longer period of well-paid parental leave which allows one of the parents (or both on a sharing basis) to stay at home for most of the first year of the child's life.

The *promotion of gender equality* in leave arrangements is *high* on the policy agenda. This is particularly true of Sweden and Iceland, with both countries putting a strong emphasis on a (non-transferable) father's quota of parental leave (2 months in Sweden, 3 months in Iceland), while in Denmark and Slovenia, we find 2 weeks of paternity leave (with 100% compensation of prior earnings) and an emphasis on the flexible gender sharing of leave. In Slovenia, for example, half of the 8 months of well-paid parental leave are for fathers even if they may be transferred to the mother; individualisation through individual entitlement to well-paid leave is therefore an important principle in this model and strongly related to gender equity in policy. Moreover, reinforcing gender equality typically leads to the introduction of mechanisms that act as incentives for fathers to take up more leave, for example, Sweden recently introduced a 'gender-equality bonus' in the form of a special tax reduction when 'equal use' of leave goes beyond the father's quota. Not surprisingly, father's take-up of parental leave is higher in the countries with a non-transferable father's quota (90%in Sweden and Iceland compared to 24% in Denmark and 6% in Slovenia).

Leave policy in these countries is also connected to governmental policies endorsing strong support for dual-earner parents through services. *Complementarity*

[4] See http://www.leavenetwork.org/ for the Annual Reviews and http://ec.europa.eu/eurostat for data on female employment in 2010.

between the 1-year leave and day care services, emphasising the idea that the majority of children after age 1 are brought into formal care, is ensured through a high availability of services adapted to parents' working hours; coverage rates for children below age 3 in 2009 are the highest in all European countries: 63% in Sweden, 73% in Denmark, 41% in Iceland and 53.3% in Slovenia.

Lastly, the economic behaviour of women and of couples with young children underlines the *erosion of the* 'male-breadwinner model' in these countries and the growing importance of women's employment and dual-earner couples. Female economic employment rates are high, including more full-time than part-time female earners, and there is a similar employment rate for women with or without children below age 6. Maternal employment has the highest levels of all European countries: in 2008, in families with children below age 15, it was equal to or above 75% in all four countries (76.5% in Denmark, 84.8% in Iceland, 75.1% in Slovenia, 82.5% in Sweden).

Division of paid labour also confirms the decline in the one-earner model: in couples with children below age 3, the full-time dual-earner model in which both parents work full time is the predominant pattern (42% in Sweden, 71% in Slovenia) (Data for 2007, Moss 2011). Nevertheless, it is far from being a fully predominant model, even in these countries. When children are very young, the one-and-a-half-earner model, based on part-time work, is important and even seems to be on the increase. The explanation may be the gradual rise in female part-time work over the last decade.[5]

The 'Parental-Choice-Oriented' Policy Model

The leave policy model that we have labelled the 'parental-choice-oriented' model emerged during the 1990s in the context of a difficult (and often heated[6]) policy debate centred on the need, advocated by some political parties and sectors of society, to allow parents to choose between caring for children below 3 years of age at home or putting them in day care. Under varied but often similar concepts – 'cash for care' (Norway), 'home care allowance' (Finland), 'cash benefit for parental education' (APE, France), 'time credit system' (Belgium)[7] – the countries that fit this model

[5] In 2010, women working part time represented 40% in Sweden, up from 36% in 2000; 39% in Denmark, up from 34% in 2000; 35% in Iceland; and 15% in Slovenia.

[6] See the article by Elin Kvande in the 2007 Review (Moss and Wall 2007) describing how the issue of long parental leave was hotly debated in Norway during the 1990s. The father's quota is also a much debated issue at present with the conservative party strongly in favour of doing away with it (Brandth and Kvande in Moss 2011).

[7] Belgium does not have a 'home care allowance' but entitlement to parental leave together with the 'time credit system' allows parents to take low-paid leave for another 18 months after the end of 4-month well-paid maternity leave.

most closely opened up their leave arrangements in order to provide parents with the *option of a long (2–3 years) paid parental leave*. However, prior to the introduction of this *low-paid* long leave (see the flat rates for each country in Table 6.2), these countries already had a well-paid leave of several months after the birth of the child (3–12 months[8]) as well as services which had expanded. In this context, the long parental leave was endorsed as an extra option for families rather than as the preferred form of care for young children.

As a result, a second characteristic of this leave policy model is a *complementary relationship between leave arrangements and childcare services*. Services are available as from the end of the initial well-paid leave so that parents who are entitled to the long parental leave can choose whether to take it or to go back to work and rely on day care. Supporting parental choice over the first 3 years after birth thus implies keeping up fairly high levels of service provision for this age group and adapting opening hours to parent's work schedules. Coverage rates in these countries in 2009 are therefore average to high: 33% in Belgium, 41% in France, 27% in Finland and 36% in Norway. Given their specific paths, France and Belgium provide services for children below age 1, thereby allowing for some 'early return to work (at the end of well-paid leave)' strategies based on the use of day care facilities, whereas Norway and Finland, as in Sweden (less so in Denmark[9]), only tend to provide services for children over age 1.[10]

Emphasis is thus on parental choice but *gender equality is also on the policy agenda*, even if less explicitly than in the previous model. In most of the countries, this implies providing well-paid paternity leave (2–3 weeks, with the exception of Norway, where paternity leave is not paid) and the possibility of gender sharing of the parental leave. Belgium has 3 days of 'compulsory' paternity leave. Finland provides 3 weeks of paternity leave (with a lower ceiling than for maternity leave, however) and an extra bonus of 4 weeks paid father's leave if the father takes the last 2 weeks of parental leave, while Norway, more in line with Sweden, has a father's quota of 10 weeks. However, although it is non-transferable, eligibility rules regarding

[8] Norway and Finland clearly have a more generous initial leave system, similar to the 'one-year-leave model', with a well-paid leave which can go up to 11 or 12 months. France and Belgium only have an initial well-paid maternity leave of 4 months.

[9] Denmark provides childcare services for children over 6 months.

[10] Even though in Finland children under one year old are 'entitled to a day care place', in practice, there are very few day care places for children of this age. As Salmi (2006) points out, parental leave ends when the baby is about 9–10 months old and the majority of mothers (80%) take home care allowance after this period and therefore rarely apply for a day care place. The average home care period lasts until the child is 1.5 years. This has led to a drop in places for this very young age group; in the 1970s, there even used to be separate sections for young babies in day care centres, but this no longer happens. As a result, if parents decide not to take the whole parental leave period, they usually consider other options, such as a private nanny at home.

the father's quota have been eased, allowing for fathers to take leave even if the mother is only working a low part time (less than half time). The change points to an emphasis on parental togetherness in leave and the 'one-and-a-half-earner' model rather than the promotion of gender equity through a father's individual entitlement to care which depends on mother's return to work.

In these countries, the economic behaviour of women and couples with young children also points to *a move away from the male-breadwinner model* but less pronounced than in the former model. Female employment rates are high in Finland (67%) and Norway (73%) and slightly lower in France (60%) and in Belgium (57%); female part-time work varies but is especially high in Belgium (42%) and Norway (43%) and somewhat lower in France (30%) and Finland (20%). However, in comparison with the countries in the previous model, maternal employment is always lower (between 64% and 69%).

On the other hand, there is a specific pattern of erosion of male breadwinning. Compared to the previous countries, the one-earner model is more important (with a third of couples in France and 46% in Finland falling into this type) in households with children under 3 years old. Although it is not a clearly predominant model as in the 'mother-centred' leave policy model (see section The 'Long-Leave' Mother Home-Centred Policy Model), it has average proportions, indicating that it is also a fairly common option in couples with young children. In summary, from the point of view of parental employment, the 'parental-choice-oriented' model still allows for a considerable amount of male breadwinning.

The 'Long-Leave' Mother Home-Centred Policy Model

A third policy model can be identified which conforms strongly to the expectation that mothers should stay at home when children are very young. During the phases of active motherhood, in particular, when children have not yet started school, it is seen as important for mothers to stay at home and to gradually take up work again as the child gets older. In the four countries (Hungary, Czech Republic, Poland and Estonia) which fall more closely into this model, leave policy is based on a *long-paid leave which emphasises maternal home care until the child is 3 years old* (Table 6.3). After an initial well-paid post-natal maternity leave (of 2–6 months), there is either a flat-rate payment for 2 (Poland) or 3 years (Czech Republic) or a more generous compensation for the first 18–24 months (see Hungary and Estonia) followed by a low flat-rate payment during the rest of the leave.

Emphasis on mother care for very young children provides linkages to three other characteristics of this model. First, there is *a low emphasis on gender equality in leave.* If women, at least when children are small, are primarily regarded as being responsible for childcare, then men are regarded as breadwinners who earn most of the income and should not be integrated into leave arrangements. Until recently, this meant that well-paid paternity leave was not provided; the Czech republic still has no paternity leave, but the other countries have introduced a short (5–10 days) well-paid paternity leave, suggesting that some building up of parental, rather than just maternal, care has also become an objective of leave policy. There are, however, no protected periods of parental leave ('quotas') or bonus months exclusively for fathers when mothers return to work. When stipulated, periods of protected leave are for mothers rather than fathers: in Hungary, the first 6 months of parental leave have to be taken by the mother.

The second characteristic is a *low availability of childcare services* as the leave system and childcare facilities are not seen as complementary. The long period of leave is seen as an alternative to service provision, in particular for children below age 3. Coverage rates for this age group are therefore low, 7% in Hungary and 3% in Poland and the Czech Republic, but higher in Estonia (25%, up from 12% in 2006); and coverage rates for the 3–6 age group are also low to average (except in Estonia[11]).

The third characteristic is *emphasis on a male-breadwinner model when couples have small children,* making for a specific configuration of parental employment. Overall, female employment rates are average or even slightly above average, but maternal employment levels are low, and there are considerable differences between the activity rates of women with or without children below age 6. The difference is as high as 41 percentage points in the Czech Republic, 33 p.p. in Hungary, 26 p.p. in Estonia and 12 p.p. in Poland in 2009 (EC 2010). As a result, the employment status of couples with children is also very different. In couples with children below age 3, the male-breadwinner model is the predominant model, representing over 70% and as high as 80% in the Czech Republic; in Poland, however, it is not as predominant (44%), suggesting that the very low flat-rate payment for parental leave does not provide an option for many working mothers.

The 'Balanced' Mother Home-Centred Policy Model

Austria and Germany, in particular West Germany (Pfau-Effinger and Smidt 2011), have been seen to closely follow the culture and policy measures underlying the long-leave mother-centred policy model. Until 2007, both countries had a short well-paid leave of a few months followed by a low-paid long leave (2–3 years, mean-tested) which was taken up essentially by mothers. There was no paternity leave, and only Austria had established entitlement to 'bonus months' in case of parental sharing of leave (3–6 bonus months, depending on the shorter or longer duration of leave). Over the last few years, concern regarding low maternal employment and the negative effects of long-term labour-market absence led to critical

[11] Estonia's leave policies thus seem to be shifting and reveal some hesitation in relation to a mother-centred model.

appraisal of the long-leave model; in particular, it was seen to provide low support for qualified women wishing to reconcile work and care through shorter well-paid leave and reliance on services.

Recent changes in leave policy introduced more emphasis on income-related payment, shorter periods of leave and services (mainly childminders for the under 3s). Not surprisingly, the well-paid one-year-leave model may be seen to have acted as a benchmark, even if this is more visible in the German 'paradigm shift' than in the Austrian. Germany introduced 1 year of parental leave at 67% of prior earnings (with a ceiling of 1,800 euros) or 2 years at 33%; if fathers share the leave, there is a bonus of 2 or 4 months (Table 6.4). The change seems to represent a compromise between a radical shift towards a well-paid 'one-year-leave' system and the former long-leave system: it allows working women to choose between a fairly well-compensated leave of 12 months or a longer low-paid leave; in either case, however, it would seem to decrease dependency on a male income model. Data on take up indicates that the longer period is only taken up by 11% of leave takers, mostly women.

Austria carried out more modest changes by introducing in 2010 two new and more generous one-year-leave options, one of which is flat rate (for those earning below 1,000 euros) and the other income related (at 80% of previous income for those earning between 1 and 2 thousand euros); the bonus months depending on gender sharing of parental leave have been kept, and policy objectives – to reach 20% take up of fathers through the two new options – have been announced. Meanwhile, neither country has introduced paternity leave. However, the issue of childcare for children below age 3 is receiving attention. Childcare is decentralised in both countries, but some regions are promoting service provision. As a result, coverage rates are still low (10% in Austria, 19% in Germany) but gradually increasing.

Considering that attitudes to full-time maternal employment are generally negative and that gender models are slow to change, we may expect divisions of work to still conform strongly to male breadwinning and female caring or part-time work. Female employment rates are average in 2010 (66% in both countries), female part time is high (46% Germany, 44% Austria) and maternal employment is therefore not as low as in the previous model. In couples with children below age 3, the male-breadwinner model is the predominant pattern but the one-and-a-half model follows closely; in other words, in contrast to the long-leave model, these countries have partially moved away from male breadwinning.

We have labelled this as the 'balanced' mother-centred model due to fundamental changes in leave policies and employment patterns which reveal that a specific process of change is underway. Historically and culturally, the impact of the male-breadwinner model and a welfare regime centred on maternal care is still visible. But there is a search for a new balance between this framework and the opening up of more options for mothers, including return to work after a well-paid shorter period of leave and outsourcing some childcare; the objective of gender equity through father's involvement in care is proposed with moderation but is now an important aspect of policy and debate.

The Short-Leave 'Part-Time Mother' Policy Model

This model strongly reflects what has been designated by some authors as a modernised version of the male-breadwinner pattern (Pfau-Effinger 1999). As in the preceding mother-centred models, women and men are to an equal degree integrated into employment as long as there are no dependent children in the household. However, rather than stay-at-home mothers, who are encouraged to use a long-leave arrangement, it is seen as adequate, during the phases of active motherhood, to combine work and childcare by working part time. The main social spheres for caring are the family and the market, with traditionally underdeveloped state provision of leave and services. Nevertheless, over the last decade, there have been some changes, in particular, in relation to the development of services.

Paid leave arrangements in the four countries (United Kingdom, the Netherlands, Ireland and Switzerland) which fit this model most closely are centred on one main type of leave: *a short, non-transferable maternity leave* which provides high compensation (70–100% with a ceiling, and a particularly low ceiling in Ireland, the only country with 6 months) for only 1–6 months (Table 6.5). In the UK and Ireland, this short paid leave is followed by some additional unpaid or low-paid maternity leave. In fact, recent extensions of maternity leave appear to be bringing these two countries nearer to the idea of an initial year of 'low-paid' or 'unpaid' home-based care by mothers as an alternative to early return to part-time work. On the other hand, there have been no significant developments in paid parental leave: Switzerland has no parental leave (under discussion at present), UK and Ireland have an unpaid parental leave of 3 months per parent, the Netherlands has a part-time parental leave of 6 months per parent (unpaid, but with tax reduction as an incentive).

Lastly, the promotion of *gender equality in leave arrangements is not high on the agenda*. Paternity leave has been introduced in the UK but with a flat-rate payment: the Netherlands has a very short paternity leave paid by the employer, and Ireland and Switzerland none at all. Moreover, the initial maternity leave is not gender flexible.

Emphasis on the need to increase female participation in the labour market in order to bring low income families out of poverty has led, over the last decades, to an *increased availability of part-time day care services.* Coverage rates for children below age 3 vary from a low 20% in Ireland (up from 15% in 2006) to 35% in the UK and 49% in the Netherlands; however, short opening hours are a key characteristic, in line with mother's part-time work. Nevertheless, in comparison with the long-leave mother-centred model, these coverage rates provide some complementarity between the leave system and care services, and promote a work-family model based on mother's part-time work.

The characteristics of female activity rates and of parental employment seem to confirm this, especially in the UK, Switzerland and the Netherlands. Female activity rates are high, close to or above the average EU value, but this includes female part-time work which has the highest levels in Europe: 77% in the Netherlands, 61% in

Switzerland and 43% in the UK; Ireland has a slightly diverging pattern within this model, with 35% of female part-time work. Maternal employment is average or high in the first 3 countries and somewhat lower in Ireland (indicating that many mothers are out of the labour market). Nevertheless, in contrast with the preceding model, it is *the one-and-a-half earner pattern*, rather than the male-breadwinner one, that is the predominant model in couples with children below age 3. In the Netherlands, 59% of couples with children this age are one-and-a-half earner couples, 19% are male-breadwinner couples and 6% are full-time dual-earner couples; in Switzerland, 39% are one-and-a-half earner and 37% male-breadwinner couples; in the UK, the proportions are respectively 35%, 33% and 21%.

The Short-Leave Modified 'Male-Breadwinner' Model

A sixth policy model can be identified that conforms more strongly to the idea of the male-breadwinner/female home-carer pattern. Although expectations and attitudes to gender roles are changing rapidly in all Southern European countries, women have traditionally been regarded as being responsible for work in the private household, not only during the phases of active motherhood but also during married life in general, irrespective of whether the couple has children or not. In the three countries (Italy, Greece, Spain) that fit this model most closely, *male breadwinning is important in couples with and without children* and emerges, even if less clearly than in the past, as the predominant employment pattern amongst couples with children below age 3: 44% in Italy, 47% in Greece and 43% in Spain. The gap between the employment rates of women in the central age group with or without children below age 6 is low – 8 percentage points in Greece, 4 p.p. in Italy, 6 p.p in Spain in 2009 – but this is due to high proportions of women, both with and without children, who are not engaged in the labour market; maternal employment rates are low, in fact similar to those of the long-leave model. Overall female employment rates continue to be amongst the lowest in Europe (46% in Italy, 52% in Spain, 48% in Greece). Part-time work is below average but is increasing in Spain and Italy, a trend which may be shifting some of the emphasis from male breadwinning to the one-and-a-half earner pattern.

Leave policy is based on *one main type of leave arrangement: a short (4–5 months) of very well-compensated leave for mothers*; the public sector in Greece, with 1 year of well-paid leave, must not be forgotten, but it is an exceptional situation, and we should be cautious in underlining overall generosity on the basis of this measure. As for parental leave, this is an unpaid or very low-paid individual entitlement. In Italy, since 2002, parents receive 30% of previous earnings when leave is taken to care for children below age 3 (unpaid when children are 3–8 years old): it is an individual entitlement (6 months per parent), but couples can only take a total amount of 10 months (Table 6.6). However, even low payment is associated with higher use: in Italy in 2005, 7.5% of men and 24.2% of women employees with at least one child below age 8 used parental leave (Addabbo and Giovannini 2011), while in Spain, parental leave takers represent 6.9% of all births and 96% are mothers.

Gender equality in leave has not been a major guiding principle over the last few decades, leading to low emphasis on father's specific entitlements. In 2010, paternity leave either is not provided (Italy, Greece's public sector) or else is very short and paid by employers (Greek private sector); the exception is now Spain which, in the context of new gender-equality objectives, introduced 2 weeks of well-paid paternity leave in 2007 (with take up increasing to 55% of fathers in 2009); however, extension to 4 weeks has been postponed (Escobedo et al. 2012).

Policies in these countries have not provided strong support for dual-earner parents through full-time services for children below age 3. The percentage of young children of this age in day care services is low to average (11% in Greece, 25% in Italy, 36% in Spain) and is often linked to short opening hours, revealing *a low integration of the leave system and the services system* and a concept of formal childcare focusing on children's rather than working parents' needs. Nevertheless, with the exception of Greece (58%), over 90% of children aged 3–6 years attend pre-school.

The 'Early Return to Full-Time Work' Gender-Equality-Oriented Leave Policy Model

The last model is what we may identify as the *early return to full-time work and gender-equality-orientated* model found in Portugal. Although Portugal's pathway is also linked to a weak welfare state and to the promotion, until the 1974 Revolution, of the male-breadwinner pattern, work-family policies emphasising the importance of female employment and gender equality have led to a specific process of change. Not surprisingly, the one-year-leave model also emerges as a template for work/family balance, but it is a trimmed-down version of the latter which has emerged, influenced by budgetary constraints as well as a preference for well-paid short leaves and the symmetrical engagement of men and women in the labour market.

From the point of view of leave arrangements, there is also one main type of leave (Table 6.7): *a short, highly compensated, post-natal leave of 4–6 months* (4 months at 100% or 5 months at 83%, plus one bonus month depending on gender sharing of leave with no ceiling). Designated as the 'initial parental leave', only 6 weeks have to be taken by the mother, the rest being gender flexible. The development of *linkages between gender-equality policy and leave policy* also led to the introduction of 5 days of well-paid paternity leave in the 1990s, later increased to 4 weeks (taken up by two-thirds of fathers), as well as a well-paid bonus month[12]

[12] Previously (since 1999), father's involvement in leave was promoted through 2 weeks of well-paid parental leave if taken up by the father.

which depends on gender sharing of leave (if fathers take at least 1 month on their own, initial parental leave increases to 5 months at 100% or 6 months at 80% of previous earnings). The introduction of the bonus month led to a rapid increase in gender sharing of leave from a previous take up by fathers of 0.6% in 2008 to 20% in 2010. The rest of parental leave (now designated as 'complementary' parental leave) – 3 months per parent – is paid at 25% of earnings and has a low take-up rate.

Another key characteristic of the 'early return to work' model is the gradual expansion of publicly subsidised services with long opening hours as well as full-time primary school. Attendance rates for children below age 3 increased to 36% (up from 12% in the early 1990s). These coverage rates are above average in the EU and are building up a *complementary relationship between the leave system and services.*

A *decline of the male-breadwinner pattern* and an increase in dual-earner couples is another characteristic of this model. Maternal employment (68%) and female employment rates in Portugal (61%) are high, women work full time (86%) and there is a similar employment rate for women with or without children below age 6. The 'dual-earner' pattern (both working full time) is the predominant model in couples with children below age 3 (66% of couples, the second highest proportion in the EU after Slovenia), and male breadwinning has a very low proportion.

In summary, Portugal's early return to full employment model does not seem to adjust to any of the preceding models. Historically, Portugal's pathway is linked to the Southern European male-breadwinner model (Wall and Escobedo 2009). However, there has been divergence in the process of change: a stronger promotion of women's employment and the dual-earner model, an emphasis on the expansion of service provision and a stronger linkage between leave and gender equality. Not surprisingly, the 'well-paid one-year-leave' model also seems to hover as a benchmark in the policy agenda for gender equality.

As we mentioned earlier, this may be an emerging model in some countries. In Spain, female employment rates, based on full-time work, are increasing rapidly, service provision is expanding and gender equality is on the policy agenda. In other countries, an 'earlier return to work' is seen once again as an interesting option. In other words, the generating principles of the 'early return to work' model may be spreading.

Conclusions

The aim of this chapter was to explore the diversity of leave policy models in contemporary European society. In contrast to other approaches, describing leave policies on the basis of leave arrangements or as connected primarily to main types of Welfare State, we have focused on the interconnections between leave systems and other policy and societal factors that shape and give meaning to leave policies. Analysis reveals three sets of conclusions.

The first is related to the issue of leave generosity and its linkages to gender equity and family well-being. Leave generosity has increased in all countries, but its meaning varies according to the leave policy model and the process of change leading to a particular model. Generosity cannot be understood *per se* with no reference to the cultural, historical and political contexts in which it emerges. Family well-being, gender equity and leave to care after the birth of a child take on different shades of meaning and have to be interpreted in the context of work/family cultures and policies. For example, generosity in the form of a longer-paid parental leave may mean that policies are shifting the leave system closer to a 'mother-centred' model or, alternatively, to a flexible 'parental choice' model aiming to include varied options of leave. The impact on gender equality of a longer, more generous leave will therefore depend not only on its design but also on its location in a specific process of change. For example, the linkage between gender equality and the introduction of father's specific entitlements depends on the model in which it is embedded: in a strongly gender-oriented model, such as the 'one year model' or the 'early return to work' models, a 'daddy month' incentivating the mother's return to work and the father's take up *alone* of leave, is likely to have a greater impact on gender equity in care than a 'daddy month' allowing fathers to take up leave when mothers are at home or working a few hours per week.

The second set of conclusions is related to the current pluralisation of leave policy models. The analytical strategy examining the embeddedness of leave systems in the complex dynamics of work-family culture and policy has helped us to understand some countries' specific and unique pathway and to identify a set of *leave policy models* in which there are similar underlying processes of change. Seven models were identified. Emphasis on gender equality, promotion of mothers' employment, support for dual-earner couples and services has tended to shape a *one-year-leave gender-equality-orientated* model in which both mothers and fathers are encouraged to combine full-time work and care for very young children. However, when gender equality and the promotion of women's employment interact with a process of change underlining the need for diverse options, the rationale of leave policy is associated with *parental choice*, a model where the state aims to provide support for working parents both through longer-paid leaves for home-based care and high availability of services for those on shorter leave.

This contrasts sharply with the *mother-centred* model in which the main policy driver has been to build up home-based care by mothers during the first years of the child's life, irrespective of whether this encourages or discourages gender equality and father's involvement in care. Family well-being in this model is seen to derive from family care and mother's specific entitlements to care for young children. However, processes of change seem to be pulling these countries into two rather different models: some have enacted a *long-leave mother-centred model* emphasising home care, low availability of services and the one-earner model when children are young while others are moving in the direction of a more *balanced mother-centred* model by offering a shorter 1-year well-paid leave as well as expansion of father's entitlements and a gradual increase in services to support some working mothers; however, they cannot be considered as ‘parental choice’ countries since their pathway is still associated with some key characteristics of the mother-centred model.

Leave policies appear to take on other meanings in the setting of traditionally underdeveloped state provision of leave arrangements and services. The *short-leave part-time mother* policy model is connected to female part-time work during the phases of active motherhood with some increase in service provision to support working parents (usually attended on a part-time basis). Lastly, developments in Southern Europe would appear to allow for two models: a *short-leave-modified male-breadwinner model* which still conforms partially to the male-breadwinning pattern and an *early return to full-time work* model where the promotion of gender equality and support for dual-earner parents through availability of services are high on the agenda.

Emphasis on gender equality is not the same in the above-mentioned models. Although entitlement to paternity leave now exists in almost all the countries under review, analysis reveals important differences in the policy effort to increase fathers’ involvement. High compensation for earnings and the use of varied policy instruments to increase fathers’ leave – gender-flexible sharing of leave, paternity leave, non-transferable ‘quotas’ and bonuses – are strongest in the *one-year-leave gender-equality-orientated* model, but they are also important, even if more modestly, in the countries with the *parental choice*, the *balanced mother-centred* and the *early return to work* models. Interestingly, in order to increase father’s use of leave, there has been a sustained policy effort in these countries to reinforce well-paid ‘father’s-only’ leave (as fathers do not seem to use either poorly paid leave or well-paid ‘family entitlement’ to leave). In contrast, emphasis in the other three models is on the care of children by mothers, while well-paid leave for ‘fathers only’ has not been on the policy agenda.

The third set of conclusions is related to the issue of convergence and divergence in leave policies across Europe during the last few decades. A first remark is that the emphasis on pluralisation must not blind us to the fact that there are some important commonalities. Seen in historical perspective, all countries have shifted away from a male-breadwinner model in which only mothers were entitled to care and to a short-job-protected leave: no country in Europe conforms today to the idea of family well-being based exclusively on female caring and staying at home throughout most of married life, and all countries have paid maternity leave, some form of parental leave and are turning to father’s specific entitlements. Historically, this is a major turning point implying state investment in both leaves and services (often for the under 3s, always for the 3–6 age group), a move away from dependency on male earning and total absence from caring, and the flagging up of policy objectives which take into account family well-being based on parental sharing and conjugal work-family balance, even if gender equality may be a secondary rather than a priority policy. That said, the direction of change over the last few decades may be seen to deflect quite strongly from the expectations launched in the 1970s, such as the idea of family well-being based on ‘dual earning/dual caring’ and almost perfect, symmetrical gender equality in couples. Overall, leave policies have moved away from the idea of this one best model: there has been a clear trend towards the recognition of the rights of mothers to more time for care, often implying strong dependency on male breadwinning or female part time when children are young as well as emphasis on flexibilisation of leave (linked to the idea that parents have the right to choose and be major actors of the leave system). Even a pioneer country such as Sweden, which often acts as a standard model for leave generosity and gender equality in work/family balance in Europe, has undergone a specific process of change, less focused on full-time dual earning than in the past, with some acceptance of female part-time work (even if a fairly 'long' part time) and male breadwinning when children are young.

At the same time, however, the processes of change analysed in this chapter suggest that this standard model undoubtedly retains some of its influence, in Europe, as a cultural norm around which to negotiate leave policies. For example, we are now seeing some Central European countries, previously focused on long leave for mothers, questioning this emphasis and drawing on the concept of a shorter, well-paid one-year-leave standard in order to open up options and roll back gender inequality in parental employment. In summary, the historical importance of state support for working parents, with its strong linkages to gender equality in parenting and employment in the European social model, has had to negotiate new and sometimes conflicting approaches to care, making for some fluidity in the concept of leave and more complexity in the processes of change. This does not mean that the possibilities of developing leave policy models are completely open. On the contrary, we can see that they are constrained culturally, politically and historically, making for continued variation in European leave policies and producing a plurality of pathways which must be constantly examined and monitored in order to understand the changing and diverse nature of leave.

Appendix – Tables

Table 6.1 Leave policy measures: Sweden, Iceland, Denmark and Slovenia

Countries	Maternity leave (months)	€	Paternity leave (during mat. leave)	€	Parental leave: Total length (months)	Parental leave: €	Parental leave: Who in family	Tot. post-natal paid leave (months)
Sweden	2 months 'mother's quota'	80% max. €3,945/month	2 weeks	80%	16 months: 11 months → 3 months → 2 months →	 80% max: €3,945/month €600 Unpaid	2-months 'father's quota'[a] 6-month per parent (trasf. with permission) +1 month unpaid per parent	*16 months* (13 months 80% with ceiling)
Iceland	3 months	75–80% max. €1,820/month	–	–	12 months: 6 months → 6 months →	 75–80% max. €1,820/month Unpaid	3 months for father, 3 months per family, 3 unpaid per parent	*9 months* (80% with ceiling)
Denmark	4.5 months (1 before)	100% max. €2,060/month	2 weeks	100% max. €2,060/month	8 months → 11 months →	100% max. €2,060/month Reduced benefit	Per family*	*14.5 months* (11.5 months 100% with ceiling)
Slovenia	4 months (1 before)	100%	3 months	15 days: 100% max €3,741/month 75 days: €165/month	8.5 months →	100% max €3,741/month	Per family	*11.5 months* (100% with ceiling)

Source: Moss (2011)

1 month=4 weeks; 1 year=52 weeks; 1 month=30 days; 1 week=7 days (except in Finland where 6 working days is considered for any type of leave)

*A father's quota has been introduced in the industrial sector

[a]A 'gender-equality bonus' in the form of a tax reduction was introduced. It offers an economic incentive for families to divide parental leave more equally between the mother and the father. The parent who has stayed at home the longest receives the bonus when she/he goes back to work if the other parent uses the parental leave for more than his or her 60-day quota period. When the two reserved months are used by each parent, for each day of more 'equal' use (typically each day the father uses), a maximum of SEK100 (€11) will be gained in tax reduction; when parents share the leave equally, the bonus is worth SEK13,500 (€1,505)

Table 6.2 Leave policy measures: Finland, France, Norway and Belgium

Countries	Maternity leave (months)	€	Paternity leave (during mat. leave)	€	Parental leave: Total length (months)		Parental leave: €		Parental leave: Who in family	Tot. post-natal paid leave (months)
Finland	4.5 months (2 weeks before)	70–90% max €4,217/month	3 weeks	70% max €2,741/ month	32.5 months:					*36 months* (11.5 months: 70–75% with ceiling)
					6.5 months + bonus of 1 month for the father (if last 2 weeks parental leave taken by father)	→	70–75% (with ceiling)		Per family (1 month father bonus)	
					25 months	→	€386/month			
France	4 months (3 weeks before)	100% max €2,946/month	2 weeks (11 working days)	100% max €2,946/ month	33 months:				Per family	*36 months* (9 months if only 1 child) (3 months: 100% with ceiling)
					If≥2 child	→	€560/month for 33 months			
					If 1 child:	→	€560 only for 6 months			
					option: if 3rd or more child:	→	€801/month for 12 months if one stops working			
Norway	2 months (3 weeks before)	100% max €4,648/month	2 weeks	Unpaid by state	34.5 months:					*36 months* (13 months: 80–100% with ceiling)
					2.5 months father's quota	→	100%;	→	2.5 months for father,	
					9 months	→	80% (ceiling)		9 months per family +	
					24 months	→	€420/month		12 months per parent	
Belgium	4 months (1 week before)	1st month: 82% 3 month: 75% with ceiling	2 weeks (3 days are compulsory)	3 days: 100%, remain: 82% with ceiling	18 months:					*22 months* (4 months: 75–82% with ceiling)
					6 months	→	€666/month	→	3 months per parent+	
					12 months of time credit system	→	€604/month	→	12 months of time credit system	

Table 6.3 Leave policy measures: Hungary, Czech Republic, Poland and Estonia

Countries	Maternity leave (months)	€	Paternity leave (during maternity leave)	€	Parental leave: Total length (months)	Parental leave: €	Parental leave: Who in family	Tot. post-natal paid leave (months)
Hungary	6 months	70%	1 week	100%	30 months: 18 months →	70% max €546/ month	Mother's quota 1st 6 months	*36 months* (24 month 70% with ceiling)
					12 months: →	€110/month	24 months per family	
*Czech Republic***	7 months (1.5 before)	70% max €1,285/ month	No	–	30.5 months	€600/month	Per family	*36 months* (5.5 month: 70% with ceiling)
*Poland***	5.5 months	100%	1 week	100%	36 months: 24 months → 12 months →	€100/month Unpaid	Per family	*29 months* (5.5 months: 100%)
Estonia	4.5 (1 before)	100%	2 weeks	Unpaid	32.5 months: 14.5 months → 18 months: →	100% max €2,157/ month €38/month	Per family	*36 months* (18 months: 100% with ceiling)

**Gender sharing of maternity leave allowed (after an obligatory period for mothers of about 6 weeks)

Table 6.4 Leave policy measures: Germany and Austria

Countries	Maternity leave (months)	€	Paternity leave (during mat. leave)	€	Parental leave				Tot. post-natal paid leave (months)
Germany	3.5 months (1.5 before)	100%	No	–	34 months:			Per family (2 months father bonus)	*30 months* (14 months: 67% with ceiling)
					12+2 months bonus	→	67% max €1,800/month		
					or 24+4	→	33%		
					6 or 20 months	→	Unpaid		
Austria	4 months (2 before)	100%	No	–	24 months[a]		€624/month	Per family (with 2 to 4 months father bonus)	*24 months* (2 months: 100%; 14 months: 80% if earnings between €1,000–2,000/month)
					20+4 months bonus or	→			
					15+3	→	€800/month		
					or 12+2 (if earnings <1,000) or	→	€1,000/month		
					12+2 (if earnings 1,000–2,000)	→	80%		

[Note: on the page, one brace groups the Austrian options from "24 months[a]" to "or 12+2 (if earnings <1,000) or" with the amounts €624/month, €800/month and €1,000/month.]

[a]In Austria, there is another payment option (€436 a month for 30 months *or* for 36 months if both parents apply for the payment – 30+6 option) which we have excluded since parental leave may only be taken until the child is 24 months. Both parents cannot take leave at the same time except for one month the first time they alternately leave. In that case parental leave ends one month earlier (i.e. one month before the child's second birthday)

Table 6.5 Leave policy measures: United Kingdom, Ireland, Switzerland and The Netherlands

Countries	Maternity leave (months)	€	Paternity leave (during mat. leave)	€	Parental leave: Total length (months)	Parental leave: €	Parental leave: Who in family	Tot. post-natal paid leave (months)
*United Kingdom***	12 months	1.5 month: 90% 8 month: €580/ month 4 month: unpaid	2 weeks	€145/week	6 months (max 1 month per year)	Unpaid	3 months per parent	*9.5 months* (1.5 month: 90%)
Ireland	10.5 months (2 weeks before)	6.5 month: 80% max €1,048/ month 4 month: unpaid	no	–	7 months	Unpaid	3.5 months per parent	*6.5 months* (80% with ceiling)
Switzerland	3.5 months	80% max €5,740/ month	no	–	No	–	–	*3.5 months* (80% with ceiling)
Netherlands	4 months (1 before)	100% with ceiling	2 days	100% (paid by employer)	12 months part time	Tax reduction of €712/ month	6 months per parent	*15 months* (3 months: 100% with ceiling)

**Gender sharing of maternity leave allowed (after an obligatory period for mothers of about 6 weeks)

Table 6.6 Leave policy measures: Italy, Greece and Spain

Countries	Maternity leave (months)	€	Paternity leave (during mat. leave)	€	Parental leave: Total length (months)	Parental leave: €	Parental leave: Who in family	Total post-natal paid leave (months)
Italy	5 months (1 before) →	80–100%	No	–	10 months	30%	6 per parent (max 10)	*14 months* (4 months: 80%)
Greece Pub. sector	5 months (2 before) →	100%	No	–	48 months →	Unpaid (if ≥ 3rd child 3 months are paid by employer) →	24 months p/parent	*12 months* (100%)
					9 months[a] →	100% →	Per family	
Priv. sector	4 months (2 before) →	100%	2 days paid by employer		7 months →		3.5 months per parent	*11 months* (2 months: 100%)
	+ 3 months[b] →	Paid by employer						
	+ 6 months (special leave) →	Min. wage						
*Spain***	4 months + 2–4 weeks[c]	100% max €3,230/month	15 days	100% max €3,230/month	Up to 36 months per parent (until child is 3)	Unpaid (flat rate in some regions per family under n conditions)		*4–5 months* (100% with ceiling)

[a]Employees are also entitled to take 'alternative use of reduced hours as leave for the care of children' lasting nine months paid as working time with no ceiling
[b]After basic leave and before special leave, employees are also entitled to take 'alternative use of reduced hours as leave for the care of children' lasting a maximum of about three months paid as working time with no ceiling
[c]Employed mothers can take reduction in working time as full-time leave for two to four weeks
**Gender sharing of maternity leave allowed (after an obligatory period for mothers of about 6 weeks)

Table 6.7 Leave policy measures: Portugal

Country	Initial parental leave (months)	€	Paternity leave (during mat. leave)	€	Parental leave: Total length (months)	Parental leave: €	Parental leave: Who in family	Total post-natal paid leave (months)
Portugal	5 months + 1 month bonus if gender sharing ('daddy month')	80% (or 4+1 at 100%)	20 days (10 compulsory)	100%	6 months → + 24 months special leave →	25% → Unpaid →	3 months per parent, Per family	*12 months* (5–6 months: 80%)

References

Aboim, S. (2010). Labour and love: The gender division of labour and caring in a cross-national perspective. In S. Aboim (Ed.), *Plural masculinities*. Aldershot: Ashgate, 83–109.

Addabbo, T., & Giovannini, D. (2011). Italy: Country note. In: P. Moss (Ed.), *International review of leave policies and research 2011*. London: Department for Business, Innovation and Skills. Available at: http://www.leavenetwork.org/

Bergman, B. (2009). Long leaves, child well-being, and gender equality. In J. C. Gornick et al. (Eds.), *Gender equality: Transforming family divisions of labor*. London: Verso books.

Crompton, R. (Ed.). (1999). *Restructuring gender relations and employment. The decline of the male breadwinner*. Oxford: Oxford University Press.

Deven, F., & Moss, P. (Eds.). (2005). *Leave policies and research. Reviews and country notes* (CBGS-Werkdocument 2005/3). Brussels: Centrum voor Bevolkings en Gezinsstudie.

EC. (2010). *Indicators for monitoring the Employment Guidelines and employment analysis. 2010 compendium.* http://ec.europa.eu/social/main.jsp?catId=101&langId=en

Escobedo, A., Flaquer, L., & Navarro, L. (2012). The social politics of fatherhood in Spain and France: A comparative analysis of parental leave and shared residence. *Ethnologie Française, XLII*(1), 125–134.

Esping-Andersen, G. (1990). *The three worlds of capitalism*. Cambridge: Polity Press.

Esping-Andersen, G. (2003). Against social inheritance. In *Progressive futures. New ideas for the centre-left policy network* (pp. 127–152). London: Policy Network.

Gauthier, A. H. (2002). Family policies in industrialized countries: Is there convergence ? *Population, 57*(3), 447–474.

Glass, J., & Riley, I. (1998). Family responsive policies and employee retention following childbirth. *Social Forces, 76*(4), 1401–1435.

Hakim, C. (2003). *Models of the family in modern society*. Aldershot: Ashgate.

Knijn, T. A., & Kremer, M. (1997). Gender and the caring dimensions of welfare states: Towards inclusive citizenship. *Social Politics, 4*(3), 328–362.

Leira, A. (1992). *Welfare states and working mothers*. Cambridge: Cambridge University Press.

McMahon, M. (1995). *Engendering motherhood*. New York: Guildford Press.

Morgan, K. A., & Zippel, K. (2003). Paid to care: The origins and effects of care leave policies in Western Europe. *Social Politics, 10*(1), 49–85.

Moss, P. (Ed.). (2011). *International review of leave policies and research 2011*. London: Department for Business, Innovation and Skills. Available at: http://www.leavenetwork.org/lp_and_r_reports/

Moss, P., & Fusulier, B. (Eds.). (2009). *International review of leave policies and related research 2009* (Employment Relations Research Series). London: Department for Business, Enterprise & Regulatory Reform.

Moss, P., & Kocourkovà, J. (Eds.). (2010). *International review of leave policies and related research 2010* (Employment Relations Research Series). London: Department for Business, Enterprise & Regulatory Reform.

Moss, P. A., & Korintus, M. (Eds.). (2008). *International review of leave policies and related research 2008* (Employment Relations Research Series No 100). London: Department for Business Enterprise and Regulatory Reform.

Moss, P., & O'Brien, M. (Eds.). (2006). *International review of leave policies and related research 2006* (Employment Relations Research Series No 57). London: Department of Trade and Industry.

Moss, P., & Wall, K. (Eds.). (2007). *International review of leave policies and related research 2007* (Employment Relations Research Series No 80). London: Department for Business Enterprise and Regulatory Reform.

Pfau-Effinger, B. (1999). The modernization of family and motherhood in Western Europe. In R. Crompton (Ed.), *Restructuring gender relations and employment. The decline of the male breadwinner* (pp. 60–79). Oxford: Oxford University Press.

Pfau-Effinger, B., & Smidt, M. (2011). Differences in women's employment patterns and family policies: Eastern and Western Germany. *Community, Work and Family, 14*(82), 217–232.
Ray, R., Gornick, J., & Schmitt, J. (2010). Who cares ? Assessing generosity and gender equality in parental leave policy designs in 21 countries. *Journal of European Social Policy, 20*(3), 196–216.
Ruhm, C. J. (1998). The economic consequences of parental leave mandates: Lessons from Europe. *Quarterly Journal of Economics, 113*(1), 285–317.
Sainsbury, D. (1999). Gender, policy regimes and politics. In D. Sainsbury (Ed.), *Gender and welfare state regimes*. Oxford: Oxford University Press.
Salmi, M. (2006). Parental choice and the passion for equality in Finland. In A. L. Ellingsaeter & A. Leira (Eds.), *Politicising parenthood in Scandinavia: Gender relations in welfare states* (pp. 145–170). Bristol: Polity press.
Thévenon, O. (2011). Family policies in OECD countries: A comparative analysis. *Population and Development Review, 37*(1), 57–87.
Treas, J., & Widmer, E. (2000). Married women's employment over the life course: Attitudes in cross-national perspective. *Social Forces, 78*(4), 1409–1436.
Wall, K. (2007a). Leave policy models and the articulation of work and family in Europe: A comparative perspective. In P. Moss & K. Wall (Eds.), *International review of leave policies and related research 2007* (Employment Relations Research Series No 80). London: Department of Trade and Industry.
Wall, K. (2007b). Main patterns in attitudes to the articulation between work and family life: A cross-national analysis. In R. Crompton, S. Lewis, & C. Lyonnette (Eds.), *Women, men, work and family in Europe* (pp. 86–115). London: Palgrave Macmillan.
Wall, K. A., & Escobedo, A. (2009). Portugal and spain: Two pathways in Southern Europe. In S. Kamerman & P. Moss (Eds.), *The politics of parental leave policies*. Bristol: Policy Press.

Chapter 7
New Social Risks and Work-Family Balance

Anders Ejrnæs and Thomas P. Boje

Introduction

The aim of this chapter is to investigate how individuals are affected by the risk of spending less time on paid work than preferred because of care responsibility. This chapter deals with the perceived risks of spending time outside paid work due to caring responsibilities for dependent children and elderly family members. Individuals' risk perception is important because it might have consequences for their decisions in economic as well as family matters. Decisions in the family concerning childbirth, education and consumption are thus influenced by the prospective for the future. This study includes both individual and institutional factors in analysing to which extend the individuals are forced to sacrifice their employment career in order to take care of family members or relatives. This question is closely related to the discussion about inequalities in the opportunities or capabilities individuals have in realising their life goals.

In periods when the male breadwinner family was the norm, care responsibility was not seen as a risk because the woman in a couple was the natural caregiver. The influx of women in the labour market, the decline of the male breadwinner system and the changing gender norms have transformed women's role as the natural caregiver. Couples where both adults are in paid work have to rely on access to public care facilities, buy care on the market or get support from relatives to remain in full-time jobs and to fulfil their career expectations in the labour market.

The risk, especially for women, of spending less time on paid work because of care for relatives has been an important issue in most European societies partly because of a political desire for more women to be in full-time employment and partly due to social

A. Ejrnæs (✉) • T.P. Boje
Department of Society and Globalisation, Roskilde University,
P.O. Box, 260, DK-4000 Roskilde, Denmark
e-mail: ejrnaes@ruc.dk; boje@ruc.dk

A. Moreno Mínguez (ed.), *Family Well-Being: European Perspectives*,
Social Indicators Research Series 49, DOI 10.1007/978-94-007-4354-0_7,

citizenship rights increasingly becoming related to the individual's position in the labour market. Inequality among social groups in the risk of spending time outside paid work is thus reproducing social inequality along gender, social status and generational lines. Welfare policies typically have been designed to provide individuals protection against these social risks and their negative consequences by offering services – right to receive care – and economic support and care leave – right to give care (see Knijn and Kremer 1997; Kremer 2007; Lister et al. 2007). In this respect, the institutional setting of welfare policies is of importance for individuals' perception of social risks in relation to care and work and their capability to realise their life goals.

The aim of this chapter is twofold. First, it investigates how different welfare and family policy regimes affect the risk of spending more time outside paid work than the individuals prefer because of care responsibilities. We want to investigate how different welfare regimes have impact on the perceived social risks related to the imbalance between work and care. The second aim of this chapter is to analyse how gender, social status and age affect the perceived risks for individuals of spending time outside paid work. The question is here to what extent the risk of sacrificing career because of care is unequally distributed because of inequality in economic and social resources. In the empirical analyses, we have chosen to compare six countries: Denmark, Germany, Poland, Portugal, Sweden, and the UK which differ when it comes to welfare and family policies (see Boje and Ejrnæs 2011).

New Social Risks in Relation to Work-Family Reconciliation

New social risks can be defined as situations where individuals experience welfare losses as a result of the economic and social changes that are associated with the transition taken place during the last three to four decades into a post-industrial society (Taylor Gooby 2008; Bonoli 2005). The most important changes are deindustrialisation of employment, the influx of women into the labour force, increased instability of family structures and the destandardisation of employment (Bonoli 2007: 498; Esping-Andersen 2009). Relevant for the theme of this chapter is the new social risks related both to changes in family and gender roles and to changes in the labour market. Concerning changes in the family, the move of women into paid work in large number and as a consequence the collapse of the traditional division of domestic work within the families has markedly changed the gender roles (Lewis 2002; Lister et al. 2007; Esping-Andersen 2009).

The expectation that women have responsibility for the unpaid care work in the private sphere while the man was responsible for wage work in public sphere has changed with women's take up of gainful employment and the changing family structure (Lewis et al. 2008). Most domestic care is however still provided by women, and twice as many women as men spend time on care tasks for children and elderly family members (Eurostat in Taylor-Gooby 2004). This division of care responsibilities has also impact on employment and income in the families. In European families with care responsibilities towards either dependent children or older people, the female employment rates are two-thirds of the male employment rates, and the poverty rates for couple households where only one partner is in paid work are up to 6 times higher than for those households where both partners are in gainful employment (Esping-Andersen 2002; Taylor-Gooby 2004).

Esping-Andersen (2009) has labelled this development the 'incomplete revolution'. Revolution refers in this context to the dramatic and rapid transformation in women's role from housewifery into a lifelong employment. The 'incomplete' refers, on the other hand, to the negative social consequences of the development in terms of lower fertility and income inequality caused by the fact that dual career norms are in large part of Europe limited to the top of the social pyramid. In the labour market, a combination of deindustrialisation and flexibilisation has tightened the link between education and employment, which again has resulted in higher risks of social exclusion of individuals with poor education and a growth in precarious low-paid jobs. Women and especially mothers are overrepresented among groups in low-paid jobs and often also among the low educated. The revolution is also incomplete because men's employment pattern has only changed slightly, while women in households with care obligations have got a double workload. The inability to combine caring for dependent children or older people with paid work can then be considered as a major new social risk in the post-industrial society and a risk which has hurt women significantly more than men and has increased the social inequality between the less educated working poor households and the educated well-paid households (Bonoli 2005).

Constraints in the Opportunities and Capabilities: Individual or Institutional Barriers

A central discussion in relation to new social risks is the extent to which the risks are triggered by individual resources or external circumstances. In other words, are the social risks experienced by the households a result of the individual's opportunities and capabilities for not being able to combine labour market involvement and care responsibilities, or are the risks determined by external circumstances such as lack of access to services for children or elderly people and possibilities for paid leave during periods with heavy care obligations? When there is lack of services or paid leave, individuals are forced to spend less time on paid work. In the literature on new social risks and work-family balance, two different approaches are often referred: social investment and social resource.

Social Investment

Due to the societal changes mentioned – individualisation, flexibilisation and polarisation of income – the conception of social security has changed. A core issue for the old welfare state was protection of people from the inequality that the market creates, while the present welfare state primarily tries to facilitate integration into the market. Instead of social protection, we are talking about social investment strategy (Jenson 2009; Esping-Andersen 2009; Ejrnæs and Boje 2011). Now social security means having the capacity to confront changes, and this acquires new skills or update of old skills in order to adapt to the new demands in a knowledge-based economy (Jenson and Saint-Martin 2006: 435; Esping-Andersen 2002).

The new social risks have thus generated new social needs. While old risks, such as accidents, illness and unemployment, are mainly covered by income-related insurance schemes for standard industrial breadwinners, reforms directed at new social risk are more service oriented and aimed at increasing labour market participation and enable parents to reconciling work and care. Investment in social services and human capital is then a precondition for combating the risk of poverty because insecurity in employment is closely linked to income insecurity (Jenson and Saint-Martin 2003; Jenson 2009). Provision of public care for dependent children and elderly people is in this context considered as a condition to stimulate women's entry into the labour market and reduce their risk of social exclusion (Knijn and Smit 2009).

In discussing social investment, Esping-Andersen is especially worried about child poverty and social exclusion of young and women. According to him, welfare policy has a huge impact on women's life income in two ways. First, it has to prevent loss of income due to work interruption because of care obligations. Second, welfare policy must be designed to prevent deprivation of human capital and loss of work experience, which is caused by the work interruption (Esping-Andersen 2009). Based on previous studies, we might assume that in welfare policy regimes which give individuals a right to receive care and a right to time to provide care, the individuals have a real choice in combining work and care and thus reduce the risk of spending less time on paid work.

Social Resource Perspective

A second approach in resisting social risks might be the social resource perspective developed by Bourdieu in this theory on capital resources (Bourdieu 1986 [1979]). Bourdieu does not talk about risks but life chances. He combines a Marxist focus on economic resources as determining people's chances with a Weberian notion of social position, such as economic, social and cultural and symbolic capitals. Resources are here not considered just as economic, but also different forms of cultural and social capital are seen as valuable resources, which can increase the individual's capability coping with social risks. It might be assumed that more affluent families have a lower risk of spending time outside paid work than less affluent families because they have the economic resources to externalise their care needs. Also social capital in terms of social networks outside the families can be seen as valuable resources in coping with risk of spending less time on paid work than preferred because of care responsibilities. In local communities characterised by frequent social contacts with neighbours, families have better possibilities of reconciling work and family life as they can get help from friends and neighbours.

The major drivers behind the changes in family and gender roles have been the increasing educational level among women and the necessity of two incomes to maintain a satisfactory family income (Taylor-Gooby 2004). This development combined with the increase in the absolute and relative numbers of elderly people has meant that the demand for social care has increased dramatically.

Hypothesis and Operationalisation

We want in this chapter to focus on two different types of risk for spending less time on paid work than preferred among individuals who have care obligation – risks which have intensified with the changes in family and gender roles (Taylor-Gooby 2004; Esping-Andersen 2009). First are the risks related to care for dependent children and second are the risks related to care for frail elderly people as a consequence of the growing older population. We define risk in relation to the work-family balance as the likelihood of spending less time on paid work than the individuals would like to do because of care responsibilities for family members and relatives. We look at both individuals in paid work who perceive that they have to reduce their involvement in employment due to care responsibilities and individuals who at the moment are out of paid work doing unpaid care work in the household and therefore have difficulties entering the labour market. Individuals that explicitly express a preference for spending time outside paid work because of care responsibilities are not included among the risk groups. In Fig. 7.1, we try to illustrate the two types of risks and the institutional and individual factors, which have influence on the transition between work and nonwork.

We closely relate inequalities in risks to inequalities in individuals' opportunities and capabilities to choose the preferred combination of work and care. The risk of individuals for being prevented from working as much as preferred is determined by a combination of institutional conditions defined by the welfare policies and individual resources measured by education, economic situation and social network. In our analysis, we differentiate between women and men due to the marked different expectations for caring responsibilities imposed on women and men, respectively. The central question is thus to what extent institutional conditions or individual resources determine the individuals' capabilities to manage the conflict between work and family responsibilities.

We measure the perceived risk of spending time outside paid work because of care responsibilities by following question in the European Social Survey 2008:

> How likely is it that during the next 12 months you will have to spend less time in paid work than you would like, because you have to take care of family members or relatives

Based on our theoretical frame, we outline 3 hypotheses:

Hypothesis 1: We expect that in countries with extensive welfare policy defined by a relatively high level of care services and care allowances, the risk of spending less time on paid work than preferred because of care for dependent children or fragile

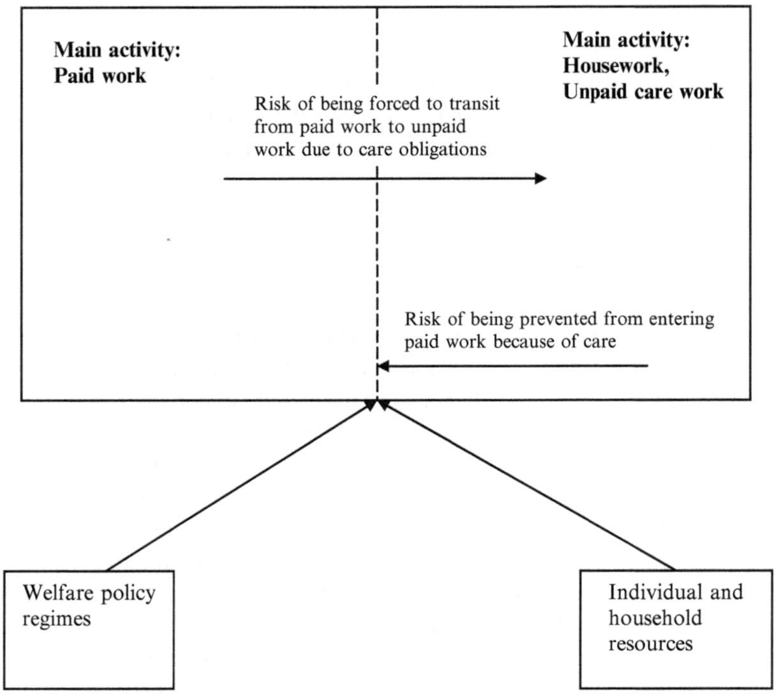

Fig. 7.1 What determines the risk of being prevented from paid work due to care responsibility

older people is low – illustrated by Denmark and Sweden. On the other hand, we expect a high risk of spending more time outside paid work than preferred because of care in countries where care services or care allowances are lacking – illustrated by Poland and Portugal.

Hypothesis 2: The accumulation of social, cultural or economic capital reduces the risk of spending less time in paid work than preferred due to care obligations. Economic capital measures the opportunities of the families to externalise their care need.[1] Social capital is defined as social contacts with friends, relatives and colleagues one time in a week or more. Cultural capital is defined as numbers of years in education.

---

[1] Because of problems in estimating the household income in different countries, we use a subjective measure of the household's economy. Economic capital is defined as the person who is living comfortably on present income or coping on present income. We use following question in the ESS 2008 to measure the economic capital:
Which of the descriptions on this card comes closest to how you feel about your household's income nowadays?
Living comfortably on present income 1
Coping on present income 2
Finding it difficult on present income 3
Finding it very difficult on present income 4

Hypothesis 3: We expect that the perceived risk of spending less time on paid work is higher for women than men because of the gendered division of unpaid work. The gendered division of paid and unpaid work within a couple means that women are much more likely to sacrifice their career in order to obtain a work-life balance than men. Therefore, the perceived risk of spending less time on paid work than they wish to do is higher for women than for men.

Institutional Settings in Selected European Countries

The impact of welfare and care regimes on women's choice in combining paid work and family work has been a core theme in the welfare policy literature for the last two to three decades. Many different approaches have been developed in understanding women's choices in reconciling work and family obligations (see Orloff 1993; Leira 2002; Lewis 2002; Lewis et al. 2008; Wall 2007; Lister et al. 2007; Gornick and Meyers 2009; Boje and Ejrnæs 2011). The typologies differ depending on the welfare policy area dealt within the analyses, but there seems to be an overall agreement about five different models or regimes defining the welfare-family policy – universal welfare model in the Nordic countries, liberal welfare model represented by the United Kingdom, continental corporatist welfare model in Germany and Austria, post-Communist welfare model represented by the Central and East European countries and a Mediterranean family-oriented welfare system in Southern Europe. In several recent studies, it has been found that this type of typology predicts fairly well the actual differences in behaviour among household members in relation to paid work, housework and care work as well as their attitudes to care obligations (see Anttonen and Sipilä 1996; Wall 2007; Gornick and Meyers 2003, 2009; Saraceno and Keck 2010; Boje and Ejrnæs 2011; Ejrnæs and Boje 2011). We have selected six countries that represent the different welfare-family policy models, and in Tables 7.1 and 7.2, an overview of provision and costs of care for small children aged 0–6 and elderly people aged 65+ is shown followed by a short description of the individual countries representing the five models.

Table 7.1 Enrolment in institutional childcare and spending on care for children

	Coverage among children in respective age groups, 2008		Expenditures in % of GDP, 2007			
	0–2 years	3–5 years	Cash	Service	Tax breaks towards families	Total
Denmark	65.7	91.5	1.48	1.80	0.00	3.28
United Kingdom	40.8	92.7	2.13	1.11	0.33	3.58
Sweden	46.7	91.1	1.49	1.86	0.00	3.35
Germany	17.8	92.7	1.09	0.75	0.88	2.71
Portugal	47.4	79.2	0.79	0.44	0.17	1.32
Poland	7.9	47.3	0.71	0.28	0.50	1.58

Source: OECD (2011)

Table 7.2 Welfare provision for elderly people

	Covered elderly people per 100 aged 65+ (2003–2004)[a]		Spending on elderly care in % of GDP[b]	Benefits kinds per person EURO PPP[b]	Spending on pensions in % of GDP[b]
	Residential care	Home help	2006	2004	2006
Denmark	8 (8)	29 (21)	1.73	512.3	10.8
The UK	5	10	0.99	155.8	10.5
Germany	4 (5)	7 (3)	0.16	48.6	12.4
Sweden	7 (7)	9 (8)	2.39	711.4	11.8
Poland	2	2	0.24	3.0	11.6
Portugal	4	7	0.26	64.4	13.1

Source: [a]Saraceno (2010) and Rauch (2007) (figures in bracket); [b]Eurostat 2008/2010

1. Denmark and Sweden represent the *universal welfare state model* where entitlement is based on citizenship and where there is a relatively high level of protection against social risk. When it comes to policies concerning care for small children, Denmark and Sweden are characterised by an extensive family policy (Boje and Ejrnæs 2011). Both countries have at least 1-year well-paid parental leave combined with high childcare coverage for children under three. This policy enables mothers to re-enter gainful employment after 1 year of paid leave. Both countries have a high level of spending on family policy. The two countries differ concerning the organisation of parental leave. In Sweden, 2 months of the leave period are reserved to the father, while it is up to the Danish families to decide the division of the leave period. When it comes to elderly care services, there are some differences between the two countries. Elderly care seems more of a universal citizen right in Denmark and given without means-testing, while in Sweden, the right to home help is more restricted and dependent on both family and financial resources (Rauch 2007).
2. The UK represents a *liberal welfare model* characterised by limited and target welfare provision. Concerning policies for dependent children, UK combines a short low-paid leave period with a high level of mothers working in part-time jobs. This model is characterised by a market-driven, highly expensive and individualised care system. During the new labour government, the availability of childcare has been improved but mostly as part-time care. In contrast to the privatised care system for small children, there has been a much larger collective involvement in services for elderly people where municipalities have been a comprehensive provider of residential care homes, while there until recently has been very little publicly organised home help (Bettio and Plantenga 2004). This has changed towards more home help combined with allowances for family carers (Saraceno 2010).
3. Germany represents the *continental corporatist welfare model* where the entitlement both to parental leave and elderly people is based on an insurance system. Concerning family policies towards small children, Germany is characterised by

long relatively well-paid parental leave but a low coverage of childcare for children under three and most formal childcare is part-time. After end of the leave period, mothers typically take up part-time jobs. During the recent years, the German family policy has been under review. The length of parental leave has been reduced, and the government has been investing massively in institutional childcare. The same improvement has not taken place in services for elderly people. Germany has been known for a largely private elderly care, which is primarily informal. (Bettio and Plantenga 2004). First with the introduction of statutory long-term care insurance in 1995, the situation improved, but still the level of both residential care and home help is low compared to the Nordic countries (Table 7.2), while the pension costs are higher and more generous (Rauch 2007). The German elderly care model can be described as a publicly facilitated, private care model, and recently, a substantial element of family allowances to be use to buy care has been introduced (Bettio and Plantenga 2004: 101; Saraceno and Keck 2010).

4. Poland represents the *post-Communist welfare regime*. Policies concerning small children in Central and East European countries, including Poland, are characterised by long periods of parental leave and poor provision of formal childcare for children below 3 years. The policy is home-centred and encourages mothers to stay home when the children are under 3 years and then return to the labour market. In Poland, the parental leave payment is lower than in several of the other Central European countries. Poland has one of the lowest rates of enrolment in Europe for both formal childcare among children aged 0–2 and for children aged 3–5 in preschool services (Table 7.1). Elderly care in Poland as in several other post-Communist countries has been a private concern after 1989. Residential care is restricted and bad, community care rarely exists, and the pensions are small. Most elderly people have to rely on their younger relatives for care and support (see Table 7.2).
5. Portugal represents *Mediterranean welfare model*. This model can also be characterised with a high level of intergenerational care (Boje and Ejrnæs 2011). The paid parental leave is short and badly paid as we find in the other South European countries, but the childcare seems to be more formalised in Portugal than elsewhere and the availability of childcare higher (Bettio and Plantenga 2004 and Table 7.1). The spending on family policy is low in Portugal partly due to the short low-paid parental leave, and also costs for childcare services are low which might indicate a low quality of services (Table 7.1). Portugal has a relatively high female employment rate but few women on part-time due to lack of this type of jobs. When it comes to care for elderly people, it is the responsibility of the family, and the care system operates through intense and diversified exchanges within the family with very fewer possibilities to rely on public care services (Bettio and Plantenga 2004). The pension system is, on the other hand, relatively generous for retired individuals who have been active in the labour market. Among the countries included in this study, Portugal thus has the highest pension costs (Table 7.2).

Combining Work and Care: Barriers to Be Employed Due to Care Obligations

From other studies, we know that care obligations only have marginal impact on the female employment in Denmark and Sweden, and for men, becoming a father even increases their rates of employment (Abrahamson et al. 2005; Plantenga et al. 2008; Ejrnæs and Boje 2011). The high female employment rates in Denmark and Sweden reflect the possibilities for women returning to the labour market after 1 year because of adequate childcare coverage for small children and appropriate public support for fragile elderly relatives. For Danish and Swedish women and men, we also find that the risk of being forced to reduce involvement in paid work due to care obligations is lower than in the other countries – see Table 7.3.

Polish women on the other hand have the highest risk of spending less time on paid work section because of care. The proportion of Polish men in paid work who think it is likely that they will spend less time on paid work is also considerably higher than the other countries. The high level of risk in Poland can be explained by a combination of low-paid parental leave, lack of facilities for both childcare and elder care and few jobs where it is possible to combine work and care obligations. We find similarly that high risk figures in Portugal especially for women despite the female employment are relatively high among mothers compared to the other Mediterranean countries. Portuguese mothers are returning to the labour market after a short maternity leave. A combination of a relatively high level of childcare coverage (Table 7.1) and intergenerational care enables women to an early return to the labour market. But they live with a constant care burden, which might explain the highly perceived risk for spending less time than preferred in paid work.

For Germany and the UK, the proportion of women in paid work who consider that they have to reduce their involvement in work due to care obligations is only slightly higher than in Scandinavia. Contrary to Scandinavian women, British and German women seem to have changed their working time to their care obligations, meaning that they do not consider reduced working hours as a risk – it has already happened. In both countries, mothers who return to work take up short part-time jobs in order to reconcile work and care and have thus accommodated their employment conditions to their care obligations. Furthermore, the German and British mothers typically are out of employment for at longer period due to motherhood than in Scandinavia. In Germany, this is the case due to a combination of prolonged period of leave and lack of adequate childcare facilities. In the UK, a short and badly compensated leave combined with shortage of affordable full-time care means that mothers are unable to return to the full-time jobs.

Among women who have housework as their main activity, more than half in the UK and Poland think it is likely that they will spend less time on paid work during the last 12 months than they wish to do. In Poland, a long parental leave, lack of affordable childcare and a culture of caring for elderly relatives in the family prevent many middle-aged Polish women from taking up gainful employment. In the UK, the barrier for transition from housework to paid work might be the combination

Table 7.3 Risk of spending less time on paid work for men and women which main activity either is paid work or housework

Main activity, last 7 days. All respondents	Country	Female: Likely to spend less time because of care (%)	Female: Total respondents	Male: Likely to spend less time on paid work because of care (%)	Male: Total respondent
Paid work	Germany	11.1	469	10.6	659
	Denmark	10.7	336	5.8	362
	The UK	11.6	483	7.3	494
	Poland	25.9	293	23.9	355
	Portugal	20.7	391	10.2	332
	Sweden	8.6	420	6.9	475
Total		14.1	2,392	10.4	2,677
Chi-square		***		***	
Housework, looking after children and others	Germany	34.4	93	29.4	17
	Denmark	28.6	21	0	5
	The UK	54.0	139	61.5	13
	Poland	55.8	43	50.0	6
	Portugal	35.0	20	100.0	1
	Sweden	36.4	11	0	1
Total		45.3	327	39.5	43
Chi-square		***			

Source: ESS Round 4
*$p<0.05$; **$p<0.01$; ***$p<0.001$

of short and badly paid maternal leave and lack of sufficient full-time childcare. The general high proportion of women doing housework or care work who consider it difficult to get into paid work illustrates the well-known barrier for entering paid work having been out of employment for longer periods. Furthermore, it also indicates that a large group of women out of gainful employment want to return if the institutional conditions were in place (Lewis et al. 2008).

We want to follow up this analysis of the risk for not being able to get into paid work as much as they want by analysing to which extent it is dependent on children or other care obligations in the household, which are the barriers. Table 7.4 shows that in all countries except in Portugal women with small children have a significantly higher risk of spending less time on paid work than they want because of care obligations.

In all six countries, the risk of spending less time on paid work is related to care for small children and not care for frail elderly. We find a high level of risk and very strong connection between presence of small children and risk perception in the UK and Germany. In both countries, about half of the women with small children under 3 years think that they will spend less time on paid work because of caring for family and relatives compared to 10% in households with no dependent children. For Polish women, we also find a strong correlation between small children and risk perception, and here, the general level of risk perception is for all groups higher than in any of the other countries. A strong familialistic care culture combined with

Table 7.4 Risk of spending less time in paid work due to small children or other care obligations in the household

		Female		Male	
		Spending less time on paid work because of care (%)	Total	Spending less time on paid work because of care (%)	Total
Germany	Children under 3	43.50	46	34.20	73
	Children above 3 living in the household	14.20	275	8.00	249
	No children living in the household	10.40	241	8.50	354
	Total	14.90	562	11.10	676
	Chi-square test	***		***	
Denmark	Children under 3	28.80	59	14.10	71
	Children above 3 living in the household	6.70	180	2.20	138
	No children living in the household	11.10	117	5.10	158
	Total	11.80	356	5.70	367
	Chi-square test	***		**	
The UK	Children under 3	45.50	132	12.30	65
	Children above 3 living in the household	18.90	238	10.30	155
	No children living in the household	10.30	252	7.00	287
	Total	21.10	622	8.70	507
	Chi-square test	***		Not significant	
Poland	Children under 3	51.90	52	23.90	46
	Children above 3 living in the household	29.50	173	24.60	167
	No children living in the household	19.80	111	24.30	148
	Total	29.8	336	24.40	361
	Chi-square test	***		Not significant	
Portugal	Children under 3	30.00	50	7.70	39
	Children above 3 living in the household	22.30	202	10.20	118
	No children living in the household	17.60	159	11.40	175
	Total	21.40	411	10.50	332
	Chi-square test	Not significant		Not significant	
Sweden	Children under 3	21.40	84	14.60	89
	Children above 3 living in the household	5.60	180	5.40	184
	No children living in the household	7.20	167	4.90	203
	Total	9.30	431	6.90	476
	Chi-square test	***		**	

Source: ESS Round 4

*p<0.05; **p<0.01; ***p<0.001

nearly no provision of institutional care for children and older people increases the risk of spending less time in paid work for both men and women. Women in these three countries thus experience a relative high child penalty defined by a loss in lifetime income due to that they have chosen motherhood instead of continuous employment (Esping-Andersen 2009). In Denmark and Sweden, women with small children also have higher risks of spending less time on paid work because of care than women without small children. However, the level of perceived risk among Scandinavian mothers is much smaller than in Poland, the UK and Germany. In Scandinavia, a comprehensive family policy in terms of 1-year employment protected leave and sufficient affordable care for both children and older relatives reduces the risk of spending less time on paid work.

In Portugal, the difference between having small children or not and the perceived risk of spending time outside paid work because of care is not significant. Portuguese women have a continuous attachment to the labour market independently of the age of their children, but they have also substantial responsibility for their dependent family members and relatives due to a strong familialistic caring culture (Saraceno 2010). The expected intergenerational care increases the risk of being forced to reduce paid work for individuals with care obligation for both young and old persons.

Among men, it is also the care of small children below aged of 3 which significantly increases the risk of being forced to reduce the paid work more than preferred in Germany, Demark and Sweden, while it in the UK also affects men in families with older children. For Germany, a remarkable high number of men say that they have to reduce their workload due to caring of small children what might be explained by a change in the German family structure related to the rapid increase of German women aiming for gainful employment (Plantenga and Remery 2005). In Poland and Portugal, we see another pattern. Here men have a higher risk of spending less time on paid work if there are older children and no children in the household. In these two countries, the caring culture implies that men are less involved in caring for small children which is the responsibility of the mothers, but they have to share the caring obligations for older relatives with their wives because of strong familialistic norms of intergenerational care and few alternatives to care for elderly within the family (Leitner 2002; Kalmijn and Saraceno 2008). Although men also are in risk of spending less time in paid work than preferred, the proportion of men in risk is much lower than for women for all six countries.

Institutional and Individual Indicators in Explaining the Risk of Spending Less Time on Paid Work Due to Care Obligations

In the previous section of this chapter, we have described how the risk of being forced to spend less time on paid work due to care obligations for men and women is related to their labour market situation and presence of small children or other dependent persons in the family. Now we will go through a multivariate logistic regression analysis and combine the institutional variation between the countries

Table 7.5 Predicting perceived risk of spending less time on paid work for men and women

		Female				Male			
		Odds ratio		Odds ratio		Odds ratio		Odds ratio	
Country	Germany	1.70	**	1.75	**	1.68	**	1.38	
	Denmark	1.30		1.46		0.82		0.84	
	United Kingdom	2.61	***	2.10	***	1.25		1.05	
	Poland	4.13	***	3.67	***	4.23	***	2.97	***
	Portugal	2.70	***	2.11	***	1.44		0.99	
	Sweden	1.00		1.00		1.00		1.00	
Age group	Below 25			.99				.10	
	26–35			.94				.59	
	36–45			.96				.10	
	46–55			1.00				1.00	
Working time	0–15			1.30				1.76	*
	16–25			1.22				1.43	
	26–35			.98				.94	
	36+			1.00				1.00	
Economic situation	Living comfortable with present income			.46	***			.38	***
	Coping with present income			.54	***			.64	**
	Difficult with present income			1.00				1.00	
Social capital	Frequently social contacts			.79	*			.76	*
	Less frequently social relations			1.00				1.00	
Household	Children under 3			4.38	***			2.21	***
	Children above 3 living in the household			1.27				.91	
	No children living in the household			1.00				1.00	
Years in education				.99				1.01	
N		2,706		2,706		2,704		2,704	

Source: ESS Round 4
*$p<0.05$; **$p<0.01$; ***$p<0.001$

and the individual characteristics in explaining the risk. The results of this analysis shown in Table 7.5 can be summarised as follows.

Among the countries, we find that Polish women are most likely to perceive a risk of spending less time on paid work followed by women from Portugal and UK, while the odds of perceived risk are much lower among women in Scandinavian countries. Only Poland stands out with a risk significantly higher than for men in the other countries. Among both women and men, the odds ratios decrease slightly when introducing the individual variables, but there is still the same ranking of countries in the perceived risk.

Together with the differences between the countries, it is the presence of small children which is most decisive in determining the risk of spending less time on paid work for women. Women with small children have thus odds of perceived risk that is more than 4 times higher than for women without children living in the household. Having small children does also increase the likelihood of perceiving a risk for men, but not to the same extent.

The household economy – subjectively evaluated – is strongly associated with the level of risk. Women and men who are living comfortable or are coping with present income have much lower odds of perceiving risks than women and men who have difficulties living with the present income. Having social networks or frequent contact to relatives and neighbours also seems to reduce the risk of being forced out of paid work. Both economic and social resources seem thus to be important resources in coping with future risks. Low-income families are more in risk of spending less time on paid work because of care responsibilities.

Explanations of the perceived risks are by and large the same for men and women except for the country variable. Institutional differences seem less important for men's risks of being forced to reduce their paid work due to care obligations than they are for women.

Conclusion and Discussion

The aim of this chapter has been to investigate how institutional and individual factors influence on the perceived risk of spending less time on paid work than preferred among women and men with care obligations in six European countries representing different types of welfare systems. Much literature has focused on the impact of welfare and care regimes on men and women's actual engagement in paid and unpaid care work. This chapter focuses on the subjective side of the incompatibility between paid work and care responsibilities.

When men and women are supposed to be engaged in both paid work and unpaid work related to care obligations, small children and fragile older relatives can be considered as a social risk because it might reduce their earning capability during the period they are caring for children, elderly or disabled at home. Uncertainty concerning the future employment and income in periods with care obligations may affect couples' decision on timing of marriage and children, as well as the number of children. The perceived risk of involuntarily spending less time on paid work due to care obligations may thus indicate, on the one hand, difficulties for individuals to fulfil the care responsibilities for family members and, on the other hand, difficulties aiming for full-time employment and earning a sufficient household income. To secure stable employment and income for citizens with care obligations is thus an important condition for combating central societal problems such as declining fertility, poverty and social exclusion. In this context, risk perception might be an indicator showing the capability of the welfare states adapting to women's new role being both carer and worker.

In the empirical analyses, we compare six European countries, which have applied different welfare strategies in establishing a balance between work and family obligations and in providing facilities for caring of dependent individuals – children or elderly people.

The major conclusion in this chapter is that there is a significant variation between the different countries in their capabilities to prevent the risk of spending less time on paid work than preferred. Hypothesis 1 assumes that the risk of reduced involvement in paid work due to care obligations is lower in countries with extensive welfare policy than in countries where the care services and the possibilities for leave are restricted can be confirmed. The perceived risks are most widespread for women in Portugal, the UK and Poland, while the risk for reduced involvement in paid work due to care obligations is slightly lower in Germany. In the Scandinavian countries, we find a significant lower risk level than in the other countries. This indicates that welfare policies matter in creating employment and economic security for the individuals who have care obligations. In countries with lack of affordable childcare facilities, paid leave and/or elderly care service, the perceived employment insecurity due to care responsibilities is more widespread. Controlling for individual resources only reduces the impact of the country differences slightly.

Care for small children has different impacts on the level of perceived risk in the different welfare regimes. In Scandinavia, the presence of small children does increase the risks significantly for women, but at a much lower level than in the other four countries. In both Denmark and Sweden, we find comprehensive and universal full-time care service for children combined with well-paid leave arrangements. In Germany and the UK, there is a stronger connection between presence of small children and the risk perception. The lack of sufficient full-time childcare facilities in both countries and a well-paid leave in the UK put women at greater risk of being forced to interrupt the employment career or to reduce the working time when their children are small.

Portugal stands out from the other countries because the presence of children has no significant influence on the perceived risk of spending less time on paid work due to care responsibilities. This can be explained by a tradition for intergenerational care, which results in sharing the risk among individuals in different stages of life. The institutional frame – badly paid leave and limited eldercare – is also an important dimension in explaining how the risks of spending less time on paid work are distributed among generations.

Hypothesis 2 assumes that accumulation of social, cultural or economic capital reduces the risk of spending less time on paid work than preferred due to care obligations. This hypothesis can only partly be confirmed. It is primarily economic capital that reduces the likelihood of perceiving a risk of spending less time on paid work. In addition to presence of children, lack of economic resources in the household is the most significant individual factor in explaining the risk. It is not very surprising as low-income households have difficulties in paying for institutional care for children or older relatives.

In countries like Portugal and the UK where institutional care is primarily market-based, low-income families are forced to familialise the care obligations, while high-income families are able to opt for a de-familialisation either through institutional care or by employing care workers. In Denmark and Sweden, the difficulties to cope with present economic situation are much lower, and we do not find any significant differences in the level of perceived risk and the household's subjective economic situation. This indicates that the universal Scandinavian welfare states with extensive family policy modify the effect of income inequality on the perceived risk, while specially the East European and Mediterranean welfare systems increase inequality in perception of risk, and the result is a society where the care obligations are familialised relying on women to withdraw from gainful employment. The tendency that low-income families are more in risk of spending less time on paid work because of care increases the economic and social polarisation between households.

Among the other individual variables, only social contact has some impact on the perceived risk, while this is not the case for education. The reason why education has no impact could be that higher education could both increase and decrease the likelihood of perceiving a risk of spending less time on paid work. On the one hand, highly educated women who expect to reduce paid work because of care obligations are more disposed to perceive it as a sacrifice than less educated women. On the other hand, more educated women have more economic and social resources to manage the conflict between paid work and family responsibilities.

As expected, women are more likely to perceive a risk of spending less time on paid work than men which confirm Hypothesis 3. However, it is surprising that a relatively high proportion of men expect to reduce paid work because of care obligations despite the presence of small children has only little effect on men's actual employment engagement. This could be an indication of the radical changes in both gender role and women's employment patterns, which have meant that men do not take it for granted that women are responsible for the care work. Also the institutional and individual factors have a different impact on the perceived risks for women and men. Differences in the institutional frame of the welfare system clearly have more importance for women than for men. Only Poland stands out with a significantly higher risk level for men. When it comes to the presence of small children, we find that the risk for men being forced to reduce their paid work more than preferred is just half the risk for women. Men are thus less affected in their labour market position by care obligations than women. This is, however, expected considering the gendered caring culture, which still exists in many European countries.

This chapter finds evidence that welfare strategies which are able to combine social investments such as regulated flexibility in the labour market and sufficient institutional care facilities with a high level of income security through paid leave for care and family benefits as we find in the Scandinavian countries will reduce the risks for especially women being forced out of paid work in periods with heavy care obligations. The opposite scenario we find in Poland and Portugal where the institutional systems for institutional care is insufficient or only available for high-income groups, which increase the risk for women being forced out of paid work. As a consequence, familialism in the caring culture is reinforced, and the society is polarised in 'work-rich, time-poor' households and 'work-poor, time-rich' households combined with widespread poverty among households with only one breadwinner. The lack of possibilities reconciling motherhood and careers in South and East Europe will create what Esping-Andersen (2009) calls a trade-off between having children, on one hand, and pursuing employment, autonomy and increasing household income, on the other hand.

References

Abrahamson, P., Boje, T. P., & Greve, B. (2005). *Families and welfare in Europe*. Aldershot: Ashgate.

Anttonen, A., & Sipilä, J. (1996). European social care services: Is it possible to identify models. *Journal of European Social Policy, 6*(2), 87–100.

Bettio, F., & Plantenga, J. (2004). Comparing care regimes in Europe. *Feminist Economics, 10*(1), 85–113.

Boje, T. P., & Ejrnæs, A. (2011). Family policy and welfare regimes. In H. M. Dahl, M. Keränen, & A. Kovalainen (Eds.), *Europeanization, care and gender, global complexities* (Social Sciences Collection). New York: Palgrave.

Bonoli, G. (2005). The politics of the new social policies: Providing coverage against new social risks in mature welfare states. *Policy & Politics, 33*(3), 431–449.

Bonoli, G. (2007). Time matters: Postindustrialisation, new social risks, and welfare state adaptations in advanced industrial democracies. *Comparative Political Studies, 40*(5), 495–520.

Bourdieu, P. (1986) [1979]. The forms of social capital. In J. G. Richardson (Ed.), *Handbook of theory and research for the sociology of education* (pp. 241–258). New York: Greenwood Press.

Ejrnæs, A. (2011). The impact of family policy and career interruptions on women's perceptions of negative occupational consequences of full-time home care. *European Societies, 13*(2), 239–256.

Ejrnæs, A., & Boje, T. (2011). Different routes to social security in Europe. Social protection or Social investment. *Comunitania. International Journal of Social Work and Social Sciences, 11*(1), 45–67.

Esping-Andersen, G. (Ed.). (2002). *Why we need a new welfare state*. Oxford: Oxford University Press.

Esping-Andersen, G. (2009). *The incomplete revolution: Adapting to women's new roles*. Cambridge: Polity Press.

EUROSTAT. (2008/2010). Statistics in Focus.

European Social Survey Round 4 Data (ESS Round 4). (2008). Data file edition 4.0. Norwegian Social Science Data Services, Norway – Data Archive and distributor of ESS data.

Gornick, J. C., & Meyers, M. K. (2003). *Families that work*. New York: Russell Sage.

Gornick, J. C., & Meyers, M. K. (2009). *Gender equality: Transforming family divisions of labor*. London: Verso.

Jenson, J. (2009). Lost in translation: The social investment perspective and gender equality. *Social Politics, 16*(4), 446–483.

Jenson, J., & Saint-Martin, D. (2003). New Routes to Social Cohesion? Citizenship and the Social Investment State. *Canadian Journal of Sociology, 28*(1), 77–90.

Jenson, J., & Saint-Martin, D. (2006). Building blocks for a new social architecture: The LEGOTM paradigm of an active society. *Policy & Politics, 34*, 3.

Kalmijn, M., & Saraceno, C. (2008). A comparative perspective on intergenerational support: Responsiveness to parental needs in individualistic and familialistic countries. *European Societies, 10*(3), 479–508.

Knijn, T., & Kremer, M. (1997). Gender and the caring dimension of welfare states: Towards inclusive citizenship. *Social Politics, 4*(3), 328–361.

Knijn, T., & Smit, A. (2009). Investing, facilitating, or individualizing the reconciliation of work and family life: Three paradigms and ambivalent policies. *Social Politics, 16*(4), 484–518.

Kremer, M. (2007). *How welfare states care. Culture, gender and parenting in Europe*. Amsterdam: Amsterdam University Press.

Leira, A. (2002). *Working parents and the welfare state*. Cambridge: Cambridge University Press.

Leitner, S. (2002). Varieties of familialism – The caring function of the family in comparative perspective. *European Societies, 5*(4), 353–375.

Lewis, J. (2002). Gender and welfare state change. *European Societies, 4*(4), 331–357.

Lewis, J., Campbell, M., & Huerta, C. (2008). Patterns of paid and unpaid work in Western Europe: Gender, commodification, preferences and the implications for policy. *Journal of European Social Policy, 18*(1), 21–37.

Lister, R., Williams, F., Anttonen, A., Bussemaker, J., Gerhard, U., Heinen, J., Johansson, S., Arnlaug, L., Siim, B., & Tobio, C. with Gavanas, A. (2007). *Gendering citizenship in Western Europe: New challenges for citizenship research in a cross-national context*. Bristol: The Policy Press.

OECD. (2011). *OECD Family Database*. Paris: OECD.

Orloff, A. (1993). Gender and social rights of citizenship: State policies and gender relations on comparative perspective. *American Sociological Review, 58*(3), 303–328.

Plantenga, F., & Remery, C. (2005). *Reconciliation of work and private life. A comparative review of thirty European countries*. Luxembourg: European Commission. Office for Official Publications of the European Communities.

Plantenga, J., Remery, C., Siegel, M., & Sementini, L. (2008). Childcare services in 25 European Union Member States: The Barcelona targets revisited. In A. Leira, & C. Saraceno (Eds.), *Childhood: Changing contexts*. Bingley: Emerald Group Publishing Limited.

Rauch, D. (2007). Is there really a Scandinavian social service model? A comparison of childcare and elderly care in six European countries. *Acta Sociologica, 50*(3), 249–269.

Saraceno, C. (2010). Social inequalities in facing old-age dependency: A bi-generational perspective. *Journal of European Social Policy, 20*(1), 32–44.

Saraceno, C., & Keck, W. (2010). Can we identify intergenerational policy regimes in Europe? *European Societies, 12*(5), 675–696.

Taylor Gooby, P. (2008). The new welfare settlement in Europe'. *European Societies, 10*(1), 3–24.

Taylor-Gooby, P. (2004). *New risks, new welfare: The transformation of the European welfare state*. Oxford: Oxford University Press.

Wall, K. (2007). Leave policy models and the articulation of work and family in Europe. A comparative perspective. In P. Moss, & K. wall (Eds.), *International review of leave policies and related research 2007* (Employment Relations Research Series no. 80). London: Department for Business.

Chapter 8
Spousal Well-Being: An Inquiry into the Links Between Household Income and Parental Task Division

Joris Ghysels

Introduction

This contribution addresses well-being through a discussion of spousal preferences regarding the task division between partners in a couple. First, it shows who of both spouses is able to realise his or her stated preferences and elaborates on potential explanations for balanced outcomes (both spouses realise their preferences) and unbalanced ones (only one spouse 'wins'). Obviously, explanations for unbalanced outcomes abound. They may refer to, for instance, power imbalances, but equally so to structural limitations like a lack of childcare facilities or more than average care needs because of the presence of a handicapped child. We confront personal, interpersonal and more widely social explanations for the gap between the actual task division and the preferred one.

In a second part, we go into the link between income security and the realisation of task division preferences. Income security functioned as the central indicator of well-being during the development phase of Western welfare states and continues to determine crucial indicators like the poverty figures of Eurostat. Nevertheless, recent developments of the welfare state mark a departure of the purely income-oriented approach with, for instance, a central role for activation in the labour market and significant efforts to facilitate the reconciliation of work and family life. Moreover, rising divorce rates coupled with a continued interest of most citizens in a successful partner relationship warrant an interest in marital happiness and one of its constituting elements, satisfaction with the actual task division in a couple. Therefore, we investigate to what extent the latter indicator adds to well-being indicators based on household income. Is satisfaction with the task division strongly associated

J. Ghysels (✉)
TIER Institute, Faculty of Humanities and Sciences, Maastricht University, Maastricht, The Netherlands
e-mail: Joris.ghysels@maastrichtuniversity.nl

A. Moreno Mínguez (ed.), *Family Well-Being: European Perspectives*, Social Indicators Research Series 49, DOI 10.1007/978-94-007-4354-0_8,

with household income (as many well-being indicators), or does it provide an independent dimension of well-being? Furthermore, we explore the potential substitution between income and task division, as one may hypothesise that dissatisfied spouses are compensated for the unbalanced outcome with a more than average household income.

For the empirical analyses of this chapter, we rely on data of the 2004–2005 Flemish Families and Care Survey (FFCS), which provides a representative sample of families with young children. Consequently, we focus on an early period in marital life, with clear challenges regarding the division of care and career responsibilities and large variation in the actual outcomes.

A Preliminary Empirical Exploration

The Source of Data and Preference Indications

We base our empirical exploration of 'contentment on the parental task division' as an indicator of well-being on the Flemish Families and Care Survey (FFCS). For the FFCS, slightly less than two thousand households with children were interviewed between November 2004 and May 2005, resulting in a survey of families with children younger than 16 representative of the Belgian region of Flanders.

As part of the interview, married or cohabiting parents (to which we will indiscriminately refer as spouses) were asked to reply various questions on their preferences regarding the time allocation of themselves and their partner. One of these questions forms the starting point of our empirical analyses:

"Often, there is talk about changing roles of men and women in households. Hereafter, we give you four types of families. What type of family would you like to have, if you did not have to care about finances or other things?

1. A family in which only the husband has a job and the wife assumes the household chores
2. A family with both partners employed, but where the wife has a less demanding job than her husband and where she assumes a relatively larger part of the household chores
3. A family in which the man and woman have an equally demanding job and time devoted household chores is equally distributed among the male and the female partner
4. A family with both partners employed, but where the husband has a less demanding job than his wife and where he assumes a relatively larger part of the household chores
5. None of these types."

We pre-structured the answers into the following five types (Table 8.1):

Table 8.1 Types of ideal task divisions (survey questionnaire)

	Full label as used in the questionnaire	Shorthand
1.	A family with only the man employed and the woman a full-time homemaker	Split
2.	A family with the woman having a less demanding job and taking care of the major part of the household work	Semi-split
3.	A family with an equal division of employment responsibilities and household work between the male and the female partner	Joint
4.	A family with the man having a less demanding job and taking care of the major part of the household work	Reversed semi-split
5.	None of the above types of families	Other

Note: When asking the question, it was explicitly noted that the answers were to reflect the preference for the personal living situation supposing no worries about money 'or other things'. We did so to invite respondents to reflect on their preferences and thus to avoid pragmatism-bias in the answers, i.e. people replying in accordance with their present situation (for a variety of reasons, e.g. 'because you have to realistic' or to avoid cognitive dissonance)

The following table (Table 8.2) compares the answers of man and women.[1] It shows that only few men and women prefer the atypical choice of women taking the lead in the labour market. Furthermore, clearly more women than men opt for a balanced division of tasks with similar job and home responsibilities for the male and the female partner. Yet, the gap between male preferences and female preferences is not extremely wide.

In Table 8.3, we represent the combination of preferences between the partners in a household. As could be expected, not all couples share the same opinion about the ideal task division in their household. On the main diagonal, we find only slightly more than half of the couples (52.9%). Another important category (12.0%) refers to women preferring an equal sharing of responsibilities while their partners prefer the 'semi-split' arrangement, which gives them the lead in the labour market. Furthermore, the reverse situation with men opting for an equal division and women preferring the 'semi-split' is also common with 7.8% of the households. However, it can be observed that disagreements tend to be small because only few couples have 'non-bordering' preferences.[2]

Preferences and Realisations

After the comparison of male and female preferences of the former section, we want to investigate to what extent preferences are realised in the observed task division. To that end, we translated the current employment situation and usual weekly working

[1] In this chapter, we focus on the available answers for heterosexual couples. In the survey, we had a too small number of homosexual couples to include them in the analysis, and the answers of single parents are not relevant for the analysis.

[2] If the category 'others' is not involved, it accounts for only 6.3% of all couples.

Table 8.2 Distribution of family type preferences among men and women (%)

	Shorthand label[a]	Man	Woman
1.	Split	19.1	15.1
2.	Semi-split	43.4	40.2
3.	Joint	30.0	37.5
4.	Reversed semi-split	1.9	2.2
5.	Other	5.5	5.0

FFCS (2004–2005)
$N=1351$
Note: The data refer to heterosexual couple families with children below 16
[a]See Table 8.1 for a full description of the types of task division

Table 8.3 The combination of family type preferences between partners (%)

		Female preference				
	Male preference	Split	Semi-split	Joint	Reversed semi-split	Other
1.	Split	8.3	6.0	3.6	0.1	1.0
2.	Semi-split	4.7	24.3	12.0	0.8	1.7
3.	Joint	1.5	7.8	19.1	0.5	1.1
4.	Reversed semi-split	0.0	0.3	0.7	0.6	0.3
5.	Other	0.6	1.9	2.2	0.1	0.8

FFCS (2004–2005)
The percentages represent the proportion of the cells in the total sample
$N=1{,}351$

hours of both spouses into a typology with the same entries as the preference typology. We were fairly lenient in the hours interval that we accepted as reflecting 'an equal division of employment responsibilities', as we accepted a difference of weekly working hours of up to 4 h. We did so because in Flanders the contractual hours of a full-time job vary between economic sectors. Additionally, the latest general reductions of the contractual working week were often introduced as additional days of holiday leave not reducing the regular working weeks. As a result, any working time between 36 and 40 h a week is a common full-time working week configuration.

Table 8.4 reveals how the tasks are truly distributed among Flemish couples with children. The most remarkable difference with the preferences in Table 8.2 is the dominance of the 'semi-split' arrangement. Hence, in reality, the equal sharing of job and household responsibilities is much less common than people would like and, instead, the arrangement with men working more hours than women is predominant. Especially women (with a 37% preference for 'joint') are thus likely to experience a gap between the preferred and the actual task division.

Table 8.4 The observed division of tasks between partners (%)

	Shorthand	Empirical implementation	Percentage
1.	Split	Man with job, woman currently without job	18.7
2.	Semi-split	Both partners have a job, but man works more than 4 h more on the job	51.6
3.	Joint	Both partners have a job, and their working hours are not more than 4 h apart from each other (in both directions)	15.3
4.	Reversed semi-split	Both partners have job, but the woman works more than 4 h more on the job	6.6
5.	Other	Any other arrangement. In practice, this often refers to unemployed men with working women	7.9

Table 8.5 Agreement on the preferences

	Woman's preference on task division				
Column %	Split	Semi-split	Joint	Reversed	Total
Disagreement	40.9	36.9	44.2	77.7	41.2
Agreement	59.1	63.1	55.8	22.3	58.8
Total	100.0	100.0	100.0	100.0	100.0
N	189	498	472	22	1,181

Note: ANOVA test of difference gives *F* value of 3.12 (>95% significance). Bonferroni test indicates that this is driven by the category 'reversed' (differs in a statistically significant way from other categories at 90–98% significance levels)

Agreement Versus Disagreement

The above confrontation of the effective task division with the preferred task division of the spouses warrants further inquiry. Whether a realisation of a task division preference is to be seen as an indicator of well-being is likely to depend on the dynamics in the couple: were both partners able to realise their preferences, or did one partner 'win' while the other did not? Conversely, one may hypothesise that the loss of well-being for not realising one's preferences be smaller when neither of the partners succeeds than when one wins and the other does not.

Before elaborating on the meaning of relative agreement, we shortly go into the empirical starting point. We should note that, for the remainder of our analyses, we leave the preference type 'other' apart because its meaning is inherently unclear.

Table 8.5 synthesises Table 8.3 and shows that, in the selected sample, 59% of partners agree on their time allocation preferences. Moreover, this agreement is equally divided among the options, except if women prefer to take a leading role in the labour market. Hence, in general, agreement in itself does not imply a choice for a specific time allocation. Yet, wanting to deviate strongly from the social norm makes it considerably harder to reach agreement. However, only very few couples are in this case (see also Table 8.2).

Table 8.6 Confronting preferences and realisations for those agreeing

Column %	Agreed preference on task division				
Actual task division	Split	Semi-split	Joint	Reversed	Total
Split	73.9	15.6	5.9	0.0	21.2
Semi-split	18.7	70.3	50.9	65.7	54.6
Joint	7.4	10.2	29.6	15.5	17.2
Reversed semi-split	0.0	3.9	13.7	18.9	7.1
Total	100.0	100.0	100.0	100.0	100.0
N	110	310	260	5	685

Table 8.7 Preference realisation of those disagreeing

Total %	Man realises preferences	
Woman does	No	Yes
No	25.1	41.0
Yes	34.0	0.0
N	293	203

Of those couples agreeing, slightly more than half (55% or 377 cases) end up in an observed time allocation that is in line with their stated preferences (cases on the main diagonal of Table 8.6). This relatively low percentage is mainly driven by the large group of couples (19% or 132 cases) stating to prefer a joint distribution of time and ending up in a semi-split arrangement. The other choices seem easier to realise, although the figures never come close to full realisation. Of those couples preferring a split and a semi-split arrangement, 74% and 70%, respectively, realise their preference.

Of the relatively large group of couples not agreeing on their time allocation preferences (Table 8.7), the majority ends up in one of the polar cases: 41% realise the preferences of the male partner versus 34% of the female partner. However, a quarter of the disagreeing couples (25%) does not realise either of the partners' preferences.

Summarising, the data indicate that 55% of partners who agree in their preferences on task division end up acting according to these preferences, while this percentage is lower for those disagreeing. Disagreeing men have only 41% likelihood of obtaining their preferred task division, while for women, this percentage decreases to 34%, more than 20% point lower than their agreeing counterparts. The above also implies that in total, in only 32% of couples (377/1,181), both spouses are able to realise their task division preference.

We hereby remind the reader that we coupled responses of two personal interviews and indicate agreement as the case where the preference voiced by the female partner equals that stated by the male partner. We did not observe and did certainly not stimulate communication about these preferences between the spouses. In fact, we made efforts to obtain a fairly clear indicator of the realisation of task division preferences through a separate interview of both spouses and separate questions on preferences and the actual task division.

Theorising Agreement and Disagreement

For a further investigation of the role of agreement in the relation between spouses and their well-being, we first develop on the micro-economic meaning of agreement. We start from a very generally formulated collective household welfare function with two decision makers, who derive (positive) utility from the consumption of private and public goods, from their leisure time and, potentially, from the utility level of their partner:

$$F(\mathbf{X}_m, \mathbf{X}_f, l_m, l_f, \mathbf{Z}) = \alpha\, U_m + (1-\alpha)\, U_f \qquad (8.1)$$

where $\mathbf{X}_i$ refers to a vector of private consumption of individual i, which we conveniently describe as either m (male) or f (female). Likewise, l_i refers to the hours of leisure time of the individual. As a final factor contributing to the utility of the collective, the vector $\mathbf{Z}$ refers to a set of household public goods, which derive from household production. In the framework of families with children whom we are addressing here, well-educated and happy children form an integral and important part of this vector $\mathbf{Z}$.

Furthermore, we assume that the collective welfare function F is a linear combination of the private utility functions of both decision makers in the household, where the constant α denotes the relative weight of the utility of the male partner in the household welfare function or, in other words, male power.

In addition to the household welfare function, we define the production function of the public goods as

$$\mathbf{Z} = Z(h_m, h_f, \mathbf{X}_Z) \qquad (8.2)$$

where h_i refers to the hours of time spent on household production and $\mathbf{X}_Z$ to a vector of market inputs for household production, including childcare services bought on the market.

Moreover, the household is characterised by the following full income constraint:

$$(w_m + w_f)T + y_m + y_f + y_h = \mathbf{P}'\left[\mathbf{X}_m + \mathbf{X}_f + \mathbf{X}_Z\right] + w_m(h_m + l_m) + w_f(h_f + l_f) \qquad (8.3)$$

where w_i refers to the market wage of the individual i, T to the total available time, y_i to various types of non-labour income of the household (either attributed to one partner or general of the household h) and $\mathbf{P}$ to the vector of market prices for all goods in vector $\mathbf{X}$.

Now, let us assume that for a non-specified, but exogenous set of prices $\mathbf{P}$ and wages w_i and for an unknown distribution of power within the household α, we know for both partners which is the mutual combination of work and household time of their preference. In other words, we know for both partners m and f what is their maximum indirect utility V^* derived from the time allocation of both partners:

$$V_i^* = \max(V_i^1, V_i^2, \ldots) \qquad (8.4)$$

with $i = m,f$ and

$$V_i^j = V_i(t_f^j, t_m^j, h_f^j, h_m^j) \quad \text{for} \quad j \in \mathrm{N}^+ \tag{8.5}$$

where V_i refers to the indirect utility function of individual i, which depends on the income generating time (paid work) t_i of both partners and their respective contribution to household work h_i. Note furthermore that the symbols with superscript j refer to the amounts of the utility providing factors in alternative j.

Apart from this, two more elements are of interest for our research question. First, we also have information about the actual time allocation of both partners and, second, we know whether partners agree in their preference or not.

These pieces of information allow us to come to the following set of predictions on the actual time allocation of the partners:

1. If partners agree in their time allocation preferences, the expected real time allocation equals their preferences (8.6), unless the household suffers from a contextual shock S:

$$V_m^* = V_f^* \wedge S = 0 \quad \Rightarrow \quad E(t_m, t_f, h_m, h_f) = t_m^*, t_f^*, h_m^*, h_f^* \tag{8.6}$$

With a contextual shock, we refer to an event that altered the constraints the household is confronted with in a way that was not foreseen when the partners determined their time allocation preferences. Examples of the latter are unemployment spells or the unavailability of childcare services at an acceptable price level.

If households do suffer from a contextual shock ($S = 1$), we predict the outcome to differ from the preferred time allocation in a way that can be rationalised within the general utility framework we elaborated before.[3] We illustrate the latter for the two examples given before.

First, (non-voluntary) unemployment of partner i (with $t_i = 0$) is likely to lead to a higher than preferred engagement in household work of partner i because this partner will want to compensate utility loss from the unexpected loss of earned income by increasing household production. Obviously, the actual increase in household efforts depends on the utility partners derive from household production and the productivity of partner i in the household production process. For the previous prediction, we only need to assume these to be strictly positive, allowing considerable variation across individuals and households.

Second, an unexpected lack of childcare services (be it for available time slots or affordable prices) is likely to drive households away from their preferred time allocation in the direction of more household time. Since we assume households to arrange their time allocation in such a way that the marginal contribution to household utility of all types of activities is equal and equals the marginal wage rate, the household that seeks to minimise the utility impact of the lack of childcare services will have its partner i with the lowest marginal wage rate increase his or her household time.

[3] We assume for now that the contextual shocks leave the power factor α unaltered.

Note from the previous that in the case of initial agreement no exertion of marital power is required. The partners agree on the goal and react to unexpected alterations of their decision framework with the common goal in mind.

2. If the partners do not agree in their preferences on time allocation, matters are more complex and power comes into play. Yet, the outcomes differ again depending on the presence of a contextual shock.

   Without a contextual shock (Eq. 8.7), we predict the actual time allocation to reflect the preference of one of the partners or lie between the two preferences. Moreover, the outcome is expected to lie closer to the preference of the individual with the highest power in the relationship:

$$V_m^* \neq V_f^* \wedge \quad S = 0 \Rightarrow \quad E(t_m, t_f, h_m, h_f) = f(V_m^*, V_f^*, \alpha) \tag{8.7}$$

   With a contextual shock, households can again be expected to adjust their time allocation in accordance with the utility framework developed before, but the direction of the adjustment is more difficult to predict because the no-shock reference situation is not fixed as in the case of initial agreement between the partners.

   Actually, outcomes become unpredictable without further information, as the following example illustrates. Suppose that unemployment strikes the more powerful partner and this partner prefers to dominate in the labour market. Under these circumstances, his or her adjustment of household time is likely to be smaller than when this individual would prefer a relatively small part in the total labour market involvement of the household and a relatively larger part in household chores. In the latter case, an increase of household time does not imply a preference conflict, while it does in the former case.

In sum, we arrive at different predictions regarding the actual time allocation of couples depending on (a) whether they agree or not on the optimal time allocation and (b) whether or not the couples are confronted with unexpected changes in their decision framework (*contextual shocks*).

Further Empirical Exploration: Testing Predictions

Empirical Strategy

We subsequently use the theoretical elaboration of the previous section as a framework of analysis. In our understanding of determinants of an actual success in realising one's preferences regarding the intra-household task division, we distinguish between three classes: preferences, contextual shocks and power indicators. Without interference of contextual constraints and power imbalances, we hypothesise that preferences are more likely to be realised in the actual task division.

As general determinants of the decision framework, we include the respondents' age and predicted wage. The latter reflects the labour market earnings that every respondent can expect given her or his age, educational level and family composition.[4]

As indicators of contextual shocks, we use the spouses' contentment on their actual working hours and on their childcare arrangement and include health indicators. Whether the individual partners are happy with their working time or not provides an indicator of a shock in the labour market. If not, this indicates a contextual shock because of rationing in the labour market due to unemployment or insufficient variation in available work schedules. For shocks related to household time, we refer to whether the individual partners are happy with the childcare services they are currently using. If not, this indicates that childcare is not organised according to the preference of the individual and, hence, is likely to disrupt the actual time allocation too. The most common case is that parents cannot rely on grandparents for childcare and therefore have to hire formal childcare services (Ghysels and Debacker 2007). Since these come at a substantial cost, the income need of the household is affected, more paid employment is required and, consequently, the degrees of freedom regarding time allocation are restricted. As indicators of health shocks, we incorporate a measure of self-assessed health in interaction with the health of the spouse. We hypothesise that a bad state of health is associated with problems to realise one's preferences, but equally a bad state of health of the spouse may hinder success.

In accordance with the hypotheses derived above, we expect that for those agreeing, marital power does not play a role in the determination of the actual time allocation, while it does for the disagreeing couples. In the empirical specification, we use two common power indicators: the relative age of the spouses and the wage ratio (male/female).

Econometrically, we will test the statistical significance of the various classes of explanatory variables in a stepwise probit regression with likelihood ratio tests between the (nested) specifications. As a test sample, we selected only cases with full and clear information on all variables needed. This implies that unclear preference indications of the type 'none of the above types' (see Table 8.1) and unclear observed time allocations of the type 'other' (see Table 8.4) were removed from the sample. The remaining sample consists of 910 observations of women and 972 observations of men.

Estimates

The Reference Specification: Model 1

In the following table, we reflect the starting estimates. The specification includes personal characteristics of the respondents which can be expected to function as preference shifters and determine the constraints of the decision set (utility possibility frontier).

[4] Wages are predicted wages from a Heckman corrected wage equation, with net hourly wages of employees as observed outcome (see Ghysels and Cornelis 2007 for more details).

Table 8.8 Probit estimates of the likelihood of realisation of task division preferences (Model 1)

	Women			Men	
Probit coefficients	Coefficient	Std. error		Coefficient	Std. error
Predicted wage	−0.12	0.04	***	−0.02	0.03
Age interval (reference = up to 29)					
30–34	0.29	0.19		0.01	0.31
35–39	0.46	0.20	**	−0.10	0.31
40–45	0.25	0.25		−0.14	0.32
46 and over	0.26	0.33		−0.05	0.35
Health interaction (reference = both spouses healthy)					
Only man unhealthy	−0.49	0.21	**	−0.15	0.19
Only woman unhealthy	−0.20	0.27		−0.10	0.23
Both unhealthy	−0.35	0.48		−0.59	0.46
Woman's working time as preferred	0.19	0.13		0.09	0.15
Having preschool and school-age children ('mix')	0.27	0.24		0.30	0.20
Out-of-school care as preferred (reference = no mix, not happy)[a]					
No mix, happy about care	−0.01	0.19		0.27	0.16
Mix, not happy about care	−0.45	0.17	***	−0.19	0.15
Preschool care as preferred (reference = no mix, not happy)[a]					
No mix, happy about care	−0.01	0.18		0.04	0.18
Mix, not happy about care	−0.08	0.16		−0.17	0.15
Triple interaction of child problem disturbing family life (1 = yes) by					
At least one child with problems (1 = yes) by					
At least one child at preschool age (1 = yes)					
0 0 1	−0.22	0.21		−0.24	0.19
0 1 0	−0.18	0.39		0.10	0.36
0 1 1	−0.19	0.30		0.01	0.29
1 0 0	−0.44	0.54		0.22	0.51
1 0 1	−0.30	0.51		−0.74	0.53
At least one child with problems, seriously disturbing family life, while all children are at school age (3+)	−1.08	0.38	**	−0.44	0.32
1 1 1	0.28	0.45		0.64	0.42
Constant	0.89	0.41	**	0.27	0.43
N		910			972
Log likelihood		−538.06			−638.56

Notes: statistical significance **>95%; ***>99%

For descriptives, see Table 8.16 (Annex)

[a]The option 'mix, happy about care' is omitted because of collinearity

Moreover, we include the indicators of contextual shocks as further determinants of the constraints of the decision framework of the parents.

The estimates in Table 8.8 indicate that for men none of these explanatory factors has a statistically significant association with the likelihood of success in the realisation of the task division. However, the estimates of women are somewhat more promising.

On the one hand, it is shown that women in the age interval of 35–39 years old are more likely to realise their task division preference than other women. On the other hand, a relatively high expected wage level is associated with a decrease in the probability of success. Specification tests with the educational level rather than the expected wage as regressors (results not shown) indicate that this negative wage effect is not an indirect indication of the variation in task division preference that is associated with various educational levels. In other words, we find no indication that the gender culture of various educational groups explains why women with higher wage levels are less likely to realise their task division preference. Apparently, it is the expected monetary reward from labour market participation in itself that explains the observed relationship.

Furthermore, the estimates of women confirm the role of several of the expected contextual shocks. Women are less likely to realise their task division preference if (a) they live together with an unhealthy spouse, (b) they were not able to realise their preference for out-of-school care (while having both preschool and school-age children) and (c) they have a child that they qualify as having problems when compared with other children of his or her age (to a degree that disturbs family life and while having all school-age children). Hence, more than average care demands of an unhealthy spouse or school-age children complicate the realisation of the optimal task division for women, but not for men.

Extended Specifications: Models 2 to 4

To test the hypotheses on the role of agreement and the relative power of spouses, we extend the basic specification in three ways. First, we add an indicator of the actual task division and the agreement of spouses on their task division preference (Model 2). We showed earlier in descriptive analyses (Section 'Agreement Versus Disagreement') that there is a direct link between the actual task division and the likelihood of preference realisation, on the one hand, and between the degree of agreement and the likelihood of preference realisation, on the other hand. Therefore, both variables are included.[5] In Model 3, we add two power indicators to the specification. We conjecture that a relative dominance in age or in expected wage may improve the likelihood of the preference realisation. In Model 4, we interact the agreement and the power indicators because we derived from theory in section 'Theorising Agreement and Disagreement' that power may only play a role when partners voiced different task division preferences (disagreement).

In Tables 8.9 and 8.10, we show a selection of estimates of these three extended specifications. We do not repeat the estimates of variables in the basic specification, because these are not significantly altered throughout the extensions, with the exception of the expected wage to which we shall return below.

[5] The variables are included in an additively separate way because an interaction effect between both proved not to improve the explanatory power (LR test) (results not shown).

Table 8.9 Probit estimates of the likelihood of realisation of task division preferences of women: model extensions

	Model 2			Model 3			Model 4		
Probit coefficients	Coefficient	Std. err.		Coefficient	Std. err.		Coefficient	Std. err.	
Actual task division (reference=split)									
Semi-split	0.02	0.19		0.10	0.18		0.10	0.19	
Joint	0.27	0.22		0.31	0.21		0.31	0.21	
Reversed	–1.97	0.36	***	–1.92	0.37	***	–1.91	0.37	***
Agree on preferences (reference=no)	0.57	0.14	***	0.60	0.13	***			
Wage ratio (reference=woman earning >10% more)									
Male/female wage in 10% range				0.40	0.22	*			
Man earning >10% more				0.84	0.25	***			
Interaction agreement and wage ratio									
Do not agree and ratio in 10% range							0.08	0.32	
Do not agree and man earning more							0.74	0.36	**
Agree and woman earning more							0.23	0.39	
Agree and ratio in 10% range							0.84	0.31	***
Agree and man earning more							1.11	0.33	***
Woman older (>2 years)				0.16	0.29		0.20	0.28	
Man older (>2 years)				–0.03	0.14		–0.03	0.14	
Constant	0.45	0.43		–0.42	0.52		–0.19	0.56	
Log likelihood	–494.60			–482.36			–479.91		
LR test on previous specification									
Ch^2 (d.f.)		86.91	(4)		24.49	(4)		4.90	(2)
Statistical significance		>99.9%			>99.9%			>91.3%	

All models also include the regressors of Model 1 (see Table 8.8). Since the estimates on these variables do hardly vary between the specifications, their estimates are not repeated here (no changes in significance, point estimates vary by <0.1)

N=910

Statistical significance *>90%; **>95%; ***>99%

Table 8.10 Probit estimates of the likelihood of realisation of task division preferences of men: model extensions

	Model 2			Model 3			Model 4		
Probit coefficients	Coefficient	Std. err.		Coefficient	Std. err.		Coefficient	Std. err.	
Actual task division (reference = split)									
Semi-split	0.06	0.17		0.07	0.17		0.06	0.17	
Joint	0.07	0.21		0.08	0.21		0.06	0.20	
Reversed	–1.68	0.35	***	–1.65	0.34	***	–1.69	0.31	***
Agree on preferences (reference = no)	0.32	0.13	**	0.33	0.12	***			
Wage ratio (reference = woman earning >10% more)									
Male/female wage in 10% range				–0.04	0.21				
Man earning >10% more				0.06	0.26				
Interaction agreement and wage ratio									
Do not agree and ratio in 10% range							–0.52	0.30	*
Do not agree and man earning more							–0.77	0.37	***
Agree and woman earning more							–0.62	0.36	*
Agree and ratio in 10% range							–0.19	0.29	
Agree and man earning more							0.12	0.34	
Woman older (>2 years)				0.22	0.30		0.24	0.29	
Man older (>2 years)				0.05	0.14		0.05	0.14	
Constant	0.02	0.46		–0.03	0.47		0.40	0.49	
Log likelihood	–590.48			–589.42			–576.81		
LR test on previous specification									
Ch² (d.f.)		96.15	(4)		2.13	(4)		25.23	(2)
Statistical significance	>99.9%						>99.9%		

N = 972

Statistical significance * >90%; **>95%; ***>99%

All models also include the regressors of Model 1 (see Table 8.8). Since the estimates on these variables do hardly vary between the specifications, their estimates are not repeated here (no changes in significance, point estimates vary by <0.1)

Table 8.9 reflects the results of women. It first confirms that women who agree on the task divisions with their spouse are more likely to realise their preferences, even when controlling for contextual shocks (Model 2) and power indicators (Model 3). Second it reiterates that the atypical situation of ‘reversed semi-split’ is unlikely to reflect the spouses’ preference. In effect, if women are actually more active in the labour market than their spouses, they are unlikely to realise their task division preferences (Models 2–4).

Third, the table shows that of the power indicators, the wage ratio is significant, but the age difference is not. Moreover, the wage ratio does not have the expected sign. The results suggest in fact that women who take the lead in expected wage (the reference group) are less likely to realise their preferences than women who can expect to earn roughly the same hourly wage as their husband or women who expect at least 10% less.[6] Apparently, women with a non-traditional position vis-à-vis their spouse have more trouble to realise their preferences than those in the more common and more culturally ‘normal’ relative position.[7]

If we interact agreement with the power indicators (Model 4), we are unable to corroborate our hypothesis. We expected power only to play a role in the case of disagreement, but the opposite seems true. The estimates on the earnings ratio indicate a stronger power surplus for those in agreement than for those in disagreement. In other words, women agreeing with their husband in their task division preferences are less likely to realise these preferences the more dominant their husband is in the labour market (i.e. as regards expected wages). This increasing effect is also found among those disagreeing, but it is less strong because it only exists for the group with the most explicit power imbalance (husband expecting to earn at least 10% more than wife).[8] Moreover, the interacted specification (Model 4) does not offer a clearly higher explanatory power than the non-interacted specification of Model 3. The bottom lines of the table show that the increase in log likelihood is hardly significant at conventional levels (>90%).

For women, we therefore tentatively conclude from the multivariate analysis that contextual shocks are very important to explain the likelihood of task division preferences. Furthermore, the mere agreement on the preferred task division provides a strong surplus, even when controlling for contextual and other parameters. Finally, the estimates suggest that deviance from the social norm comes at the cost of a decreased likelihood of preference realisation.

---

[6] A simple linear or logarithmic specification of the ratio was also tested and gives similar conclusions.

[7] It should be noted that the inclusion of the wage ratio causes the original expected wage effect to drop in size and loose statistical significance. This is due to their highly collinear nature (ANOVA test has F value of 52.13 with 2 and 1,095 degrees of freedom, >99.9 %).

[8] A Wald test indicates that the estimated coefficient 1.11 does not differ in a statistically significant way from the estimates 0.74 and 0.84. However, the estimate 0.74 does differ strongly from the estimate 0.08. As such, the wage ratio has a clearly more important effect among those agreeing than among those disagreeing.

Table 8.10 shows the estimates of a similar exercise in gradual specification extension for men. As in the case of women, the experience of a reversed semi-split task division is associated with a lower likelihood of preference realisation. Moreover, agreement on the preferences brings about a higher than average likelihood of preference realisation.

In contrast, the estimates suggest that the relative power incorporated in the wage ratio has a different meaning for men than for women. For men, agreement or disagreement makes a whole lot of difference, which is corroborated by the LR test indicating a significantly better explanation for the interacted specification (Model 4) than for the basic power specification (Model 3, see bottom lines of Table 8.10), while the simple inclusion of power indicators made no difference (Model 2 versus Model 3).

Again, however, the sign of the parameter estimates is not as expected. Without agreement, husbands are less likely to realise their task division preference if they are dominant in their expected wage or roughly on par with their wives than in the case in which their wives expect to earn more. With agreement, the reverse is true. Only in the case their wives expect to earn more, husbands are likely to be affected negatively in their likelihood of reaching their preferred task division. In effect, only the latter estimate can be reconciled with a power interpretation of the wage ratio, even though different from the hypothesised one. Apparently, agreement does not withhold men from exercising power. Conversely, in disagreement, power cannot be exercised easily. In fact, powerful women experience the same because exactly when there is disagreement and women have a stronger relative position in the labour market, men are more likely to realise their preferences. It may be that the relatively powerful are paying a price for disagreement.

The Realisation of Task Division Preferences and Income Security as Separate Indicators of Spousal Well-Being

Comparing Indicators

In the previous section, we analysed the extent of preference realisation of spouses. We argued in the introduction that satisfaction with the actual task division in the household may be seen as an indicator of well-being. Therefore, it is of interest to compare this satisfaction indicator with a traditional indicator of material well-being: disposable income. Below we will systematically refer to the equivalised household disposable income, which is the net yearly household income corrected for the composition of the family using the OECD/Eurostat equivalence scale (1 first adult, 0.5 all subsequent adults, 0.3 children up to age 13). We use two well-being indicators: the Eurostat poverty threshold for Belgium (€ 777) and the quintile distribution, which we limit to the sample population, i.e. couple households with children younger than 16 in the Belgian region of Flanders in the school year 2004–2005.

Table 8.11 The variation in poverty rate depending on the realisation of task division preferences

Percentage	None of the spouses realises preferences	Wife realises preference	Husband realises preference	Both spouses realise preferences
Poverty rate	2.4	4.6	3.1	1.7
N	377	153	175	348

Table 8.12 The income distribution (quintile of disposable equivalent household income) depending on the realisation of task division preferences

Horizontal %	1	2	3	4	5	N
None	20.4	14.4	24.0	21.1	20.2	377
Wife only	24.0	17.4	15.0	17.5	26.2	153
Husband only	20.3	25.8	15.7	22.4	15.8	175
Both	18.9	24.2	20.7	18.6	17.7	348

Note: Income quintiles are within sample and thus refer to couple households with at least one child younger than 16

Table 8.11 links the realisation of the task division preference of one or both spouses to the poverty rate. It should be noted that among couples with young children, the poverty rate is overall low (less than 3%). As the table shows, this rate does not vary with the degree of preference realisation.

Likewise, Table 8.12 compares preference realisation with the income distribution. Again no statistically significant association is found between both indicators. The intermediate conclusion is therefore that satisfaction with the task division is a well-being indicator that is independent of material well-being as measured by disposable income.

Compensating Across Spheres of Well-Being

At the end of section 'Further Empirical Exploration: Testing Predictions', we wondered whether the relatively more powerful spouse would pay a price in terms of loss of task division satisfaction. Similarly, one could wonder whether spouses realising their task division preference while their partner is not compensate for this lack of balance through a higher income. In other words, is a lack of satisfaction in one field compensated for by increased well-being of another kind? This question is particularly relevant for the relatively large group of women who are not able to secure a position in the labour market that corresponds to their aspirations. In section 'Preferences and Realisations', we already discussed that many women prefer a balanced distribution of employment and household tasks, but in practice spend less time in the labour market than their husbands ('semi-split' instead of 'joint'). In the traditional male breadwinner logic, this task division was legitimised by a career support motive. It was believed that the household as a union would gain from specialisation. It is interesting to investigate whether any income effect of an

Table 8.13 Distribution of relative imbalance by type of task division preference

Wife's task division preference	Percent of wives working less than preferred while their husband does realise his task division preference (%)
Split	0.0
Semi-split	5.7
Joint	24.8
Reversed semi-split	36.0
Total	12.9

unbalanced outcome can be seen among families with young children, whom one can expect to be at relatively early stages of career formation.

We check the existence of monetary compensation through an OLS regression of the equivalised disposable household income. We engage in four steps. First, we run the basic specification without indicators of the degree of realisation of the task preferences. This specification includes the expected wage rate of both spouses and their actual working hours as basic explanatory variables. Second, we add an indicator for the unbalanced outcome discussed above, i.e. when the wife ends up working for pay less than preferred while, on the contrary, her husband does realise his task division preference. Table 8.13 shows that imbalance is more common the higher the relative employment ambitions of the wives, as could be expected by construction. Third, we investigate whether the meaning of this indicator of relative unbalance differs according to the aspiration level of the wife because we observed in the previous section that it is harder to realise preferences that are statistically less prevalent (especially the 'reversed semi-split'; Table 8.6). In a final extension of the specification, we add the indicators of contextual shocks that we developed in the previous section. We thereby hypothesise that a monetary compensation for an imbalance will be expected by the wife only if there are no external elements that cause (or legitimise) the imbalance. Alternately, one may hypothesise that the potential of surplus of a career support arrangement can be disturbed by the contextual shocks. In both cases, the monetary compensation for an imbalance is expected to be larger in the final specification than in the third specification.

Table 8.14 shows the estimates of these specifications. The simple extension of the basic specification with the indicator of imbalance from the point of view of the wife does not add explanatory power (Model 2). However, when differentiated according to the type of task division (Model 3), the table reveals a significant estimate of compensation in specific cases. The estimates especially suggest the existence of a compensating logic in case the husband is able to realise his preference, while the wife cannot realise her preference for a 'semi-split' arrangement and is in effect not gainfully employed. In this case, the monthly disposable income is €540 higher than the average (€1,680), which accounts for an increase by one third (32%).

As we suggested above, this rise in income can be understood in two ways. First, one may suggest that husbands who prefer their wives to refrain from gainful

Table 8.14 OLS estimates of the equivalised monthly disposable household income, from wife's point of view

	Model 1			Model 2			Model 3			Model 4		
	Coef.	Std. err.		Coef.	Std. err.		Coef.	Std. err.		Coef.	Std. err.	
Wife predicted wage	18.67	16.49		18.18	16.49		14.89	16.57		24.34	19.19	
Husband predicted wage	87.79	13.16	***	87.98	13.16	***	86.63	13.15	***	97.77	15.59	***
Wife's usual weekly working hours	12.33	1.42	***	12.52	1.43	***	12.33	1.59	***	10.55	1.94	***
Husband's usual weekly working hours	8.94	1.95	***	8.75	1.95	***	9.48	1.97	***	10.94	2.44	***
Wife does not realise task division preference, while husband does ('imbalance')				86.58	69.26							
Interaction preference by imbalance (reference=prefers 'split', no imbalance)												
Prefers 'semi-split, no imbalance'							61.51	70.56		35.07	78.03	
Prefers 'semi-split, imbalance'							539.06	154.70	***	894.64	188.52	***
Prefers 'joint, no imbalance'							139.42	77.60	*	73.93	85.47	
Prefers 'joint, imbalance'							33.02	96.39		107.41	107.71	
Prefers 'reversed semi-split, no imbalance'							98.64	214.98		−118.68	225.35	
Prefers 'reversed semi-split, imbalance'							445.61	262.43	*	335.19	308.91	
Contextual shocks												
Health of spouses												
Contentment with childcare arrangement											Sign.	
Child well-being indicators											Sign.	
Constant	−116.93	151.07		−121.27	151.07		−179.16	154.83		−478.47	192.86	
Adjusted R^2		16%			16%			17%			19%	

[a]Indicators are added exactly as in section 'Further Empirical Exploration: Testing Predictions'. For lack of space, the point estimates are not shown
Sign. indicates that at least one variable is statistically significant
Statistical significance * >90%; ***>99%

employment, while their wives prefer to engage in work for pay (even to a lesser extent than their husband, 'semi-split'), compensate their wives for compliance with the husband's preference by a considerable monthly income bonus. Obviously this surplus accrues to the household, and the dataset does not allow for a breakdown to individual utility (or even more restricted to individual consumption).

Nevertheless, it can be assumed for Flemish young households that income surpluses benefit all household members to some extent and, hence, that the wife experiences some utility compensation. A second potential interpretation refers to the career bonus. Apparently, refraining from labour market aspirations can be beneficial at the household level, though only for some specific groups.

The addition of the indicators of contextual shocks in the last specification (Model 4), further clarifies the results from Model 3. When controlling for contextual elements that alter the decision framework of the household (e.g. a child with a handicap or lack of childcare services), the prior point estimate rises to almost €900. In other words, without good reason for the imbalance, the compensation for it rises.

In the previous paragraphs, we reasoned from the point of view of the wife. Obviously, one could also develop a similar reasoning from the point of view of the husband. However, we have documented in the previous sections that husband are less likely not to realise their preferences and, hence, to 'suffer' from imbalance. Moreover, an imbalance from the point of view of the husband does not have a social explanation like the imbalances from the point of view of wives. In the latter case, the resulting arrangement can be seen as 'traditional', with the compensating mechanism that is inherent in the mere concept of 'male breadwinner'. The former, however, marks a breach of social convention to which no obvious social mechanism corresponds. For both reasons, it may not come as a surprise that we do not find similar effects when estimating the income models for the husbands (see Table 8.15 in Annex).

Discussion and Conclusion

Most often the concept of well-being is reduced to an income-related measure, especially in policy circles. The 'at risk of poverty indicator' of Eurostat is perhaps the most well-known indicator of this type. Moreover, even efforts to create multi-dimensional poverty measures tend to limit their scope to material deprivation. However, recent developments of the welfare state mark a departure of the purely income-oriented approach with, for instance, a central role for activation in the labour market and significant efforts to facilitate the reconciliation of work and family life. Moreover, rising divorce rates coupled with a continued interest of most citizens in a successful partner relationship warrant an interest in marital happiness and one of its constituting elements, satisfaction with the actual task division in a couple. Therefore, we investigated in this contribution to what extent the latter indicator adds to well-being indicators based on household income.

To construct an indicator of satisfaction with the actual task division between spouses, we confronted the real task division with preferences voiced by the spouses in independent interviews, where spouses were asked to reflect on their vision on the ideal task division between them and their partner, supposing there were no worries (about money, etc.). The data on Flemish couples with young children (FFCS 2004–2005) reveal that most spouses prefer a balanced division of tasks or an arrangement with the husband taking the lead in the labour market and the wife being connected to the labour market, but to a lower extent than her husband. In general, however, the balanced arrangement is not easy to realise, which is likely to frustrate more women than men because women more often aspire to this arrangement. As a consequence, we find men to be more likely to realise their task division preferences than women.

To understand more fully the meaning of the proposed satisfaction indicator, we elaborated on explanations for success in the realisation of task division preferences. After a theoretical reflection, we grouped potential explanations in three categories (personal characteristics, contextual shocks and relative power) and tested their empirical relevance in a multivariate setting.

The estimates indicate that contextual shocks may strongly limit the probability of success for women, but not for men. More than average care demands of an unhealthy spouse or school-age children complicate the realisation of the optimal task division for women. Men, however, do not seem to be hampered by them. Apparently, our gendered care culture motivates women, not men, to curtail labour market aspirations. Furthermore, we found that women with a non-traditional position vis-à-vis their spouse have more trouble to realise their preferences than those in the more common and more culturally ‘normal’ relative positions, with men taking the lead in the labour market and women in the household. Also, the estimates show that agreement on the preferences within the couple is strongly linked with success for both men and women. Yet, only half of the couples do indeed voice the same ideal task division. Power indicators, finally, were not found to be of particular importance.

After these analyses of the meaning and explanation of satisfaction with the current task division, we compared the indicator with the household income, more specifically the equivalised monthly disposable income. Unlike many other well-being indicators (e.g. health), we found no immediate (bivariate) association between the income situation of the household and the degree of realisation of the task division preferences of the spouses.

However, when we elaborated on the nature of the relationship between both well-being indicators, we did find some evidence of a compensating logic. We wondered whether spouses realising their task division preference while their partner is not, compensate for this lack of balance through a higher income. In other words, is a lack of satisfaction in one field compensated for by increased well-being of another kind? This question is particularly relevant for the relatively large group of women who are not able to secure a position in the labour market that corresponds to their aspirations. We already discussed that many women prefer a balanced distribution of employment and household tasks, but in practice spend less time in the labour market than their husbands. In the traditional male breadwinner logic, this task division was legitimised by a career support motive. It was believed that the household as a union would gain from specialisation. Therefore, we investigated whether any income effect of an unbalanced outcome can be seen among families with young children, whom one can expect to be at relatively early stages of career formation.

The estimates indeed support the idea of a compensation, although only in the specific case the husband is able to realise his preference, while the wife cannot realise hers and is in effect not gainfully employed. This rise in income can be understood in two ways. First, one may suggest that husbands who prefer their wives to refrain from gainful employment, while their wives prefer to engage in work for pay (even to a lesser extent than their husband), compensate their wives for compliance with the husband's preference by a considerable monthly income bonus. Whether there is an active offer of compensation by the husband cannot be derived from our data and seems unlikely given the mostly implicit nature of marital bargaining. However, it may well be that male breadwinner arrangements against the preference of the wife are only chosen if the spouses feel that they can afford it or, in other words, if the wife cannot use an income argument to sustain her position. Interestingly, the compensatory logic is only found in case the wife refrains from labour market participation altogether. Apparently, the affordability/compensatory logic is no longer valid as soon as the wife works for pay, even if that is less than she prefers and indeed satisfies the preferences of her husband.

A second interpretation of the income rise relates to the specialisation logic of the male breadwinner model. Women may curtail their labour market aspirations to support the career of their husband. Empirically this only seems to work if women refrain from paid work altogether, but more analyses to create counterfactual scenarios and panel data on the career development of men and women are needed here. We leave a proper inquiry of this assumption for future research.

Summarising, we found it to be relatively rare that both spouses agree in their task division preference and are able to get what they want because this accounts for only 32% of the couples in our sample. Especially women have more trouble to realise their task division preferences. This has much to do with many women having less traditional preferences than men, combined with our gendered care culture which makes women more receptive to care demands in their household than men. Furthermore, the data do not sustain that relatively more wealthy spouses would be more likely to realise their task division preferences than the relative poor. Finally, we found only limited evidence of monetary compensation for households with an unbalanced preference outcome. Only in male breadwinner households where the homemaker role does not correspond to what the wife wants while it does comply with the husband's preference, our estimates support the idea of compensation across the two spheres of well-being. Whether this male breadwinner compensation is a remnant from the past (career support by the wife) or a compensation for what is becoming outdated behaviour is a matter for debate.

Annex

Table 8.15 OLS estimates of the equivalised monthly disposable household income, from husband's point of view

	Coef.	Std. err.		Coef.	Std. err.		Coef.	Std. err.	
Wife predicted wage	19.08	16.52		16.15	16.67		31.28	19.64	
Husband predicted wage	86.89	13.28	***	85.14	13.37	***	94.56	16.11	***
Wife's usual weekly working hours	12.39	1.43	***	11.44	1.57	***	9.34	1.97	***
Husband's usual weekly working hours	8.90	1.95	***	9.57	1.98	***	11.28	2.50	***
Husband does not realise task division preference, while wife does ('imbalance')	39.50	78.30							
Interaction preference by imbalance (reference = prefers 'split', no imbalance)									
Prefers 'semi-split, no imbalance'				63.00	63.60		17.97	73.48	
Prefers 'semi-split, imbalance'				167.45	176.30		171.38	215.17	
Prefers 'joint, no imbalance'				145.79	74.41	**	18.45	85.84	
Prefers 'joint, imbalance'				100.89	99.88		48.29	112.81	
Prefers 'reversed semi-split, no imbalance'				145.69	193.53		42.27	197.37	
Prefers 'reversed semi-split, imbalance'				–81.44	450.11		–26.37	438.95	
Contextual shocks[a]									
Health of spouses								Sign.	
Contentment with childcare arrangement								Sign.	
Child well-being indicators								Sign.	
Constant	–115.07	151.17		–147.00	154.41		–462.55	196.85	***
Adjusted R^2		16%			16%			17%	

[a]Indicators are added just as in section 'Further Empirical Exploration: Testing Predictions'. For lack of space, the point estimates are not shown
Sign. = at least one variable is statistically significant
Statistical significance **>95%; ***>99%

Table 8.16 Basic descriptive information on the explanatory variables used in multivariate analyses

	Mean	Se(mean)	Min	Max
Equivalised disposable monthly household income	1,679.46	24.50	135.14	12722.70
Wife's predicted hourly wage	9.62	0.05	6.39	16.46
Wife's usual weekly working hours	24.92	0.50	0.00	99.00
Husband's predicted hourly wage	10.52	0.07	6.74	20.14
Husband's usual weekly working hours	43.13	0.36	4.00	99.00
Wife's self-assessed health status (1 = not healthy)	0.10		0	1
Husband's self-assessed health status (1 = not healthy)	0.11		0	1
Presence of preschool child(ren) (1 = yes)	0.29		0	1
Joint presence of preschool and school-age children (1 = yes)	0.17		0	1
Wife is happy with afterschool care arrangement (1 = yes)	0.31		0	1
Wife is happy with preschool care arrangement (1 = yes)	0.11		0	1
Presence of child that seriously disturbs family life (1 = yes)	0.08		0	1
Presence of child with problems when compared with other children of his or her age (1 = yes)	0.11		0	1
Wife is more than 2 years older than husband	0.06		0	1
Husband is more than 2 years older than wife	0.49		0	1
Wage ratio (predicted wages) in intervals				
1. Wife earns more than 10% more	0.14		0	1
2. Wife and husband earn within [−10%,+10%] of each other	0.63		0	1
3. Husband earns more than 10% more	0.23		0	1

Selection: couple households with at least one child younger than 16 (FFCS 2004–2005)
N=1,055

References

Becker, G. S. (1991). *A treatise on the family* (enlarged edition, 424 p.). Cambridge/London: Harvard University Press.

Becker, G. S. (1996). *Accounting for tastes*. Cambridge/London: Harvard University Press. 268 p.

Chiappori, P. A. (1988). Rational household labor supply. *Econometrica, 56*(1), 63–90.

Chiappori, P. A. (1992). Collective labor supply and welfare. *Journal of Political Economy, 100*(3), 437–467.

Chiappori, P. A. (1997). Introducing household production in collective models of labor supply. *Journal of Political Economy, 105*(1), 191–209.

Friedberg, L., & Webb, A. (2006). Determinants and consequences of bargaining power in households (NBER Working Paper Series, No.12367). Cambridge: National Bureau of Economic Research.

Ghysels, J., & Cornelis, L. (2007). De economische waarde van zorgtijd. In J. Ghysels & M. Debacker (Eds.), *Zorgen voor kinderen in Vlaanderen: een dagelijkse evenwichtsoefening?* (pp. 237–278). Leuven: Acco. 283 p.

Ghysels, J., & Debacker, M. (Eds.). (2007). *Zorgen voor kinderen in Vlaanderen: een dagelijkse evenwichtsoefening?* Leuven: Acco. 283 p.

Kapteyn, A., & Kooreman, P. (1992). Household labor supply: What kind of data can tell us how many decision makers there are? *European Economic Review, 36*, 365–371.

Kooreman, P., & Kapteyn, A. (1990). On the empirical implementation of some game theoretic models of household labor supply. *Journal of Human Resources, 25*(4), 584–598.

Kooreman, P., & Wunderink, S. (1996). *The economics of household behaviour*. Houndmills: Macmillan. 236 p.

Vermeulen, F. (2000). Collective household models: principles and main results, *CES Discussion papers*, Leuven: CES/KULeuven, 34 p.

Chapter 9
Working Parents, Family and Gender in Spain from an European Comparative Perspective

Almudena Moreno Mínguez

Introduction

To date, empirical research into the reconciliation of work and family has chiefly been based on the comparison of work-family reconciliation policies as introduced by the various member states. Points of departure have been a series of indicators regarding parental leave, childcare services, economic benefits for families, working timetables, and so on, as well as the way these measures have contributed to fomenting gender equality in connection with the participation in the labour market of women with family responsibilities (Escobedo 2009; OECD 2006, 2011; Eurostat 2006; Moreno Mínguez 2007; Salido and Moreno 2009, etc.), but little attention has been paid to the way cultural or individual factors such as education or occupation shape the decisions and strategies concerning the organization of working and family life by the families in different welfare regimes.

The aim of this chapter is to offer a twofold analysis of the family policies (childcare services and parental leave) and family strategies to reconciling work and family, in the different European countries. On the one hand, I shall describe the extent to which the gender stereotypes rooted in a given cultural context and family policies condition the reconciliation strategies adopted by citizens in distinct institutional and cultural contexts. Then, in a second part of the study, we will use more complex statistical analysis to find out the extent to which individual factors such as professional status, education, and so on neutralise the impact of culturally assigned gender roles and consequently the expectations and strategies of work-family reconciliation.

A. Moreno Mínguez (✉)
Department of Sociology and Social Work, University of Valladolid,
Colmenares, s/n, 40001, Segovia, Spain
e-mail: almudena@soc.uva.es

A. Moreno Mínguez (ed.), *Family Well-Being: European Perspectives*,
Social Indicators Research Series 49, DOI 10.1007/978-94-007-4354-0_9,

This analysis should help us explain the extent to which, in tandem with family policies, economic factors, individual factors such as education and cultural factors, such as the 'familism',[1] typical of southern European countries, have an impact on the explanation of the different WFB arrangements adopted by Europeans in different welfare regimes. The aim of this chapter is to offer a comparative analysis of data regarding work-family balance (WFB) faced by families with children in the comparative framework of Europe's welfare regime. Accordingly, this chapter will set out some of the findings related to the comparative analysis of the data from different European surveys such as Eurobarometer and the European Labour Survey.

Theoretical Background

Definition of Work-Family Balance

Research into work-family balance (WFB) has made important contributions to the theoretical analysis of dilemmas associated with work-family reconciliation in relation to policies introduced in the various institutional frameworks. However, the measurement and quantification of WFB is rather problematic since the scales established for that purpose basically have to do with the conceptualisation of the work component in detriment of the family component, due to the difficulties of measuring the intangibles of work around the house or family responsibilities.

Many theoretical frameworks have been developed which, working from such data as the ESS survey, analyse the differences observed in work-family reconciliation strategies in the different contexts of the welfare state in Europe. One of the most complete frameworks for the explanation of these strategies is the theory of agency as defined by Hobson and Fahlén (2009), which has served to generate some indicators for the analysis of WFB in a multidimensional universe of determinants, capacities and possibilities for developing WFB-related strategies.

[1] The concept of familism has been widely used in scientific literature to explain a unique aspect of southern European societies, especially Spain and Italy (Saraceno 1995; Valiente 2010). It originated in Banfield's anthropological study of a region of southern Europe and defined familism as a form of intergenerational solidarity ('amoral familism') involving the pursuit of family interests at the expense of collective interests in the face of a precarious economic environment. Any analysis of the modern welfare state should include an assessment of the importance of norms and legitimated practices in the establishment and maintenance of welfare regimes. A moral ethos based on notions of family and family responsibility contributes significantly to the formation and legitimization of welfare regimes. Leitner (2003) identifies varieties of familism and uses a comparative perspective to describe the function of the family in child and elder care. She suggests the use of public policies as indicators of familism. In the cases of Spain and Italy, Moreno Mínguez (2007) and Naldini (2003) have referred to familism as an expression of protecting the family from risks in the social and economic environment. This is managed within the family mainly by women through solidarity between family members in response to a hostile institutional environment that threatens the safety of the family (Reher 1998).

The concept of WLB is fraught with problems. In fact, in the European Union definition of the regulatory contexts related to the adaptation of the different institutional frameworks with a view to fostering the participation of men and women in the family domain and the world of work, reference was initially made to the concept of 'reconciling work and family' (RWF) with greater emphasis on female participation in the labour market than on increased male participation in household chores (Hantrais 2000; Deven and Moss 2002; Ferrarini 2006).[2]

As a reflection of the growing criticisms regarding the incompatibility of long working hours with the time due to the family (more particularly, the time due to the family on the part of the parents) in the 1990s, a different discourse started to appear in EU documents which now spoke of work-life balance. This discourse is more inclusive than RWF in two ways: on the one hand, it refers to family and working life as an indicator of quality of life, which sets greater store by time devoted to the family; on the other, it is more gender neutral than RWF, which basically cast women in the role of main reconcilers. Symbolically, the term WLB valorises the time devoted to the family on the same level as time devoted to gainful employment. In short, WLB emphasises family interaction in connection with the time devoted by both working parents to the care of their minors and underlines the importance of work time and family time if the members of a couple are to achieve personal and professional well-being.

In this chapter, I have opted to use the concept of WFB because of its presence in the literature and in EU documentation. Nevertheless, despite the apparent terminological homogeneity in scientific and institutional documents, there is great conceptual diversity regarding the different domains and meanings of WFB, and this accounts for the lack of any analytical or empirical consensus in the processing of data (Pichler 2009: 450). In fact, as Hobson and Fahlén (2009) point out, apart from the empirical exercise of describing the costs in terms of money and/or time when choosing between work or family, there is no broad consensus on the question of how to gauge in terms of gender the balance between work and family and the consequences of that balance for the individuals involved.

Some studies carried out with that goal in mind emphasise the structural components of WFB and associate its meaning with such factors as working hours, work flexibility, demographic changes (ageing population, lower birth rate, leisure time, etc), the provision of welfare and social security; others focus on the personal circumstances of WFB, on family contexts (gender roles, care) and individual well-being. By personal circumstances of WFB are meant such factors as family situation, composition of the household and individual factors like education which may have an influence on strategies adopted in the WFB. This study, then, sets out to analyse how family contexts and individual circumstances in different cultural and institutional scenarios affect both the strategies adopted to achieve WFB and gender relations.

The empirical problem associated with this type of study has to do with the fact that the surveys conducted on the issue, such as ESS 2004, are basically concerned

---

[2] See EU Parental Rights Directive 96/34, EU Part-time Work Directive 97/81, and EU Time Directive 93/104.

with the work-related factors of WFB and how they condition family and individual life. In fact, according to most of the analyses that have come out of the data, working conditions are consider as a critical factor for variations in family life (Pichler 2009). These empirical studies emphasise the fact that work frequently has a negative impact on personal and family life and that this is consequently one of the reasons behind the problems of reconciliation. Nevertheless, the variables defined in two such major surveys as the ISSP and the ESS do not conceptualise sufficiently the ambit of 'family life', which is why, according to Pichler (2009: 465), these surveys fail to facilitate greater knowledge of the ambits of WLB.

Apart from the problems related to data, recent studies suggest that policies related to WLB may have a positive effect on birth rates (Hobson and Oláh 2006; McDonald 2000; Esping-Andersen 1999). In fact, the WFB was used as the theoretical framework for relevant research into household strategies (Wallace 2002) and female employment (Fagan 2004; Van der Lippe and Peters 2007) and for comparative analyses of welfare regime and social policies (Hobson 2006; Hobson and Oláh 2006; Pettit and Hook 2009; Guillén et al. 2009).

Work-Family Balance and Gender in Europe

In this connection, mention should be made of the extensive comparative literature about the 'welfare regime' which in recent years has tended to include different models of care, given that the conventional typology of welfare states established by Esping-Andersen (1990, 1999)[3] did not sufficiently take into account the gender inequality dimension in his attempts of classify welfare states. This classic typology, though providing important starting points for the development of theoretical model for an explanation of the differences in the institutional context of female employment, is limited in its scope to care, gender inequality and WFB.

In fact, the comparative analyses of welfare regime and of how policy regimes impact strategies adopted by householders illustrate the inconsistency and weakness of classic welfare regime typologies of Esping Andersen (Ejrnæs and Boje 2008; Lewis 2009). Numerous feminist researchers were warning as early as the 1990s that the paid work and unpaid family work should be included in comparative studies of welfare states (Arts and Gelissen 2002; Cousins 2000; Lewis 1997, 2001; Lewis et al. 2009; Orloff 1996; O'Connor 1996; Sainsbury 1994; 1999). That means creating and adding new dimensions to comparative analyses of the welfare state which would include the division of work in the family and care with a view to coming to empirical grips with the different models of WFB. For example, Walby (2004)

[3] Esping Andersen (1990, 1999) identified three distinct welfare regime (the liberal, social democratic, and corporativist) that differ in the patterns of state, market and household provision of welfare, the degree to which labour is decommodified (dependence on market and family), the degree of de-familisation (policies that lessen individuals' reliance on the family, maximizing individuals' command of economic resources independently of familial or conjugal reciprocities) and the impact of welfare state institutions on stratification.

uses the notion of 'gender regime' to refer to complex varieties of gender inequality. Our initial premise is that the WFB-related strategies adopted and choices made by members of a couple do not happen in a vacuum but in particular cultural, institutional and economic contexts. Couples make decisions in the light of the family, work and economic contexts they find themselves in. In this regard, an ample comparative typology is available of welfare state models which include these categories (family policies, division of work in the family, care types, etc.) (León 2006; Haas 2005; Wall 2007; Fux 2002; Bettio and Plantenga 2004; Ejrnæs and Boje 2008; Moreno Mínguez 2008).

The premise of these typologies is that WFB policies do not target women exclusively but members of a couple who form a family; in other words, the goal of a family policy should not only be to foment female participation in the labour market but also to enhance economic and personal well-being among the members of the family. Relevant research has shown that not only the attitudes of women impact the strategies adopted but also the attitudes and values of their companions. Indeed, it has been observed how male roles and attitudes to reconciliation and family models are important predictors of the division of work in the family (Geist 2005: 25; Fuwa 2004; Kangas and Rostgaard 2007; Cooke 2003, 2009).

We should not forget that social policies are embedded in cultural contexts which in many cases hamper or enhance the effectiveness of family policies. Numerous studies show the relationship between culture and social policy (Fux 2002; Bonoli et al. 2000; Rieger and Leibfried 2003; Van Oorschoot and Abrahanson 2003; Van Oorschoot 2007), which is tantamount to saying that cultural factors play a key role in both the implementation of social policies and the organization of citizens' lives. For example, it has been proven that differences across Europe in the degree to which children (generally daughters) look after their parents are not only a question of the regulation of the labour market and social policies but also of cultural differences in relation to the family (Dallinger 2001). It has also been shown how differences in the use of parental leave and, therefore, in WFB strategies are less a matter of the types of childcare policies and parental leave than of cultural attitudes towards the family and maternity, attitudes which are perceived to be stronger in Germany and the Netherlands than in the Nordic countries (Van Doorne-Huiskes et al. 1999). In other words, international comparative analyses have underlined the importance of the cultural variable when it comes to accounting for the effectiveness of social policy implementation and for differences between family policy models. This obliges us to include cultural factors with institutional ones in the framework for interpreting and analysing WFB variations. According to Pfau-Effinger et al. (2009: 27), the impact of welfare state policies can be modified by cultural values, other institutions, and social structures. In fact, in similar welfare state contexts, people may behave in different ways.

From the culturalist perspective, not only social policies but also social attitudes and norms (culture) have a significant effect on strategies adopted regarding work and family by gender. In this connection, Pfau-Effinger (2004, 2005) attempted to integrate cultural and institutional perspectives with a view to explaining the decisions women make about work and family named the approach of the arrangement of work and welfare.[4] However, despite the valuable contribution made by his analyses, she does not take sufficient stock of the contradictions observed between real praxis and the predominant culture. Haas (2005: 492) has tried to make good the inconsistencies of those analyses for countries like Austria by categorising countries in line with three dimensions—praxis, culture and policies introduced—and then comparing the results with those for other countries. Her hypothesis is that cultural norms and attitudes towards gender roles and family and labour policies explain WFB praxis in each country. According to Haas (2005), empirical studies have provided evidence of some inconsistency between the strategies and praxis of families embedded in particular cultural frames and political contexts. At times, the policies are not implemented adequately or go unheeded by the public because their attitudes and values differ from the political intentions and goals (Haas 2005: 489). However Haas's analysis does not give sufficient explanation for the differences observed in WFB praxis in a given institutional and cultural context since she does not take into account how individual factors like education or socioeconomic status affect the configuration of gender roles.

More recently, another argument has stressed the importance of preferences and lifestyles in the WFB arrangement. Hakim (2000)[5] has integrated in their analysis of WFB arrangements the personal practices and preferences as additional explanatory factors of the WFB strategies people adopt. According to Hakim (2000, 2003), differences in lifestyle tend to be related to differences in human capital invested and in other factors related to the individualisation process, such as the ratings given to independence and personal autonomy. Hakim (2000) considers that values and lifestyles determine stances towards work and the family rather than, together with WFB choices, reflecting or reacting to employment opportunities and personal investments in human capital.

Criticism of these analyses points out that Hakim's typification of stances and lifestyles with respect to WFB takes no account of the institutional context in which these decisions are taken and modified throughout people's lives (Crompton and Lyonette 2005; Crompton 2006). Moreover, such analyses are said not to bear in mind the way particular individual factors place people on an unequal footing with respect to lifestyle choice and preferences (Duncan 2006). Along similar lines, and in further illustration of the limitations of Hakim's theory of preferences, studies of

[4] The arrangement of work and welfares is defined by Pfau-Effinger et al. (2009) as the specific field of interrelations between cultural and institutional factors and social structures, with regard to the way work and welfare are organized in a society and how they are interrelated.

[5] Classification of women's work-lifestyle preferences in the twenty-first century according to Hakim (2000).

Home-centred: Family life and children are the main priorities. Prefer not to work. Number of children is affected by government social policy. Not responsive to employment policy

Adaptative: This group is most diverse and includes women who want to combine work and family, plus drifters and unplanned careers. Want to work but not totally committed to work career. This group is very responsive to government social policy and employment policy.

Work-centred: Childless women are concentrated in this group. Main priority in life is employment. Committed to work or equivalent activities. Responsive to economic opportunity. No responsive to social/family policies

the use made of parental leave by Swedish parents have come to the conclusion that parental choices may be understood in terms of 'adaptive preferences', which change in the course of a person's life and thus attest regulatory and cultural shortcomings, workplace demands and expectations, and economic and social pressures (Bygren and Duvander 2006; Hobson and Oláh 2006).

In sum, the cultural effects are mediated—perhaps to an extent neutralised—by individual factors such as education, income and so forth. This demonstrates that individual attitudes and capabilities, inscribed in a given cultural and institutional frame, may become agency and capacity to act in order to achieve well-being (Hobson and Fahlén 2009; Browne et al. 2004; Engster and Olofsdotter 2011). As for southern European countries, the institutional and regulatory framework partially accounts for the population's family-centred strategies for reconciling work and family, even if these strategies change when factors like education and income are considered (Rhodes 1997).

According to this theoretical framework, the present study considers that such factors as occupational status, hours of work and educational level may play an important role in individual practices and preferences concerning the gender relations which make up the different WFB models, while at the same time bearing in mind the institutional and cultural contexts in which those choices and practices regarding WFB are embedded.

Thus, the agency theory developed by Hobson and Fahlén (2009) and the approach of the arrangement of work and welfare developed by Pfau-Effinger (2005, 2009) set out a theoretical framework sufficient to explain dilemmas concerning WFB in southern European countries since it includes in the same analytical frame the impact of both institutional and cultural factors on people's capabilities and choices vis-à-vis the formulation of WFB strategies.

As for southern European countries like Spain, the history of the building and consolidation of the welfare regime—which conferred on the family a private entity as the main resolver of WFB dilemmas—have originated the configuration of gender relations based on contradictory (Meil 2006) attitudes and values in relation to WFB (Ajzenstadt and Gal 2010; Moreno Mínguez 2010). The upshot of this has been a model of privatised WFB based on the family, the scant outsourcing of family services, and the enthronement of the woman as the principle carer and person in charge of the family (Ferrera 1996). On the other hand, and as a consequence of the privatisation of family services and the limited amount of family policies designed to address the work-life balance, the effects of education and occupation may be particularly relevant for analysing the differences existing between Spanish groups in WFB strategies by gender.

Aims, Data and Methods

This chapter is an attempt to analyse how strategies of work-family reconciliation are rooted in cultural and institutional frames which, to a degree, determine individual choices and strategies—themselves mediated by such individual factors as education and income—concerning family and work. In this regard, it should be stressed that most studies have centred on the analysis of how family policies have enhanced gender equality by fostering the labour market participation of women with family responsibilities. The aim of this chapter is to analyse how WFB strategies and choices derive from individual and family contexts embedded in distinct cultural and institutional frames which originate a diversity of expectations, motivations and strategies in relation to work-family balance.

Previous empirical research conducted to date highlights the fact that family policies have different effects on female employment, the sharing of household chores, strategies of reconciliation and birth rate depending on the culture of the family and the regulatory framework of a given welfare state. As far as the southern European countries are concerned, the persistence of inequality across gender roles and the family-centredness of cultural praxis hampers the efficacy of work-family reconciliation polices since people opt for family-centred WLB strategies embedded in cultural and institutional frames which recoil at the outsourcing of family services and remain based on the figure of the male breadwinner.

Thus, the questions which underlie my study may be summarised as follows:

1. How have family policies been developed (childcare services and parental leave) to take account of the problems involved in combining work and family, and the role of the mother and father as carers?
2. How do regulatory and institutional structures (welfare regime, family policies, family culture) as well as individual factors such as education and occupation impact in the type of care and gender roles?
3. The aim of this chapter is to provide an answer to these questions by applying a comparative approach with the ultimate objective of contextualizing the Spanish case.

The first descriptive part of the analysis uses comparative aggregate data from secondary sources such as OECD family database, EU-SILC survey and Eurobarometer 247. The tables in this section present measures of family policies (childcare services, parental leave), attitudes and values to family models, care role of mother and difficulties of conciliation.

The data used in the regression analyses are based on the ad hoc module 5 on reconciliation between work and family sections of European Labour Survey conducted in 2005. The target group of the AHM 2005 consisted of all persons aged between

[6] The target group of the ahm 2005 consisted of all persons aged between 15 and 64 (16–64 for ES, UK and NO). Every respondent of this age group in the respective survey period (quarter or all quarters of the year) constituted the sample for the ahm2005 in most of the countries, with the exception of Germany, France, the Netherlands, Austria, Finland, Sweden and Norway. Germany used a 0.1% random sample of the relevant population, France restricted the sample to the last (sixth) wave of the survey in each quarter, The Netherlands restricted the sample to the first wave, Austria restricted the sample to telephone interviews and to persons who were asked for the first time in the LFS, Finland restricted the sample to the 5th wave, Sweden restricted the sample to persons from wave 2 and 7, and Norway limited the sample to persons aged 16–64 who are not the child of some other member of the household. All these countries provided special weights for the sub-samples. Participation in the ahm2005 was compulsory in Belgium, Spain, France, Ireland, Italy, Cyprus, Malta, Portugal and Slovakia. In all other countries the participation was voluntary.

15 and 64 (16–64 for ES, UK and NO).[6] The data were collected by participating countries, and it represents the residential population of the 27 European countries aged 15 and older (LFS 2005). Over 1,641,896 randomly selected citizens were interviewed. Interviews were predominantly carried out via panel reaching between 3,000 and 17,000 EU citizens depend on total population in each country.

Two analytical models were determined on the basis of the hypotheses related to gender roles. One model took as its dependent variable: 'woman cares for children/man cares for children'. The following independent variables were determined: age, number of children in household between 0 and 4 years old, number of children in household between 5 and 9 years old, father's education, mother's education, father's occupation, mother's occupation, working time of father, and working time of mother.

The lack of data for some of the countries covered by the ELS meant that only the variables for Germany, Spain, France, Greece, Italy, Luxemburg, the Netherlands, Portugal and United Kingdom could be analysed. Application of the formula of regression analyses gave the results shown in Table 9.1. The table shows a result for each country which corresponds to the order in which the predictive variables enter the analysis, based on the significance of the Wald statistic. Thus, the variable which is entered first is the one which best explains, within the dependent variable, the reference category 'woman looks after children' and so on successively. The boxes for each of the response categories show a value of the Exp (β), which enables us to know how the category varies with regard to the reference category and to quantify this variation. Only significant results are given (Sig. <0.05). In the last place, the values of $R2$ are given as well as the number of valid cases for each country.

The second model took as its dependent the type of WFB strategy adopted (see Table 9.2). Two measures on men and women are used as the dependent variables. The variables were elicited with the question 'main type of childcare used for own/spouse's children up to 14 while person is working':

- Childcare services (including paid childminders) and preschool
- Partner who is living in the household
- Relatives/neighbours/friends (unpaid)
- No childcare used

The independent variables chosen were age, number of children in household between 0 and 4 years old, number of children in household between 5 and 9 years old, father's education, mother's education, father's occupation, mother's occupation, working time of father, and working time of mother.

As in the previous case, numerous variables which were initially introduced were discarded in the process of execution, either because certain countries did not have sufficient cases or else because they are not significant or are unclear. A multinomial type of regression analyses was used in this study, as this is necessary when the dependent variable contains more than two categories. The interpretation of the results is similar to the binomial model, with the difference that instead of interpreting the probabilities as classificatory in one of the two groups of the dependent variable, in the multinomial model, a reference category must be established and the

Table 9.1 Likelihood of mother/father to look after children

	Austria	Belgium	Germany	Spain	France	Greece	Italy	Luxembourg	Netherlands	Portugal	United Kingdom
Age father				4							
Continuous variable				0.948							
Age mother	2	1									
Continuous variable	0.952	0.901									
Children 0–4 years old	4										
Two or more	11,007										
Children 5–9 years old										2	
One										0.381	
Children 10–14 years old									5		
One									0.431		
Highest level of education completed father							2				3
Upper secondary							0.629				
Third Level											3,120
Highest level of education completed mother				3							4
Upper secondary				0.488							1,175
Third Level				0.388							
Occupation (main job) father									4		
Skilled trades occupations									0.171		
Personal service occupations									0.102		
Elementary occupations									0.184		

Occupation (main job) mother									3		
Professional occupations									0.362		
Type of work father	1		1	2				2	2		1
Part-time	0.150		0.016	0.153				0.010	0.081		0.071
Type of work mother	3			1	1		1	1	1	1	2
Part-time	2,458			3,096	3,394		3,975	7,489	13,399	10,934	2,637
R2 de Nagelkerke	0.10	0.06	0.21	0.13	0.07		0.07	0.39	0.39	0.17	0.16
N	844	150	388	1.006	290	181	2.265	207	2.297	240	1.349

Source: Own elaboration from European Labour Survey, Ad Hoc Module 5, Reconciliation between work and family life, 2005
Note: Coefficients reported are hazard ratio significant at 10%, 5% and 1%. It has been included only the significant coefficients

Table 9.2 Likelihood of unpaid childcare (couple and grandparents) or paid childcare

	Austria		Belgium		Germany		Spain	
	Paid childcare	Family	Paid childcare	Family	Paid childcare	Family	Paid childcare	Family
Age father			5					
			0.958	0.941				
Age mother							4	
							1,021	0.956
Children 0–4 years old	3		1				2	
Zero		5,077	0.185				0.322	
Children 5–9 years old			3		4		9	
Zero			0.459				0.600	
One				1,957		3,381	0,629	
Children 10–14 years old	1				2		6	
Zero	2,967	2,730			4,285		1,756	2,901
One		2,212						1,957
Highest level of education completed father	6		2				1	
Lower secondly			0.405				0.638	
Upper secondly		1,837	0.507				0.728	0.703
Highest level of education completed mother	2		4		3		8	
Lower secondly	0.308		0.435		0.333		0.613	
Upper secondly	0.460		0.470	0.562	0.384		0.749	
Occupation (main job) father							5	
Managers and senior officials							1,731	
Professional occupations							2,475	
Sales and customer service occupation								
Process, plant and machine operative								
Occupation (main job) mother	5							
Managers and senior officials								
Professional occupations		3,083						
Associate professional and technical								
Administrative and secretarial								
Skilled trades occupations								
Personal service occupations	0.114							
Process, plant and machine operative								
Main labour status father								
Main labour status mother								
Type of work father					6		7	
Full time					6,054		3,966	2,477
Type of work mother	4		6		1		3	
Full time	1,972	1,484		1,650	3,887	2,654	1,898	2,438
*R*2 de Nagelkerke	0.104		0.228		0.169		0.206	
N	2,795		1,815		2,727		10,623	

Source: Own elaboration from European Labour Survey, Ad Hoc Module 5, Reconciliation
Note: Coefficients reported are hazard ratio significant at 10%, 5% and 1%. It has been included

Greece		Italy		Luxemburg		Netherlands		Portugal		United Kingdom	
Paid childcare	Family	Paid childcare	Family	Paid childcare	Family	Paid childcare	Family	Paid childcare	Family	Paid childcare	Family
		4				9		5		5	
			0.971				0.948		0.959		0.949
3						5				9	
1,046						1,043				1,033	
				1		8				2	
				0.398		0.606				0.411	
				3		3				7	
						2,386	2,346			1,612	1,653
					2,107					2,034	1,724
		3		6		2				6	
		1,606	1,973	3,673		10,563	2,809			2,645	
			1,609	2,454		2,331					
						6		4		4	
								0.474			
						0.574				0.704	
		7		3		1		3			
				0.336		0.308		0.390			
		0.731		0.489		0.411					
		0.658									
		0.597									
1		2		4		7		1		1	
						4,563		0.306	0.331	7,810	3,695
	1,853	1,880			2,951	3,277		0.431		9,899	3,655
	1,867	1,672								4,468	2,353
2,625	2,904	2,221	1,665		3,054	3,549				4,027	2,344
	1,996				2,248						
0.396		0.328						0.144	0.209		
			1,904								
		6		5						8	
		2,775	1,734	6,378	6,477					2,624	1,886
2		1		2		4		2		3	
3,725	2,857	1,494	2,598	3,380	1,810	2,551	3,003	5,236	5,913	3,464	2,301
0.132		0.091		0.271		0.232		0.216		0.283	
535		12,164		1,903		6,413		3,408		7,354	

between work and family life, 2005
only the significant coefficients

coefficients must be interpreted using this category. In this case, the reference category is 2: 'Couple living in the home' which is the category with the most cases.

Results and Discussion

Most of the comparative studies on welfare and childcare regimes have highlighted the important role of family policies as a classification criterion for dividing European countries into different typologies according to their welfare regimes. Depending on the classification criteria used, different models have been defined (Hantrais 2004) based on the scope and duration of parental leave, work times, childcare services, direct transfer to the family, etc. (Fux 2002, 2008; Bettio and Plantenga 2004, 2008; Wall 2007; Ejrnæs and Boje 2008; Haas 2005; European Foundation for the Improvement of Living and Working Conditions 2010), but very few studies have studied the gender bias implicit in the development of family policies. In this section, we present empirical evidence on the situation of family policies in the different welfare regimes from a gender perspective using some of the criteria discussed by the researchers mentioned above. We also describe how the practices for combining work and family life in Spain respond to familialist cultural strategies with an evident gender bias, which highlights the gender inequalities existing in the practices designed to resolve the work-life balance.

The data on investment in childcare services for preschool children show substantial differences between countries, as well as in the state financing of these services (see Graphic 9.1). The countries in northern Europe offer the greatest number of places and spend the most on childcare services, whereas the countries in southern Europe—including Spain—invest least in this type of services. In addition to this, in Spain, these services are privately run and thus involve a high cost for families, as shown in the table below. A certain lack of development is therefore evident with regard to state-run childcare services in countries in southern Europe. This is due to their historical background (dictatorial regime) in which traditionally these services were not provided by the state, as the family—and specifically women—were responsible for childcare. Studies on this issue have revealed that in Spain women carry out a highly disproportionate share of family work in comparison with other countries (González and Jurado 2009; Carbonero and Levin 2007; Cooke 2009) In fact, the model of the male breadwinner has for many years been a cornerstone of the Spanish welfare regime. However, recent years have seen a notable increase in women's presence in the workforce—and thus, a parallel rise in two-income families, although the provision of state-run childcare services has not kept pace. This gap can clearly be seen in the increased demand for these services and their high costs compared to other countries (Thénevon 2009).

Spain has made significant progress in legally recognising maternity, paternity and parental leave in recent years. Maternity leave now stands at 16 paid weeks, with the option of the father taking part of the leave. The European average is 14 weeks. The 2006 Equality Act between men and women extended paid paternity leave from 2 to 15 paid days. The provision for parental leave is 1 year, which can be extended

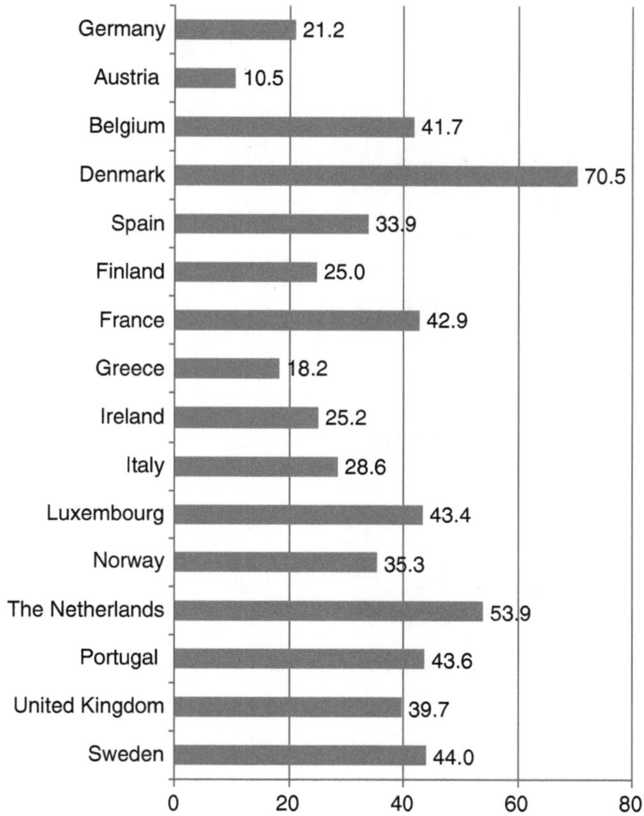

Graphic 9.1 Enrolment rates of children under age 3 in formal care or early education services, 2006 (Fuente: EU-SILC 2006)

to 2 years, with guaranteed reincorporation into the same job. The main problem with this leave is that it is unpaid, although the regional governments have put in place financial incentives to stimulate this type of leave by both fathers and mothers, with differing rates of success (Bonke and Esping-Andersen 2008; Lapuerta et al. 2009). The differences in parental leave between Spain and the rest of the European countries lie not so much in the right to leave as in the use made of this right by each sex (see Graphic 9.2). The persistence of traditional gender stereotypes may explain why it is generally women who take this kind of leave, with a very small percentage of men doing so in Spain.

The data presented below highlights the prominence in Spain of work-family reconciliation difficulties in comparison with other European countries, mainly for women (see Graphic 9.3); this in turn points to the shortcomings in the provision of services to families where both parents work. It can be deduced from the data that there is some connection between the limited development of childcare services and the reconciliation dilemmas voiced by those surveyed. Also noticeable is the high cost of such services in

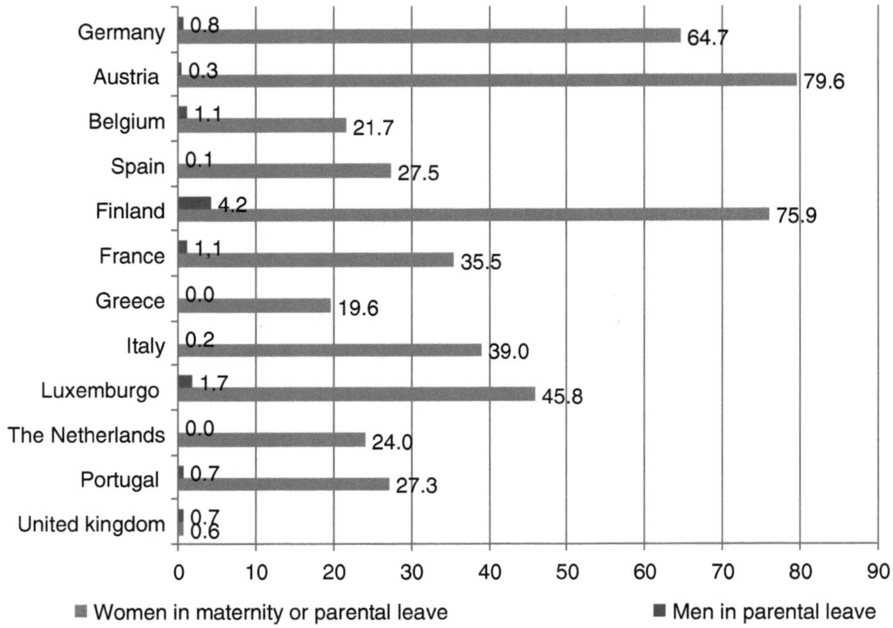

Graphic 9.2 Women in maternity or parental leave and men in parental leave (%) (Source: OECD Family Database 2011)

Spain (see Graphic 9.4). In contrast, this is a lesser source of problems in other countries where a generous, state-regulated childcare system is in place.

Yet a certain contradiction may be observed between the dilemmas voiced and the family gender roles chosen by Spaniards in order to reconcile work and family, for in comparative terms, the majority opt for a model whereby the woman takes charge of caring for the children while also stating that they experienced great difficulties when it came to reconciling family and work. It is here that the theory of gender roles becomes relevant, for these WFB strategies are inscribed in a particular cultural, family-centred context where the woman is regarded as the main carer regardless of the family policies introduced. This contradiction may also be observed in the table referring to the question of whether the female should look after the children: a very high percentage of women in Spain answered that they should look after the children as the best formula of organising childcare for preschool children (see Graphic 9.5).

These responses are rooted in a cultural context which valorises the figure of the male breadwinner and in an institutional context of stunted development of childcare services (León 2007). On the other hand, women choose to be mothers because they want to and have planned to throughout their lives, and, unlike their partners, they consider that their decision to be mothers is a fundamental piece in the construction of their personal identities and life plans. Accordingly, they assume

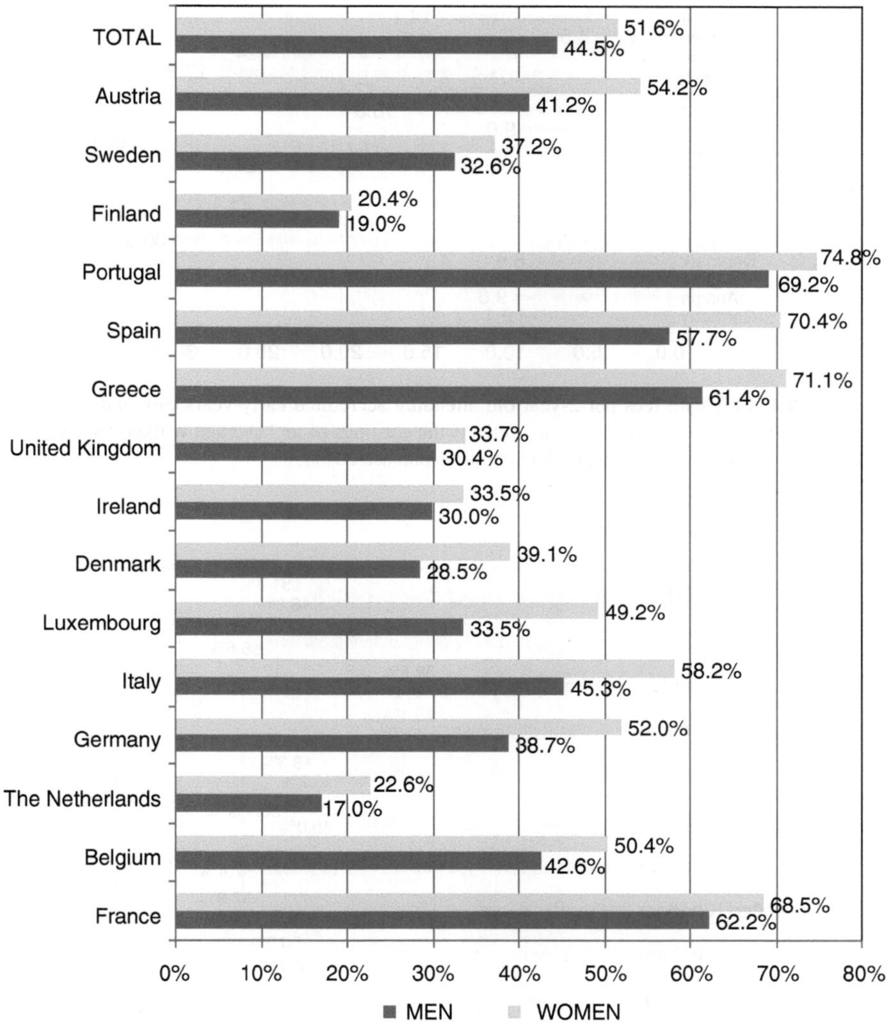

Graphic 9.3 Percent of respondents who answered "It is very difficult, fairly difficult, fairly to combine work and family life" by sex (Source: Own elaboration from Eurobarometer 2008)

that their duty is to be a 'good mother', taking charge of the care of their children. As a result, for these women, reconciliation is an unresolved contradiction embedded in a cultural context where household chores are shared unequally, where the woman believes it is her job to take care of her children, and yet where she also aspires to participate competitively in the labour market. As such, in countries like Spain and Italy it is a reconciliation dilemma with no easy solution which family policies have neither caught on to nor solved (Del Boca and Viuri 2007).

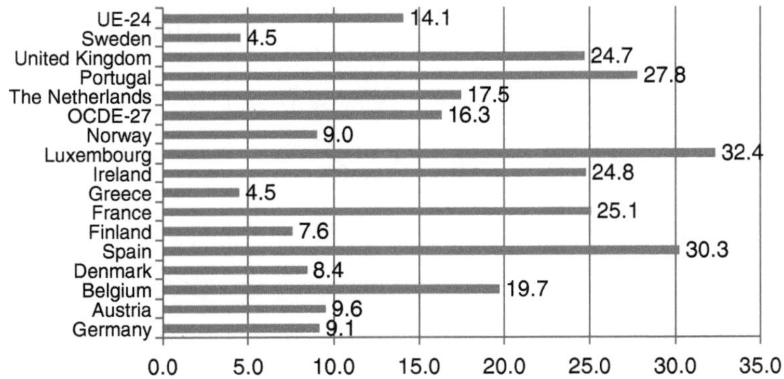

Graphic 9.4 Childcare fees per 2-year old attending accredited early-years care and education services, 2007. Note: The average wage reflects the earnings of an "average worker"; see OECD (2007): 186–7 for detail (Source: OECD Family Database 2011)

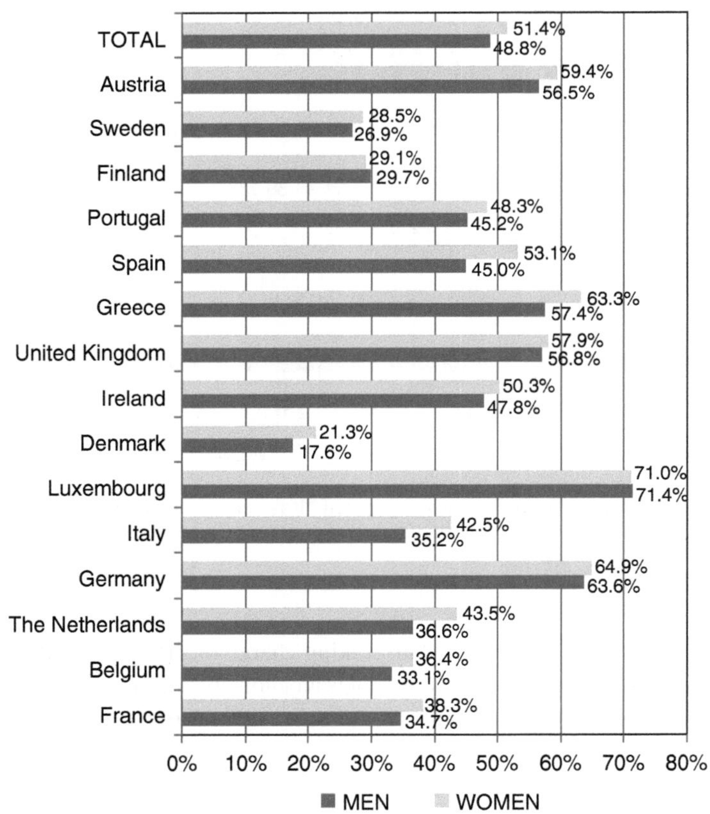

Graphic 9.5 Percent of respondents who answered "mother is the best way of organising childcare for pre-school children" by sex (Source: Own elaboration from Eurobarometer 2008)

If in earlier sections we were able to describe the cultural and institutional context of WFB arrangements in Spain in comparative perspective, we now aim to analyse the extent to which individual variables such as occupation and education influence the configuration of gender roles and the reconciliation strategies people adopt. To this end, logistical regression analyses have been performed on the basis of data from the European Labour Survey for 2005.

As may be seen in Table 9.1, the variable that best explains the probability that the mother/father cares for their children is the type of work (part- or full-time). If the woman works part-time, the likelihood that women will take care of children is greater than if you work full-time in all countries studied except Greece and Germany. As for men, if they work part-time, the probability that the woman who will take care of children is lower, particularly in Austria, Germany, Spain, the Netherlands and the United Kingdom. This outcome is especially important since it indicates that a policy that contributes to fomenting part-time work for fathers is a good means of fostering gender equality and joint responsibility for looking after children in as much as fathers are enabled to adapt and negotiate their working timetables equitably.

As for the impact of occupation on gender roles, what stands out is that this variable is only significant for the Netherlands where male employment in unskilled work reduces the chances that women take charge of caring for children. For all other countries, the fact that the woman was employed in skilled work reduced the chances that she looked after children under the age of 3 since the characteristics of her job allowed her to opt for contracting care services.

The age of children seems to be a decisive influence on gender roles given that in most countries, when the children are between the ages of 0 and 4, the chances are higher that it is the woman who looks after them.

It is important to notice how levels of education—whether the woman's or the man's—have barely any impact on the explanation of gender roles vis-à-vis caring for children. This may be due to the fact that gender roles level out increasingly as educational qualifications rise, with the male participating more in bringing up the children.

With a view to going deeper into the analysis of individual determinants related to the strategies adopted by working parents for the care of their children, another statistical model was created in order to apply a multinomial regression analysis.

As can be seen in the following Table 9.2, for all countries, the most significant variable for explaining the kind of strategy WFB used is the type of work of the mother (part- or full-time). When the mother works part-time, it is both members of the couple who mainly take charge of caring for their children. The kind of strategy adopted differs from country to country. In Austria, Belgium, Germany, Greece, Luxemburg and United Kingdom, women who work full-time opt mainly for paid services, while in Spain, Italy, the Netherlands and Portugal, they tend to entrust the care of their children to relatives and friends. As for southern European countries like Spain, Italy and Portugal, this phenomenon has been proven empirically to be the result of the cultural family-centredness characteristics of those countries, where grandparents play a key role as informal carers while the woman works (Moreno Mínguez 2008; Torres et al. 2007; Tobío 2005; Naldini 2006).

As far as the variable related to the mother's occupation is concerned, in general, when the woman works full-time, all occupation sectors follow the same pattern as before: either care services are paid for or the care of children is entrusted to relatives and friends according to the country in question. However, in the agricultural sector, when the woman works full-time, it is the couple which looks after the children, possibly because the seasonal nature of different areas of agricultural work enables caring for the children and the work to be done to be shared out according to the season or time or year.

As for the type of work of the father (part-time or full-time), the impact of this variable is smaller in comparison with the same variable in the case of the mother. In other words, in general terms, the fact that the man works full-time has no significant influences on the strategy adopted regarding the care of the children. Only a very reduced influence is to be found in Germany, Spain, Italy, Luxemburg and United Kingdom.

The variable relating to the education of the woman is of great importance in countries like Austria, Belgium, Germany, Spain, Italy and Luxemburg. The lower the level of the mother's education, the lower the probability that care services will be contracted in the market and the higher the probability that it will be the couple, more specifically the mother, who takes charge of looking after the children. This finds its explanation in the connection between educational level and kind of occupation (unskilled, skilled, etc). Women with low educational levels are employed in jobs for which few if any qualifications are required and which offer precarious salaries; consequently, when they become mothers, they opt to leave the labour market in order to take care of their children because it is not worth their while to continue working in the conditions mentioned and pay for childcare services. As earlier studies have shown (Moreno Mínguez 2008), in Spain, the education of women helps to neutralise the effects of cultural family-centredness in so far as the higher their level of education, the higher the degree of joint responsibility in taking care of the children and the higher the degree of permanence in their remunerated work. In contrast, no association is to be observed between educational level and type of care chosen.

As far as the father's education is concerned, as was the case with the type of work variable, this variable is much less important than the same one for the mother. The father's education only had some slight importance in countries like Austria, Belgium, the Netherlands, Portugal and United Kingdom. As for Spain, its importance was greater in comparative terms since the lower the educational level of the father, the higher the probability that it will be the woman who takes charge of caring for the children. This situation is of particular relevance in Spain since it confirms the thesis that the education of both partners is an indicator of gender equality in household work and bringing up the children.

As far as the variables related to number and age of children is concerned, it may be seen how in general terms, the more children there are between the ages of 0 and

4, the higher the probability that it will be couple, and more specifically the woman, who takes charge of caring for the children. In fact, as can be seen in the table, the number of children has some kind of influence on the child-rearing strategy selected when both parents work, except in Greece and Portugal. The age of the parents does not seem to be a significant variable when it comes to accounting for the probability of choosing a childcare option.

Conclusions

The aim of the study presented in this chapter was to analyse how far institutional and cultural factors linked to a particular family model, as well as individual factors such as education, work situation and occupation, affect a couple's decisions and actions with regard to the WFB depending on the cultural context of each country, with particular emphasis on the Spanish case.

The empirical analyses presented in this chapter highlight the complexity of the phenomenon of WFB arrangements in Spain. This work has used a comparative approach with the final objective of correctly contextualising the situation of the Spanish case. According to this approach, the differences with regard to WFB arrangements among the countries in the study can be explained by the dominant family model of gender roles and the degree to which the welfare state supports this model. In addition, the empirical analyses have also revealed the plurality of situations relating to the work-family balance within a specific cultural context, based on personal factors such as education, work situation and the occupation of both partners. According to our approach, the differences in relation to WFB arrangement among the countries in the study can be explained to the dominant family model of gender roles and the degree to which the welfare state support this model. In addition, the empirical analyses have also revealed the plurality of situations relating to the work-family balance within a specific cultural context, based on personal factors such as education, work situation and the occupation of both partners.

This chapter makes it clear how different cultural, institutional and individual contexts impinge on gender relations and work care, which explains why advances in equality and family policies have no substantive effect on work-family reconciliation strategies at the collective level. This study assumes that work-family reconciliation strategies are embedded in different institutional and cultural context. Thus, people's capabilities and agency relating to work-family balance strategies are a reflection of both the institutional resources available and the individual resources embedded in given cultural frames.

In the case of Spain, the limited public childcare services introduced by the Spanish Administration and high cost of private childcare service have been a key factor together with the culturally rooted family-centredness. This partly explains why Spaniards opt mostly for reconciliation formulae in which women play leading roles in caring for the children. Nevertheless, this study has made it plain that individual factors such as the woman's educational level and the formula adopted regarding working hours contribute to neutralizing the effects of family-centredness by fomenting the joint responsibility of both partners in taking care of the children and the outsourcing of childcare services. In the Spanish case, unlike other countries and as a result of the limited policies designed to address the work-life balance, the women's educational level, the work situation and occupation of both members of the couple go some way towards explaining the differences in WFB arrangements and the role played by women. For example, the results obtained show that in the Spanish case, the higher the educational level of both partners, the greater the externalisation of care services and the less likely the presence of the woman as a carer. The type of work carried out and the formula adopted (either part- or full-time) have also proved to be predictive variables with regard to WFB in Spain.

In any case, the advances which have taken place in family policy in Spain in recent years and the slow but progressive decline in the model of the male breadwinner as a consequence of the incorporation of women into the labour market may be changing the gendered WFB arrangement in Spain. In summary, this research work points out the need for further research from a plural theoretical and methodological approach in order to understand and contextualise comparatively the unequal gender relationships existing in strategies designed to address the work-life balance in Spain, in the context of the decline of the male breadwinner within the family.

References

Ajzenstadt, M., & Gal, J. (Eds.). (2010). *Children, gender and families in Mediterranean welfare states*. London: Springer.

Arts, W., & Gelissen, J. (2002). Three worlds of welfare capitalism or more? A state-of-the-art report. *Journal of European Social Policy, 12*(2), 137–158.

Bettio, F., & Plantenga, J. (2004). Comparing care regimes in Europe. *Feminist Economies, 10*(1), 85–113.

Bettio, F., & Plantenga, J. (2008). Care regimes and the European employment rate. In L. Costabile (Ed.), *Institutions for social well being. Alternative for Europe*. London: Palgrave Macmillan.

Bonke, J., & Esping-Andersen, G. (2008). *Productivities, preferences and parental child care* (Demosoc Working Paper, 29). Universitat Pompeu Fabra.

Bonoli, G., George, V., & Taylor-Gooby, P. (2000). *European welfare futures: Towards a theory of retrenchment*. Cambridge: Polity Press.

Bygren, M., & Duvander, A. (2006). Parents' workplace situations and fathers' parental leave. *Journal of Marriage and the Family, 68*(2), 363–372.

Carbonero, M., & Levín, S. (coord.). (2007). *Trabajo, familia y Estado: las transformaciones en las relaciones de género*. Rosario: Editorial Homo-Sapiens.

Cooke, L. P. (2003). *The south revisited: The division of labor and family outcomes in Italy and Spain* (IRISS Working Paper Series, 2003–12). Luxemburgo.

Cooke, L. P. (2009). Gender equity and fertility in Italy and Spain. *Journal of Social Policy, 38*(1), 123–140.

Cousins, C. (2000). Women and employment in southern Europe: The implications of recent policy and labour market directions. *South European Society and Politics, 5*(1), 97–122.

Crompton, R. (2006). *Employment and the family. The reconfiguration of the work and family life in contemporary societies*. Cambridge: University Press.

Crompton, R., & Lyonette, C. (2005). The new gender essentialism -domestic and family "choices" and their relation to attitudes. *The British Journal of Sociology, 26*(4), 601–620.
Dallinger, U. (2001). Organisierte Solidarität und Wohlfahrtskultur. Das Beispiel des 'Generationenvertrages' [Organised solidarity and welfare state culture: The example of 'generational contracts']. *Sociologica Internationalis, 39*, 67–89.
Del Boca, D., & Vuri, D. (2007). The mismatch between labor supply and child care. *Journal of Population Economics, 20*(4), 805–832.
Deven, F., & Moss, P. (2002). Leave arrangements for parents: Overview and future outlook. *Community, Work and Family, 5*, 237–256.
Duncan, S. (2006). Mothers'work-life balance: Individualized preferences or cultural construction? In D. Perrons (Ed.), *Gender divisions and working time in the new economy*. Cheltenham: Edward Elgar.
Ejrnæs, A., & Boje, T. (2008). *Family policy and welfare regimes*. Paper presented at Cinefogo conference: Gendering Theories of Citizenship: Europeanization and Care, Roskilde University.
Engster, D., & Olofsdotter, H. (2011). Do family policy regimes matter for children's well-being? *Social Politics: International Studies in Gender, State and Society, 18*(1), 82–124.
Escobedo, A. (2009). Spain. In P. Moss & B. Fusulier (Eds.), *International review of leave policies and related research 2009* (Employment relations research series, pp. 311–325). Department for Business, Enterprise & Regulatory Reform, UK. http://www.berr.gov.uk/files/file52778.pdf
Esping-Andersen, G. (1990). *The three worlds of welfare capitalism*. Cambridge: Polity Press.
Esping-Andersen, G. (1999). *Social foundations of postindustrial economies*. Oxford: Oxford University Press.
Esping-Andersen, G. (2009). *The incomplete revolution*. Cambridge: Polity Press.
European Foundation for the Improvement of Living and Working Conditions. (2010). *Second European quality of life survey family life and work*. Dublin: Eurofound.
Eurobarometer. (2008). *Family life and the needs of an ageing population*, Flash Eurobarometer n. 247, European Commission.
Eurostat. (2006). *How is the time of women and men distributed in Europe?* (Statistics in Focus, 4/2006).
EU-SILC. (2006). *Survey on income and living condition (EU-SILC)*. Luxembourg: Eurostat.
Fagan, C. (2004). Gender and working-time in industrialized countries: Practices and preferences. In J. Messenger (Ed.), *Finding the balance: Working-time and workers' needs and preferences in industrialized countries* (pp. 108–146). London: Routledge/the Institute for Labour Studies of the International Labour Organisation.
Ferrarini, T. (2006). *Families, states and labour markets. Institutions, causes and consequences of family policies in post-war welfare states*. Cheltenham: Edward Elgar.
Ferrera, M. (1996). The 'southern model' of welfare in social Europe. *Journal of European Social Policy, 6*, 17–37.
Fuwa, M. (2004). Macro-level gender inequality and the division of household labor in 22 countries. *American Sociological Review, 69*(6), 751–767.
Fux, B. (2002). Which models of the family are encouraged or discouraged by different family policies? In F.-X. Kaufmann, A. Kuijsten, H.-J. Schulze, & Strohmeier (Eds.), *Family life and family policies in Europe: Problems and issues in comparative perspective*. Oxford: Oxford University Press.
Fux, B. (2008). Pathways of welfare and population-related policies. Towards a multidimensional typology of welfare state regimes in Eastern and Western Europe. In C. Höhn, D. Avramov, & I. Kotowska (Eds.), *People, population change and policies: Lessons from the population policy acceptance study* (Vol. 1, pp. 59–90). Berlin: Springer.

Guillén, A., Moreno, N., & González, S. (2009). Conciliación de la vida laboral y familiar en España. El impacto de las políticas de la Unión Europea. *Documentación Social, 154*, 119–138.
Haas, B. (2005). The work care balance: Is it possible to identify typologies for cross national comparisons? *Current Sociology, 53*, 487–508.
Hakim, C. (2000). *Work-lifestyle choices in the 21st century: Preference theory*. Oxford: Oxford University Press.
Hakim, C. (2003). Public morality versus personal choice: The failure of social attitude surveys. *British Journal of Sociology, 54*, 339–345.
Hantrais, L. (Ed.). (2000). *Gendered policies in Europe: Reconciling employment and family life*. London/New York: Macmillan/St. Martin's Press.
Hantrais, L. (2004). *Family policy matters. Responding to family change in Europe*. Bristol: The Policy Press.
Hobson, B., & Fahlén, S. (2009). Competing scenarios for European fathers: Applying Sen's capabilities and agency framework to work—Family balance. *The ANNALS of the American Academy of Political and Social Science, 624*, 214–233.
Hobson, B., & Oláh, L. (2006). Birthstrikes? Agency and capabilities in the reconciliation of employment and family. *Marriage & Family Review, 39*, 197–227.
Kangas, O., & Rostgaard, T. (2007). Preferences or context: Opinions of child care. *Journal of European Social Policy, 17*(3).
Lapuerta, I., González, M. J., & Baizán, P. (2009). Individual and institutional constraints: An análisis of parental leave use and duration in Spain. *Population Research and Policy Review, 30*(2), 185–210.
Leitner, S. (2003). Varieties of familism, the caring function of the family in comparative perspective. *European Societies, 5*(4), 353–375.
León, M. (2006). Welfare state regimes and the social organization of labour: Childcare arrangements and the work/family balance dilemma. *The Sociological Review, 53*(2), 204–218.
León, M. (2007). Speeding up or holding back?: Institutional factors in the development of childcare provision in Spain. *European Societies, 9*(3), 315–337.
Lewis, J. (1997). Gender and welfare regimes: Further thoughts. *Social Politics, 4*(2), 160–177.
Lewis, J. (2001). The decline of the male breadwinner model: Implications for work and care. *Social Politics, 8*(2), 152–169.
Lewis, J. (2009). *Work-family balance, gender and policy*. Cheltenham: Edward Elgar.
Lewis, J., Knijn, T., Martin, C., & Osner, O. (2009). Patterns of development in work/family reconciliation policies for parents in France, Germany, the Netherlands and the UK in the 2000s. *Social Politics, 15*(3), 261–286.
McDonald, P. (2000). Gender equity, social institutions and the future of fertility. *Journal of Population Research, 17*, 1–16.
Meil, G. (2006). Welfare policies, work and family lives in modern Spain. In G. Rossi (Ed.), *Reconciling family and work, new challenges for social policies in Europe* (pp. 37–58). Milano: Franco Angeli.
Moreno Mínguez, A. (2007). *Familia y empleo de la mujer en los Estados del bienestar del sur de Europa. Incidencia de las políticas familiares y laborales* (Centro de Investigaciones Sociológicas, Colección Monografías No 246). Madrid: CIS.
Moreno Mínguez, A. (2008). El reducido empleo femenino en los Estados del bienestar del sur de Europa. Un análisis comparado. *Revista Internacional de Sociología, 50*, 129–162.
Moreno Minguez, A. (2010). Family and gender roles in Spain from a comparative perspective. *European Societies, 12*(1), 85–112.
Naldini, M. (2003). *The family in the Mediterranean welfare states*. Londres/Portland: Frank Cass.
O'Connor, J. S. (1996). From women in the welfare state to gendering welfare regimes. *Current Sociology, 44*(2), 101–118.

OECD. (2006). *Extending opportunities: How active social policy can benefit us all?* Paris: OECD.

OECD. (2011). *OECD Family Database*. Paris: OECD.

Orloff, A. S. (1996). Gender in the welfare state. *Annual Review of Sociology, 22*, 58–78.

Pettit, B., & Hook, J. (2009). *Gendered tradeoffs: Family, social policy and economic inequality in twenty-one countries*. New York: Russell Sage.

Pfau-Effinger, B. (2004). *Development of culture, welfare states and women's employment in Europe*. Aldershot: Ashgate.

Pfau-Effinger, B. (2005). Culture and welfare state policies: Reflections on a complex interaction. *Social Policy, 34*(1), 1–18.

Pfau-Effinger, B., Flaquer, L., & Jensen, P. (Eds.). (2009). *Formal and informal work. The hidden work regime in Europe*. London: Routledge Advances in Sociology.

Pichler, F. (2009). Determinants of work-life balance: Shortcomings in the contemporary measurement of WLB in large-scale surveys. *Social Indicators Research, 92*, 449–469.

Reher, S. (1998). Family ties in Western Europe: Persistent contrasts. *Population and Development Review, 24*(2), 203–234.

Rhodes, M. (1997). *Southern European welfare states: Between crisis and reform*. London: Frank Cass and Co. Ltd.

Rieger, E., & Leibfried, S. (2003). *Limits to globalization*. Cambridge: Polity Press.

Sainsbury, D. (Ed.). (1999). *Gender and welfare state regimes*. Oxford: Oxford University Press.

Salido, O., & Moreno, L. (2009). Familia y género. In L. Moreno (Ed.), *Reformas de las Políticas del Bienestar en España* (pp. 281–308). Madrid: Siglo XXI de España.

Saraceno, Ch. (1995). Familismo ambivalente y clientelismo categórico en el Estado del Bienestar italiano, en Sarasa, Sebastià y. In Luis Moreno (Ed.), *El Estado del Bienestar en la Europa del Sur* (pp. 261–288). Madrid: CSIC.

Tobío, C. (2005). *Madres que trabajan. Dilemas y estrategias*. Madrid: Ediciones Cátedra.

Torres, A., Mendes, R., & Tiago, L. (2007). Families in Europe. *Portuguese Journal of Social Science, 7*(1), 49–84.

Valiente, C. (2010). The erosion o "familism" in the Spanish welfare state: Childcare police since 1975. In M. Ajzenstadt & J. Gal (Eds.), *Children, gender and families in Mediterranean welfare states*. London: Springer.

Van Der Lippe, T., & Peters, P. (Eds.). (2007). *Competing claims in work and family life*. Cheltenham/London: Edward Alger.

Van Doorne-Huiskes, A., den Dulk, L., & Schippers, J. (Eds.). (1999). *Work-family arrangements in Europe. The role of employers*. Amsterdam: Thesis Publishers.

Van Oorschoot, W. (2007). Culture and social policy: A developing field of study. *International Journal of Social Welfare, 16*, 129–139.

Van Oorschoot, W., & Abrahanson, P. (2003). The Dutch and Danish miracles revisited: A critical discussion of activation policies in two small welfare states. *Social Policy & Administration, 37*(3), 288–304.

Walby, S. (2004). The European Union and gender equality. Emergent varieties of gender regime. *Social Politics, 11*(1), 4–29.

Wall, K. (2007). *Main patterns in attitudes to the articulation between work and family life: A cross-national analysis, in families, states and labour markets. Institutions, causes and consequences of family policies in post-war welfare states*. Cheltenham: Edward Elgar.

Wallace, C. (2002). Household strategies: Their conceptual relevance and analytical scope in social research. *Sociology, 36*, 275–292.

Chapter 10
Measuring the Past: Gender, Health and Welfare in Europe Since c. 1800

Bernard Harris

Introduction: Gender and Inequality

During the last two decades, historians and social scientists have become increasingly interested in the relationship between economic and social disadvantage, gender and health. In the case of the United Kingdom and other European countries, it has been claimed that the disadvantages experienced by women, both as children and as adults, meant that they were shorter and lighter than they might otherwise have been and that they were more likely to die prematurely. This chapter attempts to review some of the evidence in relation to a range of European countries in order to examine the extent to which differences in the circumstances of male and female lives during the nineteenth and twentieth centuries were reflected in health statistics.

It has often been argued that, in many parts of the developing world, female children suffer systematic discrimination in the allocation of either food or health care and that this is reflected in excessively high death rates (see e.g. Sen 1989). As a result, a number of historians, such as Stephen Nicholas and Deborah Oxley, have suggested that similar factors may have been at work in other countries during comparable stages in their economic development (see e.g. Nicholas and Oxley 1993). However, although there is a great deal of evidence to show that adult women were disadvantaged in the European past, it is much more difficult to find direct evidence of discrimination against female children. Several contemporary accounts show that wives and mothers often deprived themselves in order to support their families, but there is much less evidence to show that they made a conscious attempt to favour sons over daughters.

B. Harris (✉)
Division of Sociology and Social Policy, School of Social Sciences,
University of Southampton, Highfield, Southampton, SO17 1BJ, UK
e-mail: B.J.Harris@soton.ac.uk

A. Moreno Mínguez (ed.), *Family Well-Being: European Perspectives*,
Social Indicators Research Series 49, DOI 10.1007/978-94-007-4354-0_10,

Insofar as there is evidence of systematic discrimination, it tends to date from much earlier periods. Josiah Cox Russell (1948: 147–54) attributed shortfalls in the ratio of females to males in medieval Britain to selective infanticide, and Barbara Hanawalt (1993: 58–9) found evidence of 'a qualitative difference in the care and nurturing of male and female children' in medieval London. Shulamith Shahar (1990: 81–2) argued that girls were more likely to be sent to wet nurses than boys and that the care they received was inferior, but most children were nursed by their mothers, and there was no evidence to suggest that girls and boys received different treatment when they remained within the parental home.

The question of differential treatment has also been investigated by historians of the early modern period. Richard Wall (1981: 135–6) found evidence of excess mortality among later-born female infants in two English parishes between 1550 and 1800, but Keith Wrightson (1975) failed to identify any similar patterns when he examined evidence from the Essex Assizes between 1601 and 1665. Alan Macfarlane (1986: 54) concluded that there were 'few indications … in the middling ranks [that] the absence of sons was the disaster it is held to be in many Third World countries today', and Amy Erickson (1986) found no significant differences in the amounts of money allowed by the executors of modest estates for the care of boys and girls in the late sixteenth and early seventeenth centuries.

Other historians have looked for evidence of inequalities in the treatment of boys and girls in more recent periods. In early-twentieth-century Spain, one contemporary claimed that 'in general, the father and males of a family eat much better than the wife and daughters' (Vilar Ferrán 1917: 54–66; quoted in Borderías et al. 2010: 185), and Robert Kennedy (1972; cited in Johansson 1977: 175) claimed that girls growing up in rural Ireland received less food than their brothers because they had poorer employment prospects. In Britain, the working-class autobiographer, Robert Roberts (1971: 109), recalled that 'in the apportioning of food, small girls often came off very badly indeed; mothers felt that they didn't need much – "not the same as lads"'. However, such direct evidence of 'male-favouring' behaviour is comparatively rare.[1] As Rachel Fuchs (2005: 49) has argued, 'there is little evidence that women sought to limit their family size by selective neglect, favouring the survival of male children. Parents were not indifferent to their children, but saw them in both economic and emotional terms'.

Jane Humphries (2010: 180–3) has recently claimed that there was a small but significant decline in the average age at which children entered the workforce in Britain during the late eighteenth and early nineteenth centuries. If this decline affected boys more than girls, it may have increased the bargaining power which boys exercised within the family (*ibid.*: 243–4). However, even if this was the case, working conditions were extremely arduous and these boys may have paid a high price for any advantages they incurred. It is also important to remember that the

[1] There is some evidence which suggests that fathers were more likely to sacrifice some of their resources with their sons, but mothers were more likely to share their resources with their daughters (see Klasen 1998: 455–6).

incidence of child labour declined during the second half of the nineteenth century, and this was true of both sexes (Harris 1998: 416).

Although there is little evidence of discrimination against younger girls, it is possible that the health of girls may have been placed under greater stress during their teenage years. In Britain and many other European countries, the most common form of employment for teenage girls was domestic service, and contemporary accounts leave little room for doubt as to arduous nature of the conditions under which they worked (Harris 1998: 419, 2008: 175–6, Fuchs 2005: 118–22).

In recent years, historians have devoted particular attention to the employment of women in agriculture. In Britain, it seems likely that female participation in agriculture declined during the course of the nineteenth century, but in other parts of Europe, men and women continued to work alongside each for much of the period (Harris 2008: 172–5; Fuchs 2005: 86–95). However, even when men and women were both employed, the division of labour was often highly gendered, and even when the two sexes were engaged in the same work, women's pay was often lower. The gap between men's and women's earning capacity was probably exacerbated by industrialisation and the rise of the 'male breadwinner family'. Although the majority of women were engaged in paid employment before marriage and continued to make a significant contribution to the economic well-being of the family after marriage, their bargaining position within the household remained relatively weak (Oren 1974: 221; Fuchs 2005: 110–6).

Although the disadvantages which women faced in the labour market may not have had a direct impact on the relative welfare of boys and girls during childhood, there seems little doubt that they did have an effect on the welfare of women in adulthood. According to Cristina Borderías et al. (2010: 185), 'the practice of women serving men and eating only after men' was widespread in the Spanish countryside during the nineteenth and early twentieth centuries, and British observers often reported that women ate less than men in order to preserve the strength and earning capacity of the principal breadwinner (see e.g. Harris 1998: 418). In Hamburg, the Union of Construction Workers reported that 'in working-class families … [t]he man, the one who after all has to work, consumes the largest share of the available food. The children too have as much as possible. In most cases the mother … has to be satisfied with one or two mouthfuls if there is not enough to go around, and lives on bread, coffee and potatoes. A working man's wife … is happy if nobody shouts for more, even [if] she is still hungry herself' (quoted in Fuchs 2005: 117).

During the second half of the nineteenth century, some contemporaries sought to justify the allocation of less food to women on physiological grounds. One French writer argued that women 'need to eat less and different food [to] men' because of 'the size of their stomach and liver', and a Spanish writer deduced that women needed less food *because* they 'lack the ability to perform … work demanding high energy levels' (Borderías et al. 2010: 186–7). Modern nutritionists would also argue that women require less food than men, on average, because their bodies are smaller (Floud et al. 2011: 46). However, a great deal of the work which women performed both inside and outside the home was physically very demanding, as several contemporary accounts attest (see e.g. Harris 1998: 418–9, 2008: 177–8; Fuchs 2005: 116–35).

Many writers have also drawn attention to the physical demands of pregnancy and motherhood. During the 1890s, according to Richard Titmuss (1987: 89), the average working-class woman in Britain might expect to spend 15 years of her life either pregnant or nursing a child under the age of 1 year, but there is little evidence to suggest that this was reflected in increased nutritional allocations. In 1905, a Spanish observer noted that ‘a woman’s deficient condition during the period of her pregnancy due to hard agricultural work and bad and insufficient food leads to difficult deliveries, in which generally the innocent being pays with her life, as does sometimes the poor mother’ (López-Palacios 1905; quoted in Borderías et al. 2010: 184). As Rachel Fuchs (2005: 45, 157) has argued, ‘the worn-out bodies and poor nutrition of pregnant poor mothers contributed to premature births and infant deaths’, but they may also have impaired the mother’s own health as well.

Whilst many observers recognised the extent of women’s health problems, particularly around the time of pregnancy, these may have been compounded by a lack of access to health care. As James Riley (1997) and others have pointed out, the number of workers who belonged to friendly societies and other mutual-aid organisations increased quite sharply during the course of the nineteenth century. These associations were designed to provide compensation for loss of earnings due to ill health, together with a range of other benefits including pensions and death benefits, but many societies also provided access to a limited range of health services (see Harris and Bridgen 2007: 3–4). However, the vast majority of members were male, and rights to medical provision were not normally extended to their dependants. Moreover, many friendly societies specifically excluded women from their health assurance schemes because of concerns about the extent of their health needs (see e.g. Harris et al. 2012).

Although historians of gender have tended to concentrate on the extent to which the economic and social disadvantages of women may have been reflected in their health statistics, it is also important to consider the extent to which sex-specific differences may have influenced male statistics. One of the ways in which we might try to assess the impact of women’s disadvantages on their health is by comparing the relationship between female health and male health in the past with the relationship between female health and male health today, but just as some factors may have had a particularly adverse effect on the health of past generations of women, others may have contributed to a relative deterioration in the health of men. In the twentieth century, three factors may have been particularly important: first, the disproportionate exposure of young men to deaths from accidents and violence; second, the extent of male participation in war; and, third, the greater exposure of men to death from cancer and coronary heart disease as a result of differences in the incidence and intensity of smoking behaviour (Harris 1998: 422, 2008: 195–6).

The Contribution of Anthropometry

Since the late 1970s, an increasing number of historians have used information about the height, and to a lesser extent weight, of past generations to measure changes in human well-being. As the majority of the records on which this research has been based are derived from the attestation papers of military recruits, the main focus has inevitably been on men, but we also possess a limited amount of information about female heights, and some writers have used this information to draw conclusions about differences between the two sexes.

Although the main causes of variation in individual height may be genetic, it has long been recognised that variations in the heights of different groups of people owe much more to economic and social circumstances. As Louis-René Villermé observed in 1829, 'human height becomes greater and growth takes place more rapidly, other things being equal, as the country is richer; comfort more general; houses, clothes and nourishment better; and labour, fatigue and privation during infancy less' (quoted in Tanner 1981: 162). The auxologists, Phyllis Eveleth and James Tanner (1990: 1), summarised modern thinking in the following terms:

> A child's growth rate reflects, better than any other single index, his [or her] state of nutrition and often, indeed, his [or her] psychological situation also. Similarly, the average value of children's heights and weights reflects accurately the state of a nation's public health and the average nutritional status of its citizens, when appropriate allowance is made for differences, if any, in genetic potential. This is especially so in developing or disintegrating countries.... Indeed, as infant mortality goes down in a country's development, so the importance of monitoring growth rate increases.

As we have already seen, the majority of anthropometric records relate to the heights (and sometimes weights) of male military recruits, but we also possess some data on the heights of other groups which can be used to examine gender differences. So far as the eighteenth and nineteenth centuries are concerned, the majority of these data relate to particular subgroups, such as the impoverished boys who joined the Marine Society in London between 1770 and 1873 (Floud and Wachter 1982; Floud et al. 1990), orphans, factory children, convicts and prisoners. In the twentieth century, national governments became far more aware of the extent to which anthropometric records could be used to monitor the health of the population as a whole, and this led to a substantial increase in the volume of data collected through school surveys and national health surveys (Harris 2009: 62–4).

One of the main methodological problems associated with the analysis of height data is the problem of comparing the heights of people of different ages and sexes. In earlier work (Harris 1988, 1989, 1994, 1998), I attempted to address this issue in the case of British children by comparing the average heights of boys and girls in the past with the distributions of boys' and girls' heights in London in 1965. However, in 1995, Richard Steckel published a new set of height standards based on figures compiled by the United States National Center for Health Statistics in 1977, and these standards have since been accepted for use in historical analysis by other workers in the field (see e.g. López-Alonso 2000; Komlos 2003: 40).

Although it seems reasonable to compare the heights of past generations of boys and girls with those of more recent generations, this approach incorporates two important assumptions. In the first place, it assumes that the same standards can be applied to all populations, and takes little account of any potential differences in what Eveleth and Tanner (1990: 1) called 'genetic potential'. However, a number of studies have shown that international differences in height owe far more to social, economic and environmental variations than to differences in 'race' or ethnicity

(Steckel 1983; Schmitt and Harrison 1988). Eveleth and Tanner (1990: 179–90) suggested that some differences persisted even when people from different ethnic backgrounds were brought up under comparable circumstances, but the differences were not great, and they did not suggest that there were any significant 'ethnic' differences between populations of European origin.

The second key assumption is that differences between the heights and rates of growth of males and females in the standard population are not themselves the consequence of persistent patterns of gender discrimination. One might argue that this assumption is ultimately untestable under 'natural' conditions, but it seems unlikely that gender discrimination exercised a greater influence on the heights and weights of US children in 1977 than on the heights of European children in the more distant past (see also Harris 1998: 428).

Another important problem, from the point of view of gender-based comparisons, concerns the existence, or otherwise, of physiological differences in the reactions of males and females to adverse circumstances. Many auxologists have argued that males are more vulnerable to the effects of undernutrition and that girls show greater powers of resistance (Thomson et al. 1967; Tanner 1962: 127). These arguments are reinforced by evidence which suggests that the average heights of males increased more rapidly than those of females over the course of the twentieth century (Harris 1998: 425–8). However, some commentators have argued that this may not necessarily have been true in all countries (see Silventoinen et al. 2000; Silventoinen 2003: 274–5), and others believe that the evidence for female resistance has been overstated. According to Guntupalli and Baten (2009: 46), 'the female robustness argument … suffers from lack of good data' and Tanner's arguments for the existence of female robustness in the face of undernutrition and radiation suffer from a 'dearth of information about sample size and physiological mechanisms'.

Anthropometric Indicators of Gender Disadvantage

Although most of the available data relate to adult males, we do possess some information about the heights of both boys and girls and can use these data to examine differences in the welfare of the two sexes during their growing years. Table 10.1 shows the average value of the heights of children in different European countries at the ages of 9 and 13 between 1865 and 1940. The original data were derived from a variety of published surveys (for more information, see Harris 2009: 66) and have been converted into centiles of the NCHS distribution using information supplied by Richard Steckel (1995).

In Oslo, the average value of the heights of 9-year-old girls lagged behind that of 9-year-old boys in 1925, 1930, 1935 and 1940, and in Jena, the average value of girls' heights was lower than that of boys' heights in 1932. However, in every other case, including Oslo in 1920, and Jena in 1880 and 1921, the girls were taller, in comparison with the NCHS height standards, than their male counterparts. Taken together, these data provide little support for the view that girls experienced

Table 10.1 Average heights of children in different European countries, 1865–1940

			Boys		Girls	
	Year of measurement	Age	Height (cm)	Percentile	Height (cm)	Percentile
England (London)	1905	9.5	125.2	5.39	124.7	6.60
	1938	9.5	130.9	25.68	130.3	24.10
Germany (Jena)	1880	9.0	123.2	5.85	122.3	7.18
	1921	9.0	128.1	23.75	127.6	24.84
	1932	9.0	130.5	38.35	129.7	35.32
Greece (Athens)	1920	9.0	120.0	1.68	122.4	7.39
	1928	9.0	127.1	18.71	126.2	18.77
	1931	9.0	126.8	17.34	126.2	18.77
Hungary	1910–1920	9.0	124.2	8.28	123.5	9.96
Italy	<1939	9.0	124.7	9.51	123.8	10.44
Netherlands	1865 (Orphans)	6.5	102.0	0.05	102.9	0.34
	1865 (Schoolchildren)	6.5	106.0	0.60	105.9	1.56
Norway (Oslo)	1920	9.0	126.1	14.40	125.3	15.41
	1925	9.0	128.6	26.53	127.8	25.79
	1930	9.0	130.6	39.02	129.7	35.60
	1935	9.0	132.1	49.31	131.3	44.71
	1940	9.0	133.3	57.60	132.6	52.36
Sweden	1883	13.0	142.0	4.40	145.5	4.57
	1938/1939	13.0	153.6	36.65	155.0	37.99

Sources: Cameron (1979): 515, Harris (2009): 66

systematic discrimination in the past, and are consistent with the suggestion that they showed greater resilience than boys, when subjected to the same conditions. However, this was not always the case. In the German city of Jena, the average heights of girls declined between 1932 and 1944 whereas those of boys increased. In Oslo, the average heights of 13-year-old girls declined, in comparison with those of 13-year-old boys, between 1940 and 1945. These differences may have reflected variations in the actual ages of the children being measured or, in the case of the Oslo girls, the different ages at which boys and girls reached adolescence, but they may also have reflected differences in the treatment of boys and girls during the war years (Harris 2009: 67–70).

We possess rather more information, over a longer period, about the heights and weights of adults. However, it is important to remember that even though the height measurements were taken during adulthood, they nevertheless reflect the cumulative impact of conditions during the growing years.

The most common sources of data on the heights of adult females are derived from convict records. Nicholas and Oxley (1993) examined the records of 2,926 English-born and 3,370 Irish-born women who were born between 1790 and 1820 and transported to Australia between 1826 and 1840, and compared their heights with each others' and with the heights of 19,886 men who were transported between 1817 and 1840. They found that the average heights of rural-born women declined more sharply than the average heights of both urban-born women and rural-born men, and attributed this to a perceived decline in employment opportunities for women in rural areas during the Napoleonic period.

These findings have provoked considerable debate. One important reservation concerns the relationship between the timing of changes in the average heights of female birth cohorts and the decline in female employment opportunities. As we have already seen, there is little consensus about the exact nature of the extent and timing of the decline in female employment opportunities in rural areas, but many commentators believe that it did not begin in earnest until rather later in the nineteenth century, and many women continued to make an important financial contribution to the economic welfare of labouring families in agricultural areas for much of the period (Verdon 2002: 196–7).

Other writers have questioned the statistical basis of Nicholas and Oxley's findings. Jackson (1996) argued that the decline in women's heights was largely attributable to changes in the average age of women being measured and claimed that Nicholas and Oxley had 'attribut[ed] long-run significance to what is essentially a short-run movement in a fluctuating series'. Nicholas and Oxley (1996) denied that their results were affected by variations in average age, but they failed to refute Jackson's larger point – namely, that they had attributed too much importance to short-term changes (see also Johnson and Nicholas 1997: 209–10).

In view of the doubts which have been raised about these findings, it is interesting to compare Nicholas and Oxley's original work with the results published by Nicholas and Johnson on the basis of their subsequent examination of the heights of a sample of 'habitual criminals' who had been born between 1812 and 1857 and who were incarcerated in Newgate Gaol in 1877. When Nicholas and Johnson compared their results with the earlier figures produced by Nicholas and Oxley, they found that the average height of male criminals born in 1812/1813 (166.65 cm) compared very closely with the average height of male convicts (166.19 cm) (Johnson and Nicholas 1995: 478). However, when they compared the average heights of female criminals with female convicts, the convicts were substantially shorter (Nicholas and Oxley 1993: 734, 1996: 597; Johnson and Nicholas 1997: 211, 218, 221). The differences between the average heights of male convicts and male criminals and the average heights of female convicts and female criminals imply that at least one of these series is less representative than the others, and this in turn implies that conclusions regarding the differential impact of economic development on the welfare of males and females before 1815 should be treated with considerable caution.

Whilst it is interesting to note that Nicholas and Oxley's original findings suggested that the average heights of rural-born females declined more rapidly than those of rural-born males, Nicholas and Johnson's subsequent research into the heights of Newgate criminals showed that male and female heights moved 'roughly in unison' after 1815 (Johnson and Nicholas 1995, 1997: 222). These findings are broadly consistent with the results obtained by Floud during his analysis of the trends indicated by a range of published datasets during the course of the nineteenth century. Whilst Floud was rightly cautious about drawing too many conclusions from some extremely limited samples, he was able to observe a rough similarity between the trends for males and females during those periods for which comparisons were possible (Floud 1998: 10–5).

Although neither Johnson and Nicholas nor Floud detected any significant differences in the main trends in the heights of men and women born after 1815, Riggs (1994) argued that differences did exist in the average heights of men and women who were born between 1800 and 1849 and incarcerated in Glasgow between 1840 and 1880. He claimed that the average heights of both men and women declined between the birth cohorts of the early 1800s and the 1830s, but the average heights of women continued to decline with the birth cohorts of the 1840s, whereas those of men improved. He speculated that this might reflect the impact of changes in the labour market for men and women in Glasgow during the 1840s, but he also conceded that the results for this decade 'could ... be an artefact of the data, perhaps stemming from subtle changes in policing and, therefore, in the initial sampling of the population from which this dataset is derived' (p. 73, note 47). It may therefore be premature to argue that these data provide unequivocal evidence of sex-specific differences in the welfare of the Scottish population during this period (cf. Komlos 1994: 217; Komlos and Coll 1998: 231–3; Komlos and Baten 2004: 202).

Floud also investigated the absolute value of differences in height, weight and body mass index when these figures were compared with modern standards. In some respects, these results were rather more surprising. As we have seen, it is now generally accepted that women and children often deprived themselves in order to ensure that the father of the household was adequately nourished, but Floud found little evidence of these differences in the anthropometric record. If anything, his figures suggested that adults were more likely to be underweight than children and that men were more likely to underweight than women (Floud 1998: 16). However, these findings have been called into question by Horrell, Meredith and Oxley's study of the heights and weights of nearly 33,000 men and women who were incarcerated in the London House of Correction between 1858 and 1878. They found that the average BMIs of female prisoners were typically much lower than those of male prisoners and that the difference increased with age. Their overall conclusion was that 'as girls became adults and mothers – the ones responsible for dishing out the food – they discovered just how hard it was to make those decisions about scarce family resources … when families grew, women shrank' (2006: 19; see also *ibid.* 2009: 114–5).

Although much of the information which is currently available with regard to the heights of adult women is limited to the United Kingdom, Baten and Murray (1997, 2000) have extended the discussion by examining the heights of approximately 2,500 women who were born between 1819 and 1886 and incarcerated in Wasserburg prison in Bavaria.[2] In 1997, they showed that there were no significant differences between the heights of women who were born illegitimately in cities or to middle-class families, but there was a significant difference between the heights of legitimately and illegitimately born women from peasant families, especially among those born in the 1840s. In 2000, they compared the heights of these women with those of 1,596 male prisoners who were incarcerated at Kaisheim. Their most striking finding was that 'economic factors in early childhood had more systematic influence on girls' than boys' heights, and were more important than disease factors for both sexes' (Baten and Murray 2000: 351).

At the present time, it is difficult to reach any definite conclusions about the extent to which these differences provide any clear evidence about the extent or nature of anti-female discrimination. As we have already seen, there is little direct evidence to show that parents actively discriminated against female children during this period, and, therefore, it is difficult to see why 'economic factors in early childhood' should have led to differences in the pattern of adult heights. Baten and Murray rejected suggestions that the differences may have been attributable to sampling variations but suggested that boys may have had more opportunity to benefit from 'catch-up' growth in later childhood. Although they did not pursue this point in any detail, it may be worth exploring more fully in the future (see Baten and Murray 2000: 355, 358, 363, 368).

Gender and Mortality

Historians have also looked for evidence of female disadvantage in mortality patterns. This work has tended to emphasise three particular issues. Some writers have argued that the declining role of women within agriculture weakened their bargaining

[2] According to Baten and Murray (1997: 52), their sample comprised 1,672 legitimately born women and 829 illegitimately born. In their later paper, they said that the number of women was 2,546 (Baten and Murray 2000: 354) or 2,549 (*ibid.*: 357–8).

position within the household and led to disproportionately high levels of female mortality, especially in agricultural areas (see e.g. Johansson 1977; Klasen 1998). Other writers, such as Arthur Imhof (1981: 172), have attributed high rates of female mortality to 'the diversity of simultaneous burdens on women as wife and mother, in the household and in special duties'. A third group, including Dominique Tabutin (1978; but see also Eggerickx and Tabutin 1994), Louis Henry (1987, 1989) and Tony Wrigley et al. (1997: 299–300), have argued that the disproportionately high rates of mortality experienced by past generations of women were largely attributable to the fact that women were more susceptible to the effects of tuberculosis and other infectious diseases during a period in which the prevalence of these diseases was much greater.

The main aim of this section is not to ask how we should explain changes in the ratio of female mortality to male mortality over time but to ask how far disproportionately high rates of female mortality can be linked to underlying patterns of female disadvantage. The remainder of the section uses a technique known as shift-share analysis to help address this. The analysis enables us to estimate the extent to which changes in the female mortality rate (m) can be attributed to changes in the national mortality rate (M), the incidence of particular causes of death (i), or the particular circumstances of female lives.[3]

The following tables show the impact of different factors on the decline of female mortality in four broad age groups in England and Wales between 1851/1860 and 1979/1995. Table 10.2 shows that more than 98% of the decline in mortality between the ages of 0 and 14 was attributable to factors which influenced both male and female death rates and that only a very small proportion of the decline in female mortality in this age group was directly associated with 'being female'. However, 'being female' accounted for a somewhat larger proportion of the decline in mortality among women between the ages of 15 and 44. Table 10.3 shows that the majority of the decline in this age group was also caused by factors which were common to both sexes and by a decline in the relative importance of infectious diseases, but 'being female' accounted for 5.38% of the decline in total mortality and more than 6% of the decline in infectious-disease mortality. Although these proportions are not in themselves very large, they do provide some indication of the ways in which the particular hardships faced by women during the 1850s may have contributed to higher mortality rates within this age group.

The last two tables (Tables 10.4 and 10.5) present the results for women between the ages of 45 and 64 and for women aged 65 and over. Although Table 10.4 provides further evidence of the additional extent of the decline in female mortality from infectious diseases, both tables reveal the importance of twentieth-century trends in mortality from cancer (neoplasms) and circulatory diseases. In each case, the increasing importance of these diseases had the effect of raising both male and female mortality, but the increase in male mortality was much greater, and this led to a further reduction in the ratio of female-to-male mortality within these age groups.

---

[3] For more information, see Harris 2008: 185.

Table 10.2 The contribution of different factors to the decline of female mortality at ages 0–14 between 1851/1860 and 1979/1995

1851/1860–1979/1995	Deaths per million				%			
Age group 0–14	Whole population	Cause of death	Female mortality	Total	Whole population	Cause of death	Female mortality	Total
1. Infectious diseases	−10,514	−1,517	−119	−12,150	86.54	12.48	0.98	100.00
2. Neoplasms	−25	52	−3	25	−97.05	207.65	−10.60	100.00
5. Mental disorders	−1,517	−2,317	1	−3,834	39.58	60.44	−0.02	100.00
6. Diseases of the nervous system and sense organs	−889	−56	34	−912	97.49	6.19	−3.67	100.00
7. Diseases of the circulatory system	−373	79	24	−270	138.28	−29.38	−8.90	100.00
8. Diseases of the respiratory system	−4,647	919	−46	−3,774	123.13	−24.35	1.21	100.00
9. Diseases of the digestive system	−1,040	495	−5	−550	189.07	−89.98	0.91	100.00
10. Diseases of the genito-urinary system	−94	48	15	−31	300.84	−153.92	−46.93	100.00
11. Complications of pregnancy, childbirth and the puerperium	−408	974	−566	0	–	–	–	100.00
12. Diseases of the skin and subcutaneous tissue	−82	24	−7	−64	127.85	−38.04	10.19	100.00
13. Diseases of the musculoskeletal system and connective tissue	−39	−14	−2	−54	71.30	25.72	2.97	100.00
17. Injury and poisoning	−691	100	38	−552	125.06	−18.18	−6.87	100.00
18. Other	−6,317	1,682	−205	−4,840	130.51	−34.74	4.23	100.00
Total	−26,635	470	−841	−27,006	98.63	−1.74	3.11	100.00

Source: Harris (2008): 189

Table 10.3 The contribution of different factors to the decline of female mortality at ages 15–44 between 1851/1860 and 1979/1995

1851/1860–1979/1995	Deaths per million				%			
Age group 15–44	Whole population	Cause of death	Female mortality	Total	Whole population	Cause of death	Female mortality	Total
1. Infectious diseases	–4,108	–1,189	–377	–5,674	72.40	20.96	6.64	100.00
2. Neoplasms	–341	456	–69	45	–757.98	1,012.29	–154.31	100.00
5. Mental disorders	–329	–226	–9	–565	58.30	40.07	1.63	100.00
6. Diseases of the nervous system and sense organs	–157	180	–5	19	–844.24	970.89	–26.66	100.00
7. Diseases of the circulatory system	–903	450	–101	–554	163.11	–81.33	18.23	100.00
8. Diseases of the respiratory system	–641	112	–58	–587	109.12	–19.02	9.90	100.00
9. Diseases of the digestive system	–522	–14	–14	–550	94.95	2.48	2.57	100.00
10. Diseases of the genito-urinary system	–461	183	89	–190	243.13	–96.35	–46.78	100.00
11. Complications of pregnancy, childbirth and the puerperium	–507	–168	–1	–676	75.01	24.89	0.10	100.00
12. Diseases of the skin and subcutaneous tissue	–10	–3	1	–13	81.77	23.40	–5.17	100.00
13. Diseases of the musculoskeletal system and connective tissue	–43	–9	8	–44	97.14	20.25	–17.38	100.00
17. Injury and poisoning	–183	111	65	–7	2,594.44	–1,573.31	–921.13	100.00
18. Other	–210	–32	–14	–256	81.95	12.45	5.60	100.00
Total	–8,416	–149	–487	–9,051	92.98	1.65	5.38	100.00

Source: Harris (2008): 190

Table 10.4 The contribution of different factors to the decline of female mortality at ages 45–64 between 1851/1860 and 1979/1995

1851/1860–1979/1995	Deaths per million				%			
Age group 45–64	Whole population	Cause of death	Female mortality	Total	Whole population	Cause of death	Female mortality	Total
1. Infectious diseases	−2,458	−802	−239	−3,500	70.24	22.93	6.83	100.00
2. Neoplasms	−1,490	1,330	−406	−566	263.51	−235.23	71.71	100.00
5. Mental disorders	−1,056	−755	−9	−1,820	58.03	41.50	0.47	100.00
6. Diseases of the nervous system and sense organs	−138	142	14	18	−782.45	803.98	78.47	100.00
7. Diseases of the circulatory system	−2,752	1,327	−454	−1,879	146.50	−70.66	24.16	100.00
8. Diseases of the respiratory system	−1,986	−209	−72	−2,267	87.60	9.23	3.18	100.00
9. Diseases of the digestive system	−1,169	−312	−26	−1,507	77.59	20.71	1.70	100.00
10. Diseases of the genito-urinary system	−515	169	−41	−387	132.93	−43.53	10.59	100.00
11. Complications of pregnancy, childbirth and the puerperium	−19	−11	0	−30	63.05	36.73	0.22	100.00
12. Diseases of the skin and subcutaneous tissue	−31	−6	3	−34	91.77	17.14	−8.90	100.00
13. Diseases of the musculoskeletal system and connective tissue	−80	15	19	−45	175.54	−34.04	−41.50	100.00
17. Injury and poisoning	−223	7	28	−188	118.70	−3.62	−15.08	100.00
18. Other	−707	−327	−10	−1,045	67.69	31.31	1.00	100.00
Total	−12,625	567	−1,192	−13,250	95.28	−4.28	9.00	100.00

Source: Harris (2008): 191

Table 10.5 The contribution of different factors to the decline of female mortality at the ages of 65 and over between 1851/1860 and 1979/1995

1851/1860–1979/1995	Deaths per million				%			
Age group ≥65	Whole population	Cause of death	Female mortality	Total	Whole population	Cause of death	Female mortality	Total
1. Infectious diseases	−11,804	−4,129	−282	−16,214	72.80	25.46	1.74	100.00
2. Neoplasms	−8,783	8,700	−2,684	−2,766	317.54	−314.57	97.03	100.00
5. Mental disorders	−12,414	−9,863	−3	−22,280	55.72	44.27	0.02	100.00
6. Diseases of the nervous system and sense organs	−1,370	1,624	−94	160	−857.26	1,016.05	−58.79	100.00
7. Diseases of the circulatory system	−30,828	19,552	−2,994	−14,270	216.03	−137.01	20.98	100.00
8. Diseases of the respiratory system	−27,684	1,868	−153	−25,970	106.60	−7.19	0.59	100.00
9. Diseases of the digestive system	−7,828	−1,453	−139	−9,419	83.11	15.42	1.47	100.00
10. Diseases of the genito-urinary system	−2,888	753	701	−1,433	201.44	−52.56	−48.88	100.00
11. Complications of pregnancy, childbirth and the puerperium	0	0	0	0	#DIV/0!	#DIV/0!	#DIV/0!	#DIV/0!
12. Diseases of the skin and subcutaneous tissue	−514	12	39	−463	111.14	−2.64	−8.50	100.00
13. Diseases of the musculoskeletal system and connective tissue	−714	416	196	−102	703.11	−410.10	−193.00	100.00
17. Injury and poisoning	−2,334	112	−10	−2,232	104.57	−5.01	0.43	100.00
18. Other	−58,415	−18,057	−1,427	−77,899	74.99	23.18	1.83	100.00
Total	−165,574	−464	−6,849	−172,887	95.77	0.27	3.96	100.00

Source: Harris (2008): 192

Conclusions

This chapter has explored the extent to which the particular hardships experienced by the female population may have been reflected in the size and shape of women's bodies and in their mortality rates. Although these are important dimensions of welfare in their own right, the chapter has been particularly concerned to examine the extent to which they can be associated with underlying differences in the circumstances of male and female lives.

A number of authors have argued that the decline in female employment opportunities in agriculture led to a deterioration in the life experiences of both girls and women, but there is comparatively little historical evidence to suggest that parents discriminated actively against their female children in either the early modern or modern periods. In view of this, it may not be so surprising that we have found relatively little evidence of any systematic differences in the relative values of male and female heights in either the nineteenth or twentieth centuries. However, differences may have emerged in later childhood, and some authors have found evidence of quite sharp differences in the body mass indices of male and female adults. This suggests that there is considerable scope for further research into the anthropometric characteristics of older girls and adult women, if such data can be obtained.

The chapter has also examined the extent to which underlying differences in the welfare of males and females may have been reflected in mortality rates. Although there has been a decline in the ratio of female-to-male mortality at all ages since the mid-nineteenth century, our analysis of changing mortality patterns in England and Wales showed that much of the decline at younger ages can be attributed to changes in the incidence and lethality of infectious diseases. However, changes in the circumstances of female lives may have been reflected in the mortality experience of women between the ages of 15 and 44. This analysis therefore reinforces the importance of using cause-specific mortality rates to investigate the relationship between gendered patterns of disadvantage and mortality experience in other European countries.

References

Baten, J., & Murray, J. (1997). Bastardy in south Germany revisited: An anthropometric synthesis. *Journal of Interdisciplinary History, 28*, 47–56.

Baten, J., & Murray, J. (2000). Heights of men and women in nineteenth-century Bavaria: Economic, nutritional and disease influences. *Explorations in Economic History, 37*, 351–369.

Borderías, C., Pérez-Fuentes, P., & Sarasúa, C. (2010). Gender inequalities in family consumption: Spain 1850–1930. In T. Addabbi, M.-P. Arrizabalaga, C. Borderías, & A. Owens (Eds.), *Gender inequalities, households and the production of wellbeing in modern Europe* (pp. 179–196). Farnham: Ashgate.

Cameron, N. (1979). The growth of London schoolchildren 1904–66: An analysis of secular trend and intra-country variation. *Annals of Human Biology, 6*, 505–525.

Eggerickx, T., & Tabutin, D. (1994). La surmortalité des filles en Belgique vers 1890: une approche régionale. *Population, 49*(3), 657–684.

Erickson, A. (1986). *The expense of children and maternal management in early-modern England.* Paper presented to the Ninth International Economic History Congress. Berne.
Eveleth, P., & Tanner, J. (1990). *Worldwide variation in human growth* (2nd ed.). Cambridge: Cambridge University Press.
Floud, R. (1998). *Height, weight and body mass of the British population since 1820.* National Bureau of economic research working paper series on historical factors in long run growth (Historical Paper 108).
Floud, R., & Wachter, K. (1982). Poverty and physical stature: Evidence on the standard of living of London boys, 1770–1870. *Social Science History, 6*, 422–452.
Floud, R., Wachter, K., & Gregory, A. (1990). *Height, health and history: Nutritional status in the United Kingdom 1750–1980.* Cambridge: Cambridge University Press.
Floud, R., Fogel, R., Harris, B., & Hong, S. C. (2011). *The changing body: Health, nutrition and human development in the western world since 1700.* Cambridge: Cambridge University Press.
Fuchs, R. (2005). *Gender and poverty in nineteenth-century Europe.* Cambridge: Cambridge University Press.
Guntupalli, A., & Baten, J. (2009). Measuring gender wellbeing with biological welfare indicators. In B. Harris, L. Gálvez, & H. Machado (Eds.), *Gender and wellbeing in Europe: Historical and contemporary perspectives* (pp. 43–58). Farnham: Ashgate.
Hanawalt, B. (1993). *Growing up in medieval London: The experience of childhood in history.* New York: Oxford University Press.
Harris, B. (1988). Unemployment, insurance and health in interwar Britain. In B. Eichengreen & T. Hatton (Eds.), *Interwar unemployment in international perspective* (pp. 149–183). Dordrecht: Kluwer Academic Publishers.
Harris, B. (1989). *Medical inspection and the nutrition of schoolchildren in Britain, 1900–1950.* Ph.D. thesis, University of London.
Harris, B. (1994). The height of schoolchildren in Britain, 1900–1950. In J. Komlos (Ed.), *Stature, living standards and economic development: Essays in anthropometric history* (pp. 25–38). Chicago: University of Chicago Press.
Harris, B. (1998). Gender, height and mortality in nineteenth- and twentieth-century Britain: Some preliminary reflections. In J. Komlos & J. Baten (Eds.), *The biological standard of living in comparative perspective* (pp. 413–448). Stuttgart: Franz Steiner Verlag.
Harris, B. (2008). Gender, health and welfare in England and Wales since industrialisation. *Research in Economic History, 26*, 157–204.
Harris, B. (2009). Anthropometric history, gender and the measurement of wellbeing. In B. Harris, L. Gálvez, & H. Machado (Eds.), *Gender and wellbeing in Europe: Historical and contemporary perspectives* (pp. 59–83). Farnham: Ashgate.
Harris, B., & Bridgen, P. (2007). Introduction: The "mixed economy of welfare" and the historiography of welfare provision. In B. Harris & P. Bridgen (Eds.), *Charity and mutual aid in Europe and North America since 1800* (pp. 1–18). New York: Routledge.
Harris, B., Gorsky, M., Guntupalli, A. M., & Hinde, A. (2012). Long-term changes in sickness and health: Further evidence from the Hampshire Friendly Society. *The Economic History Review, 65*, 719–745.
Henry, L. (1987). Mortalité des hommes et des femmes dans le passe. *Annales de Démographie Historique*, 87–118.
Henry, L. (1989). Men's and women's mortality in the past. *Population, 44*, 177–201.
Horrell, S., Meredith, D., & Oxley, D. (2006, August 23). *Measuring misery: Body mass among Victorian London's poor.* Paper presented to Session 50 (Anthropometrics, markets and disease in historical standards of living: Eurasian and American countries) of the Fourteenth International Economic History Congress, Helsinki.
Horrell, S., Meredith, D., & Oxley, D. (2009). Measuring misery: Body mass, ageing and gender inequality in Victorian London. *Explorations in Economic History, 46*, 93–119.
Humphries, J. (2010). *Childhood and child labour in the British industrial revolution.* Cambridge: Cambridge University Press.

Imhof, A. (1981). Women, family and death: Excess mortality of women in child-bearing age in four communities in nineteenth-century Germany. In R. Evans & W. R. Lee (Eds.), *The German family: Essays on the social history of the family in nineteenth- and twentieth-century Germany* (pp. 148–174). London: Croom Helm.

Jackson, R. (1996). The heights of rural-born English female convicts transported to New South Wales. *The Economic History Review, 49*, 584–590.

Johansson, S. R. (1977). Sex and death in Victorian England: An examination of age- and sex-specific death rates, 1840–1910. In M. Vicinus (Ed.), *A widening sphere: Changing roles of Victorian women* (pp. 163–181). London: Methuen.

Johnson, P., & Nicholas, S. (1995). Male and female living standards in England and Wales 1812–57: Evidence from criminal height records. *The Economic History Review, 48*, 470–481.

Johnson, P., & Nicholas, S. (1997). Health and welfare of women in the United Kingdom, 1785–1920. In R. Steckel & R. Floud (Eds.), *Health and welfare during industrialization* (pp. 201–249). Chicago: University of Chicago Press.

Kennedy, R. (1972). The social status of the sexes and their relative mortality rates in Ireland. In W. Peterson (Ed.), *Readings in population* (pp. 121–135). New York: Macmillan.

Klasen, S. (1998). Marriage, bargaining and intrahousehold resource allocation: Excess female mortality among adults during early German development, 1740–1860. *Journal of Economic History, 58*, 432–467.

Komlos, J. (1994). On the significance of anthropometric history. In J. Komlos (Ed.), *Stature, living standards and economic development: Essays in anthropometric history* (pp. 210–220). Chicago: University of Chicago Press.

Komlos, J. (2003). On the biological standard of living of eighteenth-century Americans: Taller, richer, healthier. *Munich Economics* (Discussion Paper 2003–2009).

Komlos, J., & Baten, J. (2004). Looking backward and looking forward: Anthropometric research and the development of social science history. *Social Science History, 28*, 191–210.

Komlos, J., & Coll, S. (1998). The biological standard of living and economic development: Nutrition, health and well-being in historical perspective. In C. E. Núñez (Ed.), *Debates and controversies in economic history* (pp. 219–282). Madrid: Fundación Ramon Areces/Fundación fomento de la historia económica.

López-Alonso, M. (2000, November 17). *An anthropometric approach to the measurement of living standards, Mexico*. Paper presented to the LACLIO Conference, Stanford University.

López-Palacios, F. (1905). *Apuntes para el estudio medico topográfico de Cantalojas-Guadalajara*. Unpublished manuscript.

Macfarlane, A. (1986). *Marriage and love in England: Modes of reproduction, 1300–1480*. Oxford: Basil Blackwell.

Nicholas, S., & Oxley, D. (1993). The living standards of women during the industrial revolution, 1795–1820. *The Economic History Review, 46*, 723–749.

Nicholas, S., & Oxley, D. (1996). Living standards of women in England and Wales, 1785–1815: New evidence from Newgate prison records. *The Economic History Review, 49*, 591–599.

Oren, L. (1974). The welfare of women in laboring families. In M. Hartman & L. Banner (Eds.), *Clio's consciousness raised: New perspectives on the history of women* (pp. 226–244). New York: Harper Torchbooks.

Riggs, P. (1994). The standard of living in Scotland, 1800–1850. In J. Komlos (Ed.), *Stature, living standards and economic development: Essays in anthropometric history* (pp. 60–75). Chicago: University of Chicago Press.

Riley, J. C. (1997). *Sick, not dead: The health of British workingmen during the mortality decline*. Baltimore/London: Johns Hopkins University Press.

Roberts, R. (1971). *The classic slum: Salford life in the first quarter of the century*. Harmondsworth: Penguin.

Russell, J. C. (1948). *British medieval population*. London: Macmillan & Co.

Schmitt, L., & Harrison, G. (1988). Patterns in the within-population variation of stature and weight. *Annals of Human Biology, 15*, 353–364.

Sen, A. (1989). Women's survival as a development problem. *Bulletin of the American Academy of Arts and Sciences, 43*, 14–29.
Shahar, S. (1990). *Childhood in the middle ages*. London: Routledge.
Silventoinen, K. (2003). Determinants of variation in adult body height. *Journal of Biosocial Science, 35*, 263–285.
Silventoinen, K., Kaprio, J., Lahelma, E., & Koskenvuo, M. (2000). Relative effect of genetic and environmental factors on body height: Differences across birth cohorts among Finnish men and women. *American Journal of Public Health, 90*, 627–630.
Steckel, R. (1983). Height and *per capita* income. *Historical Methods, 16*, 1–7.
Steckel, R. (1995). Percentiles of modern height standards for use in historical research. *NBER working paper series on historical factors in long-run growth* (Historical Paper 75).
Tabutin, D. (1978). La surmortalité féminine en Europe avant 1940. *Population, 33*(1), 121–148.
Tanner, J. (1962). *Growth at adolescence, with a general examination of the effects of hereditary and environmental factors upon growth and maturation from birth to maturity* (2nd ed.). Oxford/Edinburgh: Blackwell Scientific Publications (first published 1955).
Tanner, J. (1981). *A history of the study of human growth*. Cambridge: Cambridge University Press.
Thomson, A., Billewicz, W., & Holliday, R. (1967). Secular changes in the height of Aberdeen women. *British Journal of Preventive & Social Medicine, 21*, 137–140.
Titmuss, R. (1987). The position of women. In B. Abel-Smith & K. Titmuss (Eds.), *The philosophy of welfare: Selected writings of Richard M. Titmuss* (pp. 87–101). London: Allen & Unwin.
Verdon, N. (2002). *Rural women workers in nineteenth-century England: Gender, work and wages*. Woodbridge: Boydell Press.
Vilar Ferrán, J. (1917). *Topografía médica del distrito municipal de Villanueva de la Cañada*. Unpublished manuscript.
Wall, R. (1981). Inferring differential neglect of females from mortality data. *Annales de Démographie Historique*, 119–40.
Wrightson, K. (1975). Infanticide in earlier-seventeenth century England. *Local Population Studies, 15*, 10–22.
Wrigley, E. A., Davies, R., Oeppen, J., & Schofield, R. (1997). *English population history from family reconstitution 1580–1837*. Cambridge: Cambridge University Press.

Part IV
Youth, Elder, Migration and Social Work

Chapter 11
Support and Success in Youth Transitions: A Comparative Analysis on the Relation Between Subjective and Systemic Factors

Andreas Walther, Barbara Stauber, and Axel Pohl

Introduction

> Declining birth rates and rising life expectancies have brought about dramatic changes in the size and age structure of Europe's population ... Young people have a significant contribution to make to ... growth and to sustainable development, as they make up the future work force, and are the future source of much-needed research capabilities, innovation and entrepreneurship. These goals can only be achieved if young people are properly equipped with knowledge, skills and competences through high quality, relevant education and training. (European Commission 2005)

This exemplary quote from a recent policy document of the European Commission refers to difficulties young people meet in their transitions to work and adulthood. The suggested policy perspectives imply a general and shared meaning of success with regard to youth transitions across Europe defined from the systemic perspective of societal institutions: entering the workforce, contributing to reproduction and avoiding welfare dependency. One can argue that this and other policy documents implicitly rely on assumptions of standard life courses with a quite linear sequence of education–training–employment–family building–retirement (cf. Walther et al. 2009).

Martin Kohli (2009) reminds us that the modern life course is a result of the institutionalisation of age-based roles (and the transitions between them) in early

A. Walther (✉)
Institute für Social Pedagogy and Adult Education, University of Frankfurt, Robert-Mayer-Straße 1, D-60054 Frankfurt, Germany
e-mail: A.Walther@em.uni-frankfurt.de

B. Stauber
Institute of Education, Tübingen University, Muenzgasse 22-30, D 72070 Tübingen
e-mail: Barbara.Stauber@uni-tuebingen.de

A. Pohl
Institute for Regional Innovation and Social Research (IRIS), Tubingen, Germany
e-mail: axel.pohl@iris-egris.de

A. Moreno Mínguez (ed.), *Family Well-Being: European Perspectives*, Social Indicators Research Series 49, DOI 10.1007/978-94-007-4354-0_11,

modernity, restructuring the societal division of labour under conditions of individualisation. This institutionalisation on the one hand depended on individuals who accepted this predefined life course as orientation for the subjective construction of their biographies. On the other hand, it was interrelated with the process of nation state building, whereby different normalities of the life course have evolved. Both the coincidence of systemic and social integration and the sovereignty of the nation state in securing standard life courses seem to have been weakened in the process of modernisation, whereby the assumptions of success and support with regard to youth transitions are being questioned. Yet, persisting assumptions of normality are reflected by a terminology focussing on the deviance of young people from the timing of the standard life course: prolongation of transitions, early school leaving, teenage pregnancy or postponed parenthood.

Our chapter aims at reflecting the meaning of success and support in youth transitions from a life course perspective. This has a comparative dimension with regard to different ‘transition regimes’ and a biographical dimension asking for the subjective views of young men and women. We start from the assumption that late modern life course trajectories consist of frictions and paradoxical constellations while the life course ideology still implies consistency, linearity and manageability. There is a simultaneity (and at the same time discrepancy) of a de-standardisation of life courses and institutions, policies as well as individual life plans continuously referring to the ‘normal’ life course. These simultaneities can be shown with regard to the areas of family and work, the classical cornerstones of the status of adulthood:

- *Transitions to work* have become increasingly complex and precarious, even for young people with higher education and even in countries apparently less affected by the economic crisis. There is a sustainable mismatch on youth labour markets reflected by long searching periods for an adequate job, high rates of fixed-term jobs and high levels of youth unemployment. Activation policies at the same time reinforce the ideology of the possibility of self-responsibility, full employment and economic independence – padded by discourses on human capital and lifelong learning (Walther and Pohl 2005; Schoon and Silbereisen 2009).
- *Family transitions* are interrelated with transitions to work. This is true for both the transition to independent living and the foundation of an own family which are being prolonged and postponed, but sometimes also anticipated. The issue of reconciliation of work and family refers to the fragmentation of de-standardised life courses which confronts individuals with biographical dilemmas (Walther et al. 2009) that have to be solved individually (Lewis and Smithson 2006; Stauber 2010).

Transitions to work and family reveal the interrelatedness of individualisation and social inequality. Inequality is no longer limited to differences in social mobility but extends to risks of social exclusion, and it can no longer be ascribed to monocausal relationships but requires the analysis of intersecting gender, class, ethnic and other differences (cf. Phoenix 2009).

Our argumentation is based on the findings of three EU-funded comparative studies which have been carried out in the framework of the EGRIS network (European Group for Integrated Social Research):

- The *Youth Policy and Participation* (YOYO) project analysed the relevance of participatory approaches in supporting young people – especially so-called disadvantaged youth – in their transitions to work. One key focus was young people's motivation in actively engaging in their transitions, their acceptance and use of available support. The project involved nine countries (Denmark, Germany, Ireland, Italy, Netherlands, Portugal, Romania, Spain and the UK). Methodologically, it consisted of 28 project case studies including qualitative interviews with 365 young people (70% interviewed a second time within 1 year) and 141 expert interviews (see Walther et al. 2006).
- The *Families and Transitions in Europe* (FATE) project analysed how young people mobilise support for prolonged transitions to the labour market especially from their families. The project combined a quantitative survey (N=1,600) and in-depth interviews with young people (N=360) and their parents (N=270) at the end of their educational trajectories on strategies, experiences and impact of family support on decision-making processes. The study allowed for insight into the way intergenerational support varies across welfare regimes (Biggart and Kovacheva 2006; Stauber and du Bois-Reymond 2006).
- The project *Youth – Actor of Social Change* (UP2YOUTH) consisted of a comparative review of research literature aimed at analysing the double relationship between young people's agency and social change: the impact of social change on young people's actions and the active role of young people in social change. The focus lay on three dimensions of transitions to adulthood: young parenthood, transitions to work of immigrant and ethnic minority youth and youth participation (Walther et al. 2009).

This chapter evolves as follows: Throughout the three projects, a model of transition regimes has been developed which will be presented with regard to the support mechanisms different transition systems foresee and the definitions of successful transitions they imply. The next introduces the biographical perspective which, theoretically, relates to the interplay between life course and biography or between structure and agency. Before this background, empirical findings from the FATE and YOYO studies are presented and discussed to analyse how individuals negotiate meanings of success and support in interaction with institutional (and socio-economic) structures. The final section concludes by outlining consequences emerging from the combination of a comparative and a biographical perspective on success and support in youth transitions.

Definitions of Success and Mechanisms of Support Across Different Transition Regimes

Young people's transitions to adulthood are a crucial moment in both individual biographies and the process of social integration. They represent a period in which the linkage between individual lives and social contexts are renegotiated and redefined in terms of occupational, family and citizenship roles. Inasmuch as these roles have been shaped by – not only but decisively – public institutions, especially education and welfare, one may expect that nation states play a major contextual role in defining what means success in youth transitions and what kind of support individuals need and can expect from the public. In this section, we want to show that subjective constructions and interactive negotiations of success and support between individuals, families, peers and institutions are framed, informed and influenced by what we call *transition regimes*. This concept refers to constellations of socio-economic, institutional and cultural factors that contribute to different 'normalities' of being young and growing up, of which aspirations (meaning of success) and expectations (of support) are held legitimate.

A starting point in developing the model has been the typology of *welfare regimes* of Esping-Andersen (1990; modified by Gallie and Paugam 2000) which distinguishes welfare states according to access and level of social security. The notion of 'regime' refers to the power of such constellations. They influence both the rationales of institutions and policies and the individuals' biographical orientation. In fact, the regime concept implies a dialectic interrelation of structure and agency in articulating, reproducing and modifying social relationships.

The model of transition regimes has evolved over a series of studies on youth transitions including YOYO, FATE and UP2YOUTH involving the analysis of institutional arrangements, document analysis of policy programmes, statistical analysis, expert interviews, project case studies, in-depth interviews and focus group discussions with young people across different educational levels as well as with parents (Biggart and Kovacheva 2006; Walther et al. 2006, 2009). Apart from structures of welfare and the question to what extent young people are entitled to benefits and services from the state, the following dimensions of the model can be seen as structuring transition-related *support*:

- Structures of education and training and the extent to which they channel pupils to different educational pathways with unequal outcomes (Allmendinger 1989)
- Structures of 'open' versus 'close' labour market entry and the degree of flexibility for transitions within labour market careers (Shavit and Müller 1998; Müller and Gangl 2003)
- Orientations of policies against youth unemployment towards general education, vocational training or employability including different interpretations of activation (cf. van Berkel and Hornemann Møller 2002; McNeish and Loncle 2003; Harsløf 2005; Walther and Pohl 2005)
- Mechanisms of doing gender allocation of young men and women to different trajectories (Sainsbury 1999)
- Levels and patterns of public expenditure for education, active labour market policy, family and children (Walther and Pohl 2005)

Behind these institutional structures aimed at facilitating transitions to work and adulthood, there are cultural patterns – values, meanings and discourses – which imply what is held as a *success*ful transition. This refers especially to:

- Dominant institutional representations of youth and the respective institutional demands and expectations addressed to young people
- Interpretations and ascriptions of disadvantage to individual deficits (such as a lack of employability) or to structural deficits (a lack of jobs or adequate education and training opportunities (Walther 2006))

The regime typology resulting from assessing national transition systems according to these dimensions must not be misunderstood as descriptive. It clusters different groups of national transition systems according to their guiding rationales – or the dominant meanings of success and support in regulating youth transitions. This implies that institutional details may diverge considerably within one regime type while contributing to a similar rationale in regulating youth transitions. For the time being, four regime types have been modelled (Table 11.1):

- The *universalistic* transition regime of the Nordic countries is based on inclusive education systems in which general and vocational education are largely integrated and reflect the individualisation of life courses. Youth is first of all associated with individual personal development providing young people a status of 'citizens in education'. This is reflected by an education allowance for all who are over 18 and still in the education system which contributes to a partial independence from their families. Education, training and activating labour market policies allow for individual choice to secure motivation and provide multiple counselling services. Gendered career opportunities are highly balanced due to the integration of general and vocational education, a broad public employment sector and available public child care (Os 2002; Bechmann Jensen et al. 2005).
- The *liberal* transition regime in Ireland and the UK is best characterised by the notion of individual responsibility in which young people without work face major pressure to enter the workforce. Youth is regarded as a basically transitory life phase which should be turned into economic independence as soon as possible. Both the labour market and education and training are structured by a high degree of flexibility. While this provides multiple entry options, it also implies a high level of insecurity. Although female employment is high, it tends to be of part-time nature and in low-skilled or unskilled service occupations. Activation policies are interpreted in terms of workfare, implying pressure and control of jobseekers and confronting young people with considerable risks of precariousness and social exclusion (Biggart 2005; Furlong and Cartmel 2006).
- In the Mediterranean countries, transition regimes are *sub-protective* or *under-institutionalised*. Due to a lack of reliable training pathways into the labour market, transitions often involve a waiting phase until the mid-1930s, with unequal outcomes. As they are not entitled to any kind of social benefits, young men and women depend to a large extent on their families who are referred to as 'social amortisator' for the sociopolitical vacuum. Long family dependency indicates that youth do not have a formal status and place in society – with consequences ranging from considerable freedom to experiences of 'forced harmony', affecting especially young women's opportunities (Leccardi and Rusmini 2004). Current

Table 11.1 Transition regimes across Europe

Dimension	Dimensions of 'support' (in a broad sense)								Criteria of 'success'	
Regime	Country	School	Training	Social security	Employment regime	Female employment	Focus of transition policies	Public expenditure for education/families and children/active labour market policies[a]	Concept of youth	Concept of disadvantage
Universalistic	Denmark Finland	Not selective	Flexible standards (mixed)	State	Open Low risks	High	Education Activation	DK: 7,*8/3,7/1,0* FI: 5,9/2,9/0,7	Personal development, citizenship status	Individualised and structure-related
Employment-centred	Austria Germany France Netherlands	Selective	High standards (dual)	State/family	Closed Risks at the margins	Medium	(Pre-)vocational training	A: 5,4/2,7/0,5 D: 4,5/2,8/ 0,5 F: 5,6/2,5/0,7 NL: 5,3/1,6/0,7	Socialisation for occupational/social positions	Individualised
Liberal	Ireland UK	Principally not selective	Low standards (mixed)	State/family	Open High risks	High	Employability	IE: 4,9/2,6/0,5 UK: 5,4/1,5/0,1	Early economic independence	Individualised
Sub-protective	Italy Portugal Spain	Not Selective	Low standards and coverage (school)	Family	Closed High risks (Informal work)	Low	'Any status' (work, education or training)	IT: 4,3/1,2/0,4 PT: 5,3/1,2/0,4 ES: 4,3/1,3/0,6	Without distinct status	Structure-related
Post-socialist transformation societies										
	Bulgaria Poland Romania Slovakia Slovenia	Principally not selective	Standards in process of transformation (mixed)	Family/state	Closed High risks	Low (except Slovenia)	Mixed	BG: 4,1/1,2/0,3 PL: 4,9/0,8/0,1 RO: 4,2/1,7/0,1 SK: 3,6/1,5/0,1 SI: 5,2/1,8/0,1	Mixed	Mixed

[a]Eurostat data on expenditures for education/families and children/active labour market policies in 2007 as % of GDP

policies aim at providing young people any kind of status also if precarious without clear priorities. Often young people opt for a recognised status in higher education while gaining limited economic independence through informal work.

- The *employment-centred regime* of continental countries is characterised by a differentiated (and partly highly selective) school system connected to a rigidly standardised and gendered system of vocational training. Different tracks separate pupils from age 10 or 12 according to performance. The dominant expectation towards youth is to be socialised for a set occupational and social position – through training. This is reflected through the provision of a two-tiered division of social security, favouring those who have already been in regular training or employment, while others are entitled to stigmatised social assistance. Those who fail entering regular vocational training are referred to as 'disadvantaged' in terms of individual deficits and channelled into pre-vocational measures which most often imply adaptation and reduction of aspirations.

It is obvious that this picture is limited inasmuch as it represents the so-called Western world. In fact, Central and Eastern European countries have been analysed according to the same dimensions, but the pace of transformation and the diverse mixtures between an apparently uniform past and increasing heterogeneity do not allow for simply subsuming them under the regime types or creating a single post-socialist one.

- The *post-socialist* countries at first sight appear rather close to the under-institutionalised regime type with public institutions being rather unreliable. Yet, differentiation is needed in a double sense: first, an increasingly sub-protective presence merges with the experience of the (socialist) past in which life courses were structured by a mixture of a universalist and an employment-centred logic, and second, social positions were tied to employment to which everyone entitled was respectively obliged. Female employment was high and secured by availability of child care. However, Pascall and Manning (2000) have identified women as the losers of transformation. Due to the conditions imposed by trans-national actors like the EU or the World Bank, processes of transformation imply orientation towards existing (Western) models, yet leading to particular mixtures and still open for change. According to Kovacheva (2001), one particular feature of youth transitions is that life conditions either leap from premodern constellations into postmodern fragmented ones or combine both.

As the model is primarily heuristic, it does not replace further comparative analysis especially as differences *within* regime types are neglected and as it has to be constantly reassessed with regard to social change. One open question is also to what extent and how different regime types are reflected by performance – i.e. the success of transitions. For example, there is no clear relation between transition regimes and youth unemployment which is low in Denmark and high in Finland and Sweden as far as the universalistic regime is concerned or low in the Netherlands and Austria, medium in Germany and high in France in the employment-centred regime. Obviously, the relationship between economies and transition regimes is not yet fully understood. The rationales of transition regimes and their

Table 11.2 Most important source of income (in %) indicated by young people (15–30) in 2007

	Denmark	Germany	Italy	UK
Regular job	*57*	35	37	56
Benefits	5	6	0	*11*
Allowances/grants	22	13	2	11
Relatives, partner	5	26	*50*	14
Casual work	5	*15*	9	5
Others, don't know	5	4	1	3

Source: Eurobarometer (2007)

differing support mechanisms become more relevant regarding the duration of youth unemployment: long-term unemployment is lower in the countries of the liberal and the universalistic regime types than in those of the employment-centred and the under-institutionalised one (Walther and Pohl 2005). Effects of transition regimes are even more visible in a long-term perspective. If one compares the living situation of young people aged 15–29 according to their main source of income, young people in Denmark display the highest level of independence from their parents and the welfare state. They are those with the highest rate living from own job-related income or from education allowances – which however is not seen as support but as a right. In the UK, the rate of job-related income is similar but welfare dependency is much higher. In Italy, not surprisingly, a majority depends on their parents while Germany holds a position in between (see Table 11.2; Eurobarometer 2007).

This picture suggests that different rationales in regulating youth transitions affect young men's and women's trajectories. This implies that contextual factors intervene with individual decision-making. The next section introduces a biographical perspective on young people's active construction and negotiation of success and support in their transitions to adulthood.

Doing Transitions: Success and Support in Young Men's and Women's Biographies

If one understands youth transitions as a dialectic relationship between the institutional structures of the life course and the agency of individuals constructing their subjective biographies, this implies that institutionalised normalities of success and support are constantly interpreted, negotiated and eventually modified in interaction between individual and institutional actors. Individual agency does not represent linear realisations of subjective wishes and goals but complex processes of compromise and negotiation. According to Alheit und Dausien (2000), the 'latent biographicity of the social' implies that 'there is no mere structural influence which determines directly the individual's reaction but social structure is both constitutive of and constructed by individuals' (p. 410). Most of the existing research on youth transitions focuses either on young people's attitudes, orientations and values with regard to key aspects of adulthood such as work, family and citizenship – which may be referred to as the input-variable of agency – and the outcome-variable of concrete discernible actions: educational investment, occupational choices, family foundation or voting in elections. This perspective leaves out the decision-making processes in between. The obvious discrepancy between young people's wishes and orientations and the actions they actually take indicates that (unequal) structural conditions and contexts are being reworked and negotiated individually or collectively in the course of decision-making which so far has been largely neglected by research on youth transitions.

We situate decision-making in the context of biographical agency. Emirbayer and Mische (1998) conceptualise agency as the

> ... temporally embedded process of social engagement, informed by the past (in its habitual aspect), oriented towards the future (as a capacity to imagine alternative possibilities) and 'acted out' in the present (as a capacity to contextualise past habits and future projects with the contingencies of the moment). (p. 963).

Applying this to the decision-making of young people in their transitions to adulthood, one may argue that situations framed by different or unequal possibilities are evaluated and addressed according to different anticipations and imaginations of the future which in turn are influenced by past experiences. However, inasmuch as the future is increasingly uncertain, it can be anticipated less and less but requires subjective imagination of being a parent or of working in a segmented and potentially precarious labour market. Indeed, the dominance of an 'extended present' in young people's orientations can be read as a deprivation of future. Decisions and actions appear as more reactive because subjective meaning cannot be developed through imaginations of the future but needs to be actualised in the present (Leccardi 2005).

A key dimension of how young people make decisions and act is the *meaning* they give to specific goals and the actions necessary to achieve them. The dimension of meaning is the biographical complement to the institutional notion of *success* in transitions. However, in contrast to assumptions of success which are often taken for granted, the interactionist perspective implies that meaning-making is a constant process embedded in individual (and collective) decision-making and action. One focal point in which the interaction between dominant criteria of success and individual meaning-making is reflected is young people's work orientations. In the YOYO project, young people were asked in qualitative interviews on their work orientations and life plans. Across different contexts, work was associated with both instrumental and self-oriented aspects:

> When I think of work, I see money. (male, 18, Netherlands)

> It has to be a job that I am looking forward to when I wake up in the morning, looking forward to doing my work again, like that. (male, 23, Germany).

In many cases, their accounts mirrored the difficult negotiation between institutional criteria, socio-economic possibilities and subjective meaning:

> I don't mean life without work. But everybody should do what he can and not that I have to do something which I don't want. (male, 18, Germany)

> … that they respect me and pay me when they have to, that they make a legal contract. (female, 16, Spain).

On a more general level, work orientations are related to young people's translations of the normal life course into individual life plans:

> Afford a house, afford food and what you have, afford to put clothes on your kids' back. (male, 17, UK)

Difficulties in achieving the institutionalised status of adulthood are reflected in young people's attempts of reconstructing or 'inventing' adulthood (Henderson et al. 2006) around the notions of responsibility, autonomy and decision-making:

> … making decisions on your own. Assuming responsibility, knowing how to manage yourself. (female, 24, Portugal)
>
> Above all it is a matter of mind… just standing up saying 'here I am' and responding like 'what's up?' (female, 21, Germany)

The biographical meaning-making in transitions to adulthood is related with the process of constructing the own identity. The UP2YOUTH project analysed *how* young people 'do' family, work and citizenship 'differently' by negotiating dominant images with youth cultural styles and symbols and creating new practices. While images and meanings which are institutionalised and/or transmitted by the media constitute powerful forces, they often fail in providing biographical meaning for those who are expected to act within these institutions. It has therefore been argued that much more attention should be paid to the actions young people actually perform and to analyse their implicit meaning rather than focussing on what young people do not do, do not do enough, too early or too late. Especially under conditions of late modernity, it has been suggested that transitions to parenthood, work and citizenship need to allow for *visibility* of the individual person. While this seems obvious in expressive youth cultural lifestyles, under conditions of late modernity, these practices need to be interpreted as reflexive lifestyles and as mobilisation of recognition in concrete individual – and potentially dilemmatic – biographical situations (Walther et al. 2009).

The perspective of biographical agency conceives of decision-making in youth transitions as socially contextualised and interactive. Decision-making in youth transitions is often referred to (both affirmatively and critically) in terms of 'choice'. The assumption of choice as 'constrained' (Folbre 1994) and socially embedded does not mean discarding the concept of choice as such but differentiating between 'free' choice and choice in terms of decision-making – to act or not or feeling forced to choose despite of a lack of meaningful options.

The differences in young people's choices and actions according to socio-economic background, education, gender, ethnicity or labour market structures tend to be interpreted as evidence for the structural determination of young people's agency through *social contexts*. These differences are obvious, e.g. in the coincidence of early pregnancy with low education, or of demotivation for education with low socio-economic status, but they are far from being absolute. While in many cases outcomes of agency appear predictable according to the social position of the actors, the existence of minority constellations and exceptions suggests that also other factors are at work which are mediated with each other in the course of individual decision-making. This means to take into consideration especially those choices which do not fit into dominant concepts of activity: new forms of family and family formation, changing gender relationships including forms of apparent re-traditionalisation against the modern normalities of 'new' motherhood or fatherhood; concepts of work and career beyond existing occupational profiles; or alternative forms of political engagement including the changing meaning of what is political and how individual needs and interests connect with collective affairs in the public. These decision-making processes are far more complex than suggested by deterministic approaches, according to which social positions generate specific actions. Rather than a 'middle ground position' between structure and agency (Woodman 2009), this implies that the focus must lie on understanding and explaining the subjective interpretation and the interactive negotiation of contextual conditions and situations.

Obviously, social contexts provide young people with different resources and opportunities which influence their capabilities of exerting specific choices and actions. Structured choices and the inequality of realising meaningful and successful transitions reflect the possibilities of young men and women in mobilising *support* – either informally from their families and peers or formally from public institutions. Comparative analysis shows that societal institutions 'filter' socio-economic forces to different extent (Blossfeld and Klijzing 2005). This includes different welfare and education systems, family and integration policies and the concrete institutional actors by which they are set into practice. In the YOYO and FATE studies, young people's narratives on their experiences with public institutions reflect the implications of the different transition regimes in terms of realities in which they have to and actually do negotiate their transitions.

In *Denmark* (universalistic), individualised education and welfare option encourage and support young adults in experimenting with yo-yo transitions – as long as they do this within the system. Most young people realise and appreciate this freedom of choice and, as the following quotation shows, are ready to defend this against the expectations of educational institutions:

> It is *my* education, and *I* have to use it for something, so *I* have to work it out ... *it is me* who decides... A lot of students did that: changed their plans. This shows that you have matured and developed ...and then it is good that you can change it. (female, 19, Denmark)

In the *UK* and *Ireland* (liberal), young people apparently have internalised the rationale of the liberal regime of assuming self-responsibility as soon as possible. This reflects experiences of youth unemployment programmes where straight labour market entrance is still the main aim:

> Being on benefits for three years I had begun to lose sight of my personal goals. I was afraid to come off benefits; to go back to work; afraid to set goals, but most of all afraid to fail. (female, 23, UK)

While the underlying frame of normality is not challenged here, education and training options are often criticised as short-term and for their lack of reliable quality standards:

You fill in forms … and then you hear nothing, unless they have a poxy job going where there's no money and you're treated like a slave. (male, 18, Ireland)

In *Germany* (employment-centred), young people have to relate to a rigid occupational structure implying far-reaching decisions regarding their subjective identity. The fact that all those who do not enter regular training directly are classified as disadvantaged due to individual deficits is experienced as soon as they are confronted with the employment service and channelled into remedial schemes. One young woman put the permanent pressure that this creates like this:

In secondary school you get pressure:…. training, training, training; without it you will never make it … Many only because of pressure … take up some vocational training. (female, 21, Germany)

The subjective alienation of these relatively sharp assumptions of what is 'normally' expected of those who need support is reflected by the following statement:

[Employment Service] is an administration after all. They are not in the mood for working. Just staring into your file, going bah, bah, treating you like a cow. (male, 23, Germany)

Finally in *Italy* (under-institutionalised), yo-yo transitions do not develop against dominant assumptions of youth but rather emerge from a social vacuum. One might state that neither choice nor flexibility nor security are provided by the transition system. Depending on the extent of family support, young people try to use the existing spaces for individual trajectories:

We are alone … If you have friends, fine, otherwise … (female, 19, Italy)

The more proactive way of dealing with this 'normality' is not to have any expectations for state support but to believe in one's own inventiveness:

Keeping complaining and day-dreaming about the 'permanent job' seems to me a waste of time … You have to create your job yourself, inventing new professions, considering your own wishes. (female, 21, Italy)

So, these insights into young people's subjective meaning-making of the expectations and structures in the respective transition system show that support in youth transitions does not occur automatically but is transmitted through interaction. Therefore analysing the meaning and effect of support from a biographical perspective implies distinguishing the structural and the interactive dimension of social context in concrete relationships with intermediate institutional actors or with peers and families in everyday life. The analysis of FATE and YOYO interviews suggests that especially relationships with 'significant others' are experienced as supportive, i.e. with persons who are emotionally close, present in everyday life with a high density and frequency of interaction and who are capable of opening options for agency. Symbolic interactionism (Mead 1934) assigns the quality of 'significant others' primarily to family members which is also evidenced by our data – and not only in the context of the under-institutionalised regime:

Most important in terms of support has been, that they [the parents] represented a kind of security net for me, not in the sense of economic and of practical support; but this kind of security net, a general feeling of support, of understanding, of giving good advice and so on. (male, 28, Germany)

Such experiences are associated with *trustful relationships* as a kind of basic support structure. In institutional contexts, this kind of relationships is much more difficult to develop. However, youth workers or social workers who invest an advance of trust in young people may not only become significant others but also represent another type of adult than teachers, employment officers or parents. This ‘otherness’ does not only derive from professional habitus but also from sociocultural orientations relying more on personal authority and trust than on power.

> I can’t talk about certain things with them [parents]... He [the project worker] made me see what it really means to listen to somebody. (female, 21, Italy)
>
> If there is nobody who cares for a person, this person will think automatically that it does not a make a difference whether or not she has a job. That’s what I thought at that time. But then there was the change. I saw there is somebody who cares. (21, female, Germany)

While it is not surprising that peers can be ‘significant others’, especially if sharing important biographical and everyday life experiences, this is not only the case among friends but can also emerge in projects or schemes, primarily if organised in a participatory way:

> We were very supportive of each other all the time. There was a few of us went through different things during the project, you know, outside of work, and suppose everyone was always involved in supporting each other. (female, 19, UK)

A good deal of support young people receive in institutions, schemes and projects may be categorised as *learning*. The dimension of learning in youth transitions is normally limited to knowledge and competencies required by the labour market and/or to qualifications, i.e. to formal learning. However, formal learning is characterised by the double-bind situation of preparing for a future which may never take place. Coping with uncertainty and with disadvantage in youth transitions therefore requires also biographical learning: learning can qualify agency if it contributes to a reflexive recomposition of an individual’s agentic orientations towards the own past (iteration) and future (projectivity) (Biesta and Tedder 2007).

On the one hand, young people learn informally not to trust public institutions while they may also learn ‘by doing’, i.e. experimenting with new practices. In some areas like young parenthood, this has led to a professionalisation of everyday life based on information from a mixture of informal support networks and youth cultures or the Internet. From a pedagogical perspective, this is self-evident as learning is an activity or social practice of the individual learner relating to and appropriating his or her social (and material) context through ‘communities of practice’ (cf. Wenger 1998). On the other hand, this may happen non-formally in the context of youth work or integration schemes where young people have the opportunity of experimenting and reflecting own ideas in a safe environment:

> Nobody should tell you: ‘do this and that’ but it’s you in the first place who has to take decisions... a sort of self-experimentation. We realised that we had made some mistakes during this project but it was nice, even making mistakes, growing up, it was like self-training. (female, 21, Italy)
>
> ... having freedom in choices... having the courage and the self-confidence to stand up and say, ‘this is the choices I want to make and these are the right choices’. (female, project worker, UK)

Young people in these measures develop biographical *reflexivity* (or biographicity, cf. Alheit and Dausien 2000) with regard to their subjective meaning-making and thereby to what they define as success with regard to their own biographical transitions. They take a reflexive attitude towards their goals and possibilities in the process of social positioning – and under conditions of the de-standardisation of the life course, they are more and more forced to do so. Reflexivity however also means that young people's decision-making and coping strategies are not only structured by but contribute to structuring changing patterns of social integration in terms of 'sub-politics' (Beck 1992; cf. Giddens 1984). They learn informally from each other and organise informal networks in terms of both bridging and bonding social capital. This learning and support may not be successful from an institutional perspective but relevant from an individual one such as networks of young parents sharing child care or transport of children or migrant networks, 'ethnic business' and re-ethnicised subcultures.

Success and Support in Transition: Negotiated and Compared

In this chapter, we have tried to enlarge a dominant institutional perspective which reduces success in transitions to work and adulthood to entering the labour market, founding a family and avoiding poverty and which informs policy measures aimed at supporting young people in their transitions to work. First, we have shown that assumptions of success and support held as generally valid actually do differ across different contexts and constellations of youth transitions. Different meanings of youth and disadvantage have been reconstructed as variations in what is referred to as successful transitions while different institutional structures represent different forms of and entitlements to support in coping with transitions to work and adulthood that have become increasingly uncertain and precarious. Second, we have found that successful transitions for them include not only stable and well-paid jobs – although this remains important – but also trajectories they can identify with. The same accounts for support – whether being absent, conditional, ambivalent or universally accessible – which needs always to be made fit into the own biography and its narrative of an agentic self.

While institutional transition structures only are actualised by individual agency, different structural qualities biographically make a difference. Our findings suggest that research which up to now has concentrated on input and output of young people's agency needs to put more stress on analysing the complex interpretation and negotiation processes that underlie individual decision-making. Thereby it may contribute not only to a better understanding of young people's agency but also to the analysis of social change and – through a reflection of what makes successful transitions – its implications for the status of adulthood. These negotiations and struggles about subjectively relevant meanings of success and forms of support reflect the interplay between structure and agency. Inasmuch as structures differ across transition regimes, also these spaces are framed differently. The combination of a biographical and a comparative perspective therefore has a potential of contributing to theorising the relation between structure and agency in youth transitions – or better: the 'spaces between structure and agency' (Settersten and Gannon 2005).

This has also consequences for policy and practice inasmuch as the findings suggest that participatory settings of support are more likely to be experienced as support – as young people can make them fit to their lives and needs. This implies choice and flexibility, trustful relationships, times and spaces for experimenting with own life plans while policy and practice need to be open for negotiating what may be success in the individual case. This implies an increased level of reflexivity of institutional actors concerned with supporting young people in their transitions to adulthood in terms of what Fraser (1989) has termed 'politics of needs interpretation', whereby welfare and the identities of welfare recipients are balanced through participation. This reflexivity seems to be higher in transition regimes centred around the rights of individual citizens. While in the liberal regime the individual is mainly addressed in terms of self-responsibility, the universalistic regime dominant in the Nordic countries seems most advanced in securing support through social rights in balance with recognising the individual.

References

Alheit, P., & Dausien, B. (2000). 'Biographicity' as a basic resource of lifelong learning. In P. Alheit (Ed.), *Lifelong learning inside and outside of schools* (pp. 400–422). Roskilde: Roskilde University/Universität Bremen/Leeds University.

Allmendinger, J. (1989). Educational systems and labour market outcomes. *European Sociological Review, 5*(3), 231–250.

Bechmann Jensen, T., Weltz, C., & Jorgensen, L. (2005). *Denmark. National report for the thematic study on policy measures for disadvantaged youth.* Annex to the final report. Tübingen: IRIS.

Beck, U. (1992). *Risk society. Towards a new modernity*. London: Sage.

Biesta, G., & Tedder, M. (2007). Agency and learning in the life course. Towards an ecological perspective. *Studies in the Education of Adults, 39*(2), 132–149.

Biggart, A. (2005). *Families and transitions in Europe.* Final report of the research project FATE. Coleraine: University of Ulster.

Biggart, A., & Kovacheva, S. (2006). Social change, family support, and young adults in Europe. *New Directions, 113*, 49–61.

Blossfeld, H.-P., Klijzing, E. & Mills, M. (Eds.). (2005). *Globalization, uncertainty and youth in society: The losers in a globalizing world.* London: Routledge.

Emirbayer, M., & Mische, A. (1998). What is agency? *The American Journal of Sociology, 103*(4), 962–1023.

Esping-Andersen, G. (1990). *The three worlds of welfare capitalism.* Princeton: Princeton University Press.

Eurobarometer. (2007). *Young Europeans. A survey among young people aged between 15–30 in the European Union.* Analytical report. Brussels: Eurostat.

European Commission. (2005). *Addressing the concerns of young people in Europe – Implementing the European youth pact and promoting active citizenship.* Communication from the Commission to the Council. Brussels: Commission of the European Communities.

Folbre, N. R. (1994). *Who pays for the kids? Gender and the structures of constraint.* London: Routledge.

Fraser, N. (1989). *Unruly practices. Power, discourse and gender in contemporary social theory*. Minneapolis: University of Minnesota Press.
Furlong, A., & Cartmel, F. (2006). *Young people and social change. Individualization and risk in late modernity* (2nd ed.). Buckingham: Open University Press.
Gallie, D., & Paugam, S. (Eds.). (2000). *Welfare regimes and the experience of unemployment in Europe*. Oxford: Oxford University Press.
Giddens, A. (1984). *The constitution of society. Outline of the theory of structuration*. Cambridge: Polity Press.
Henderson, S., Holland, J., McGrellis, S., Sharpe, S., & Thomson, R. (2006). *Inventing adulthoods – A biographical approach to youth transitions*. London: Sage.
Harsløf, I. (2005). 'Integrative' or 'Defensive' youth activation in nine European welfare *states. Journal of Youth Studies, 8*(4), 461–483.
Kohli, M. (2009). The world we forgot. A historical review of the life course. In W. R. Heinz (Ed.), *The life course reader* (pp. 64–91). Frankfurt am Main: Campus.
Kovacheva, S. (2001). Flexibilisation of youth transitions in Central and Eastern Europe. *Young, 9*(1), 41–60.
Leccardi, C. (2005). Facing uncertainty. Temporality and biographies in the new century. *Young, 13*(2), 123–146.
Leccardi, C., & Rusmini, G. (2004). Life plans. In A. Biggart & D. Cairns (Eds.), *Families and transitions in Europe. Comparative report of qualitative interviews*. Coleraine: University of Ulster.
Lewis, S., & Smithson, J. (2006). *Gender, parenthood and the changing European workplace. Young adults negotiating the work-family boundary*. Final report 5th framework program of the European Union. www.workliferesearch.org/transitions
McNeish, W., & Loncle, P. (2003). State policy and youth unemployment in the EU. Rights, responsibilities and lifelong learning. In A. López Blasco, W. McNeish, & A. Walther (Eds.), *Young people and contradictions of inclusion. Towards integrated transition policies in Europe* (pp. 105–126). Bristol: Policy Press.
Mead, G. H. (1934). *Mind, self & society*. Chicago: University of Chicago Press.
Müller, W., & Gangl, M. (Eds.). (2003). *Transitions from education to work in Europe. The integration of youth on EU labour markets*. Oxford: Oxford University Press.
Os, L. (2002). Denmark. *National report for the families and transitions in Europe project* (Working Paper). Copenhagen: University of Copenhagen.
Pascall, G., & Manning, N. (2000). Gender and social policy. Comparing welfare states in Central and Eastern Europe and the former Soviet Union. *Journal of European Social Policy, 10*(3), 269–296.
Phoenix, A. (2009). De-colonising practices. Negotiating narratives from racialised and gendered experiences of education. *Race Ethnicity and Education, 12*(1), 101–114.
Sainsbury, D. (1999). *Gender and welfare state regimes*. Oxford: Oxford University Press.
Schoon, I., & Silbereisen, R. (Eds.). (2009). *Transitions from school to work. Globalisation, individualisation and patterns of diversity*. Cambridge: Cambridge University Press.
Settersten, R. A., & Gannon, L. (2005). Structure, agency, and the space between. On the challenges and contradictions of a blended view of the life course. In R. Levy, P. Ghisletta, J.-M. LeGoff, D. Spini, & E. Widmer (Eds.), *Towards an interdisciplinary perspective on the life course* (pp. 37–57). London: Elsevier.
Shavit, Y., & Müller, W. (1998). *From school to work. A comparative study of educational qualifications and occupational destinations*. Oxford: Clarendon.
Stauber, B. (2010). *Transitions into parenthood. Expertise for the European family platform*. Download from http.//www.familyplatform.eu/
Stauber, B., & Du Bois-Reymond, M. (2006). Familienbeziehungen im Kontext verlängerter Übergänge. Eine intergenerative Studie aus neun europäischen Ländern. *Zeitschrift für Soziologie der Erziehung und Sozialisation (ZSE), 26*(2), 206–221.
Van Berkel, R., & Hornemann, M. I. (Eds.). (2002). *Active social policies in the EU. Inclusion through participation?* Bristol: Policy Press.

Walther, A. (2006). Regimes of youth transitions. Choice, flexibility and security in young people's experiences across different European contexts. *Young, 14*(1), 119–141.
Walther, A., & Pohl, A. (2005). *Thematic study on policies for disadvantaged youth in Europe.* Final report to the European Commission. Tübingen: IRIS.
Walther, A., du Bois-Reymond, M., & Biggart, A. (Eds.). (2006). *Participation in transition. Motivation of young adults in Europe for learning and working*. Frankfurt a. M: Peter Lang.
Walther, A., Stauber, B., & Pohl, A. (2009). *UP2YOUTH. Youth – Actor of social change.* Final report. Tübingen: IRIS. Download. http.//www.up2youth.org. 1 May 2011.
Wenger, E. (1998). *Communities of practice. Learning, meaning, and identity. Learning in doing*. Cambridge: Cambridge University Press.
Woodman, D. (2009). The mysterious case of the pervasive choice biography. Ulrich Beck, structure/agency, and the middling state of theory in the sociology of youth. *Journal of Youth Studies, 12*(3), 243–256.

Chapter 12
Policies to Support Carers

Frédérique Hoffmann, Manfred Huber, and Ricardo Rodrigues

Introduction

Care provided to older people by their spouses, adult children, relatives or friends, i.e. informal care, remains ever more important today despite all societal transformations, changing demographics and public policies in European countries. Unlike health care, which has been increasingly professionalised and removed from the realm of the family, for the most part, long-term care maintains the characteristics of a 'cottage industry', easily substitutable between the family, the market and the state (Anttonen et al. 2003).

Informal care is frequently unpaid and provided within the household, thus making it difficult to measure both within and across countries. Nevertheless, the OECD (2011) has recently estimated that one in ten persons provides care to older relatives that require help with activities of daily living (ADL).[1] The importance of informal carers to the satisfaction of care needs is further exemplified by the potential financial impact that a reduction in their availability would have on the public expenditure of long-term care (see, e.g. European Commission and ECFIN 2009).

There has been an increased recognition of the need to conciliate the social, economic and financial well-being of carers with that of care recipients and the need to adequately support the former through health and social services. Nonetheless,

[1] Activities of daily living consist of everyday tasks of bathing, dressing, moving around in the house, eating, using the bathroom and controlling bladder and bowel. This personal care may be provided together with medical services, i.e. nursing care, such as medication, wound dressing, palliative care, monitoring of health condition and rehabilitation.

F. Hoffmann (✉) • R. Rodrigues
European Centre for Social Welfare Policy and Research (ECSWPR), Vienna, Austria
e-mail: hoffmann@euro.centre.org; rodrigues@euro.centre.org

M. Huber
World Health Organization (WHO), Copenhagen, Denmark
e-mail: mhu@euro.who.int;

A. Moreno Mínguez (ed.), *Family Well-Being: European Perspectives*,
Social Indicators Research Series 49, DOI 10.1007/978-94-007-4354-0_12,

caregivers are coming under increased pressure, particularly in light of the fact that there is a preference among OECD countries for older people to ‘age in place’, which puts additional pressure on the carer as a result of demographic and societal changes. Indeed in the context of an ‘increased female labour market participation and anxieties about future dependency ratios, the key issue is not so much whether women’s labour market participation threatens the supply of informal care, as whether there is adequate social and financial protection from the labour market-related consequences of providing substantial amounts of informal care’. (Kemp and Glendinning 2006: 135). Furthermore, the post-crises public budget deficit in a number of EU countries suggests that reform of long-term care systems as well as policies to support carers may be postponed or come under threat.

The present chapter will seek to provide an overview of the challenges facing informal carers today and in the near future, while also presenting a critical appraisal of the public policies in place to support them. The questions this chapter tackles are the following: is the current picture of informal caregiving in Europe likely to hold in the future, and how may the different public policies impact carers? In order to answer these questions, we will employ a wide range of sources, including the publication *Facts and Figures on long-term care: Europe and North America* (Huber et al. 2009), which was a part of the United Nations Economic Commission for Europe mandate for the Europe Centre Vienna to monitor the progress of public policies tackling demographic ageing. The first section of this chapter discusses the division of responsibilities between the family and the state in the provision of care and portrays informal caregiving in Europe as being in a state of flux. In the second section, we turn to some of the main policies that exist to support carers, namely cash benefits, care leaves and in-kind benefits, and analyse whether they sufficiently meet the challenges caregivers are faced with. The final section concludes by summarising the main findings and policy trends.

Informal Care in Europe: How Long Can the Current Picture Hold?

The Profile of Informal Carers in Europe

Although some of the dependent old-age people facing more complex care needs receive elaborate care, most are in need of help with tasks that, although fundamental for their well-being or independent living (such as eating or personal hygiene), do not necessarily involve a great degree of complexity. What is more, unlike the case of health care, the quality of care provided by informal carers does not necessarily have to compare unfavourably with formal care services (Jensen 2008). In part, this arises from the fact that long-term care encompasses the bonding between the carer and the person cared for (e.g. Himmelweit 1999; Jochimsen 2003). Such factors illustrate why informal care can more easily substitute for the state or the market in the long-term care system and therefore remain the backbone of care across Europe and beyond.

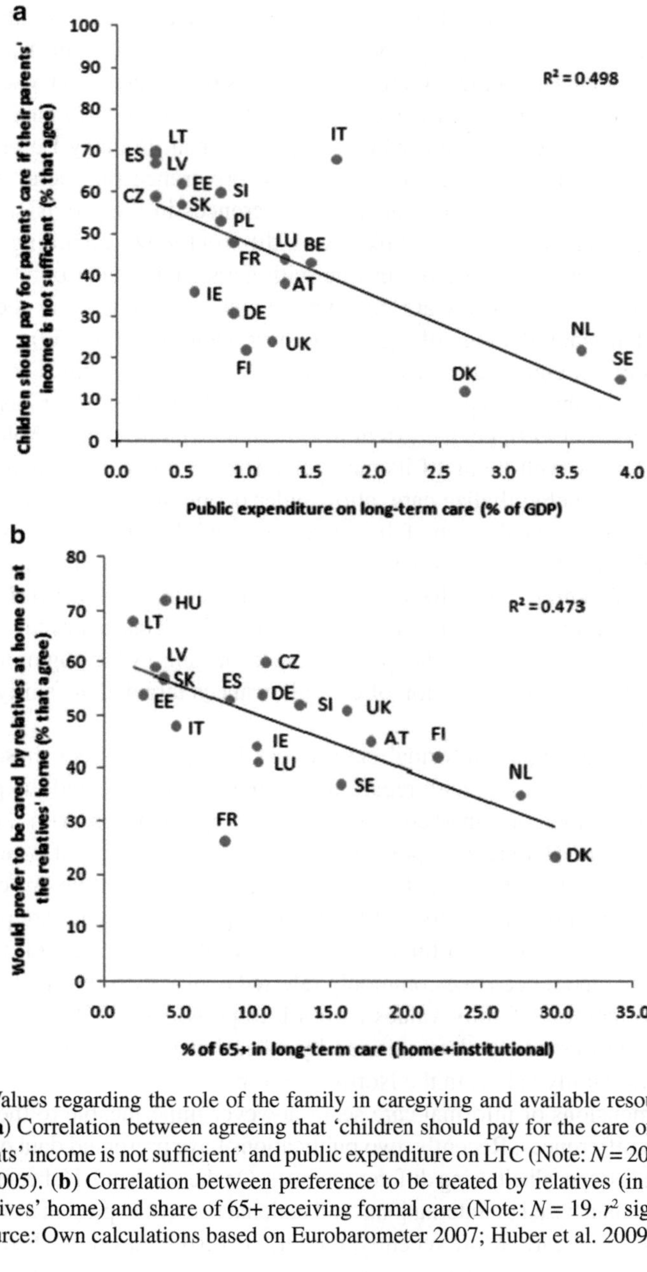

Fig. 12.1 Values regarding the role of the family in caregiving and available resources in long-term care. (**a**) Correlation between agreeing that 'children should pay for the care of their parents if their parents' income is not sufficient' and public expenditure on LTC (Note: $N = 20$. r^2 significant at a $p < 0.0005$). (**b**) Correlation between preference to be treated by relatives (in own home or in their relatives' home) and share of 65+ receiving formal care (Note: $N = 19$. r^2 significant at a $p < 0.05$) (Source: Own calculations based on Eurobarometer 2007; Huber et al. 2009)

Using a recent Eurobarometer survey on Europeans' attitudes and views regarding long-term care (Eurobarometer 2007) and comparing some of the responses with data on available care services or public expenditure on long-term care (Huber et al. 2009), both sources demonstrate interesting correlations between the perceived role of the family and the resources devoted to long-term care (Fig. 12.1). Thus, taking the statement 'children should pay for the care of their parents if their parents' income is not sufficient' as a sign of stronger family values, countries where the share of respondents agreeing with this statement is higher are also those where the state devotes less resources (in percentage of GDP) to long-term care. Similarly, although the preference for informal care is predominant in many European countries, there is a negative correlation between this preference and the availability of long-term care services. It thus seems that differences in the provision of formal care in Europe may somewhat be linked with different views regarding the role of the family in meeting care needs, in line with Carsten Jensen's point that social services such as long-term care are 'much more conformable to other social forces, such as the dominant ideology of a given country' (Jensen 2008: 159).

Furthermore, country differences may also reflect dissimilarities in the policy settings across countries, in particular the degree of 'defamilialization' as coined by Esping-Andersen (1999), i.e. the extent to which the welfare system holds families responsible for the well-being of its members. Thus, welfare systems that provide care services, i.e. defamilialize care, allow older people to become independent of their families for the satisfaction of their care needs, while simultaneously providing family members with enhanced possibilities to be employed in the labour market. The opposite, meaning familialization or the strengthening of the traditional caring role of the family, may also be pursued by public policies. This can occur 'implicitly' when formal care services and other public benefits are simply lacking or 'explicitly', for example, through the provision of care allowances targeted at family members (Leitner 2003).

One could thus expect informal care across Europe to reflect these different attitudes and values. In fact with regard to the intensity of care and the prevalence of informal care, there are marked differences among countries, with a number of studies based on SHARE data pointing towards the existence of a north–south gradient (Bolin et al. 2008; OECD 2011). Therefore more people are engaged in informal care in Northern Europe but higher average hours of care are provided in Southern European countries (Table 12.1). This would be in line with the portrait depicted above, and indeed one commonly referred explanation for these differences has been the nature of family values across Europe (Reher 1998), with Southern European countries being characterised by 'ties that bind' as opposed to more individualistic family values in the North of Europe.

Other dimensions of informal care seem however impermeable to these alleged value-driven differences. Recently, two publications have presented data on informal caregiving in Europe, albeit using different sources. On the one hand, Huber et al. (2009) have gathered data based on international and national sources to present a comparative picture of informal care. More recently, the OECD (2011) has published indicators on informal care based on the European Survey on Health and Ageing (SHARE) and national household surveys in the UK. Both reveal a strong gender dimension in the provision of informal care. Women constitute the majority of carers, particularly among the 45–64 age groups where most informal carers are concentrated, and they also seem to shoulder a disproportionate share of the heavier care tasks

Table 12.1 Prevalence and intensity (number of hours) of informal care among 50+ in Europe

	Providing informal care				Weekly hours of informal care (for those providing informal care)			
	Men		Women		Men		Women	
	Mean	SD	Mean	SD	Mean	SD	Mean	SD
Austria	0.31	0.46	0.26	0.44	6.65	13.63	11.29	20.47
Germany	0.39	0.49	0.31	0.46	5.48	13.72	8.17	20.26
Sweden	0.44	0.50	0.39	0.49	3.32	8.33	3.98	9.64
The Netherlands	0.44	0.50	0.40	0.49	5.40	17.18	7.00	17.56
Spain	0.14	0.35	0.17	0.38	12.10	22.87	22.99	34.19
Italy	0.25	0.43	0.25	0.43	9.10	20.17	19.96	35.31
France	0.30	0.46	0.26	0.44	4.56	9.34	9.21	18.39
Denmark	0.50	0.50	0.41	0.49	3.60	9.21	4.30	9.15
Greece	0.15	0.36	0.19	0.39	6.21	15.11	15.40	25.59
Switzerland	0.32	0.47	0.32	0.47	4.22	13.28	6.57	14.72
Belgium	0.42	0.49	0.39	0.49	6.28	17.19	8.84	21.60
Czech Republic	0.32	0.46	0.33	0.47	9.94	20.70	11.74	23.92
Poland	0.20	0.40	0.17	0.38	5.81	14.13	15.33	30.13

Source: Own calculations based on SHARE data (2nd wave)
Notes: Weighted results
SD standard deviation

(Huber et al. 2009). The predominance of women as informal carers is a common feature across Europe, regardless of the characteristics of the welfare system. Although the share of informal carers is higher among women of working age, this picture is inverted among carers aged 65 and older, where men have a greater probability of providing informal care (OECD 2011). The gender dimension of care thus seems to shift with age.

Informal care may however be more complex than the above portrait, and the impact of other factors in explaining country differences in informal care should not be ruled out, namely the role played by different living arrangements and public policies. Glaser et al. (2004) and Dykstra and Fokkema (2011), for example, argue that differences in the provision of informal care between countries hide more than simple cultural differences. Demographics and living arrangements are as likely to impact informal care provision. For example, the intensity of caregiving seems to be correlated with differences in the provision of informal care to co-resident or non-co-resident relatives (Huber et al. 2009).

Regarding the higher probability of older men providing care, Del Bono et al. (2009) present contrasting evidence for the UK, highlighting again the importance of living arrangements. According to their research, differences in the provision of informal care among older carers simply reflect gender differences in marital status: married persons are more likely to provide care and men are more likely to be married at later stages of their lives. After controlling for household size, health and marital status, older women continue to have a higher chance of providing informal care and provide on average more hours of care.

A Preview of Future Informal Care

The current picture of informal care may also be changing, and informal caregiving as depicted above may be in a state of flux as demographic and societal pressures are likely to bring about changes in the profile of caregivers.

Demography will most likely impact the profile of informal carers through the reduction in the support ratio of the oldest old, i.e. the ratio of those aged 45–65 to those aged 80 or older (Table 12.2). Although there is some degree of discretion in building such indicators (Robine et al. 2007), it nevertheless provides a striking indication of the reduction in the number of people that nowadays make up for a large share of informal carers in comparison to those who stand a higher chance of needing care.[2] Furthermore, as fertility rates have plummeted, this suggests that informal care tasks will most likely be shouldered by fewer adult children, which could deprive them from the benefits of sharing care tasks that being part of a wider caring network encompasses (Tolkacheva et al. 2011). This is likely to be further exacerbated by the increased participation of women in the labour market, which could lead, to some extent, to a greater commodification of care as some of the employment gains among women could come from jobs created in the care services (Rodrigues and Schmidt 2010).

A possible outcome could be that informal carers will themselves become increasingly older and spouses will take up some of the care provided nowadays by daughters and daughters-in-law of working age. However, this replacement effect could be mitigated if past trends observed in living arrangements of older people continue to hold, for example, if more older people live alone (Huber et al. 2009). As carers become older, this might also raise issues regarding the extent to which their health condition will allow them to care for their spouses and the effects that caring could have on their well-being and health.

Another potential transformation derived from the changes in demographics and living arrangements could be the emergence of new types of solidarity beyond the duties of kinship (Rodrigues and Schmidt 2010) or shifts in the apparent nature of familialism in some welfare states.

Francesca Bettio and colleagues (Bettio et al. 2006) and Annamaria Simonazzi (2009) point towards such transformations occurring in the Southern European countries. Using Italy as an example, Bettio et al. (2006) argue that 'female migrants met unsatisfied needs for care while ensuring the continuity of a family-based long-term care model' (p. 278). Migrant carers are perceived by families as a cost-effective solution that facilitates the conciliation of family responsibilities towards older relatives and the employment aspirations of family carers. In Italy at least, the sheer number of migrant workers that applied for the regularisation procedure attest

[2] One important caveat to this concerns the uncertainties surrounding the evolution of disability trends in old age, which would impact the number of dependent older people and the health status of older carers.

Table 12.2 Evolution of support ratio and female employment rates

	Support ratio (45–64/80+)			Female employment rates (15–64)		
	1990	2010	2030	1990	2000	2010
Austria	6.47	5.59	3.81	–	59.7	66.4
Belgium	6.52	5.46	3.90	40.8	51.9	56.5
Bulgaria	11.61	7.27	4.54	–	47.2	56.4
Cyprus	8.10	8.51	4.76	–	53	63
Czech Republic	8.94	7.68	4.59	–	56.8	56.3
Denmark	6.03	6.54	3.53	70.7	72.1	71.1
Estonia	9.33	6.32	4.25	–	57.2	60.6
Finland	7.84	6.23	2.95	–	65.2	66.9
France	–	4.99	3.27	50.9	54.8	59.9
Germany	6.95	5.46	3.31	54	57.8	66.1
Greece	8.32	5.63	4.42	37.5	41.8	48.1
Hungary	9.49	6.71	4.76	–	49.4	50.6
Ireland	8.09	8.17	5.63	35.5	53.2	56
Italy	7.72	4.63	3.52	36.4	39.3	46.1
Latvia	9.00	6.63	4.57	–	53.3	59.4
Lithuania	8.47	7.04	4.78	–	58.2	58.7
Luxembourg	7.76	7.11	5.42	41.4	50	57.2
Malta	10.36	8.59	3.42	–	33.4	39.2
Netherlands	7.19	7.13	3.49	46.7	63.4	69.3
Poland	10.06	8.31	5.11	–	49.3	53
Portugal	9.07	5.79	4.20	53.3	60.5	61.1
Romania	13.11	7.98	6.19	–	59	52
Slovakia	9.50	9.76	6.44	–	51.1	52.3
Slovenia	10.32	7.14	4.56	–	58.5	62.6
Spain	7.66	5.11	4.44	30.7	41.2	52.3
Sweden	5.24	4.87	3.16	–	69.7	70.3
United Kingdom	5.97	5.49	3.54	61.7	64.5	64.6

Source: Eurostat

to their importance for the provision of care (see Bettio et al. 2006: table 4). It seems therefore that the face of informal care in countries with a more familialistic approach to care is changing towards a greater reliance on migrant carers, and such carers also make for a substantial part of care provided in countries such as Germany and Austria (Simonazzi 2009).

Public Policies to Support Carers

It is not only the profile of informal carers that is currently undergoing transformation. Public policies on long-term care have also changed as governments have begun to realise the pivotal role that carers play within our society and their potential contribution to the fiscal sustainability of long-term care systems. As a result, addressing the needs of carers and recognising them as key stakeholders have been one of the defining characteristics of recent policy developments in long-term care. These policies have been developed along the following broad lines:

- Providing cash benefits to carers, thereby at least partly compensating their foregone income
- Recognising their role as carers, for instance, by setting up services aimed at facilitating their caring tasks (e.g. counselling, respite care, day centres, etc.)
- Providing carers with leaves that could, to some extent, improve the conciliation of their care tasks with gainful employment

In view of this, what policies are in place – and how much do they vary across Europe and impact carers – and to what extent do they support caregivers in the critical role they perform in society? The analysis is very much policy oriented and takes on a comparative view, focusing mostly on countries of the European Union.

(a) Providing Cash to Carers

One set of policies aimed at supporting carers that has gained momentum in recent years has been cash-for-care benefits. The latter are either paid directly to carers in the form of care allowances or to those in need of care with attendance allowances, which may then be used to compensate informal carers. The increasing role that these benefits play goes hand in hand with the development of policies aimed at increasing user choice in access to long-term care, as informal care becomes one of the 'options' available for those in need of care.

But this development also has a clear 'cost containment' motivation. Supporting informal care or the family in their traditional caregiving role may be seen as a cheaper option for the public purse, even if from a societal point of view it may be more expensive to have people out of the labour market. The amount of social benefits available to family carers is usually small in relation to the cost of providing professional care services – as Fig. 12.2 depicts, the average amount of these benefits in many countries is inferior to 30% of the average wage. Some of the cash benefits available to those in need of care provide lower amounts if informal care is the selected option (e.g. in the case of Germany or the Dutch Personal Budget), thus discounting for overhead costs. Nevertheless, they may still be sufficient to maintain dependent people in their homes if no severe disability arises, which in turn avoids or considerably reduces the expensive admission into institutional care (OECD 2005). This goes hand in hand with the preference for older people to 'age in place', which can nevertheless not occur at the expense of the carer's financial and physical well-being.

However clear the trend towards providing *cash for care* may be, such policies may involve trade-offs that policymakers ought to bear in mind when weighing in their options. One of these is to balance the financial support for carers while limiting

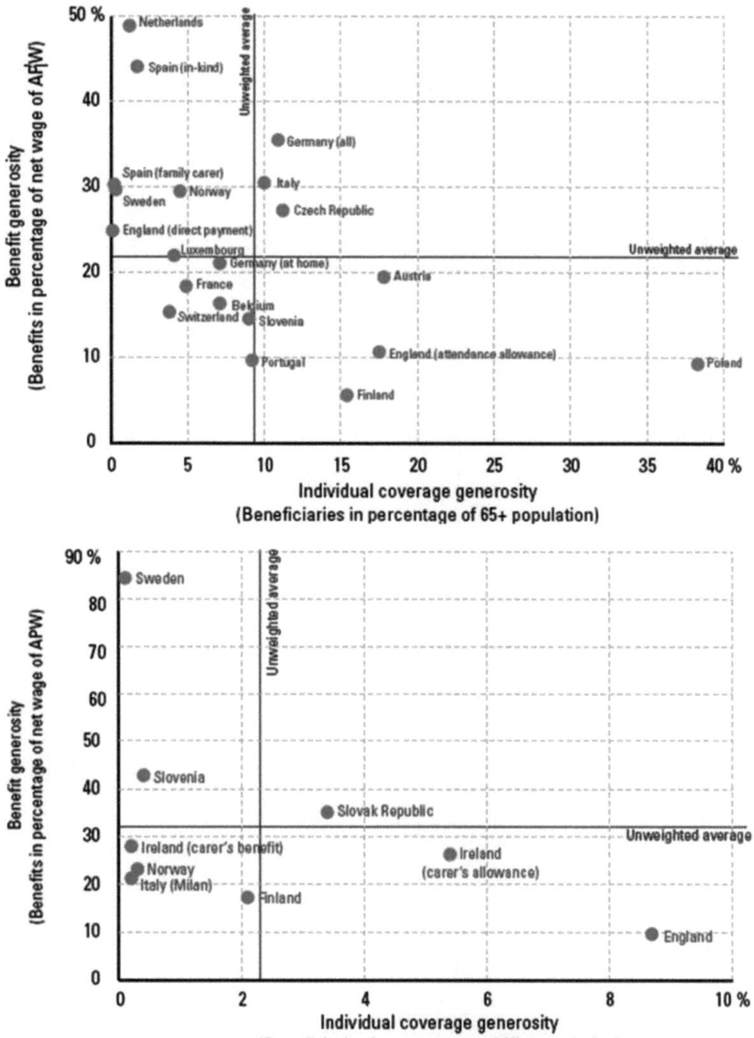

Fig. 12.2 Providing cash to carers. Relative generosity of cash benefits (care allowances and attendance allowances) from which carers may benefit (Source: Reproduced with authorization from Huber et al. 2009: 115–116)

the disincentives to gainful employment and the impact of cash benefits on the labour supply of carers. Balancing the goals of the European Commission's 2020 Strategy on employment while supporting informal carers need not be conflicting social policy objectives, but their conciliation may prove challenging. In countries where care allowances are in place, these usually come with the condition that caring becomes a full-time activity, or close to one (Table 12.3).

Table 12.3 Hurdles in the conciliation of care allowances with employment

Country	Benefit	Means testing	Other benefits	Limitations on paid or full-time employment
Ireland	Carer's allowance	Yes		Full-time care required (cannot be accumulated with more than 10 h employment/training per week)
Ireland	Carer's benefit	No	Supplement benefit for children.	Full-time care required (cannot be accumulated with more than 10 h employment/training per week) Maximum duration of 65 weeks
Finland	Care allowance or informal care allowance/ support for informal care	No	Leave and support services to relatives Respite care (2 days per month) Pension credits (limited) and accident insurance Quasi-contract	May be accumulated with paid work
Luxembourg	Carer's allowance	No	Pension credits (based on minimum wage) Paid social contributions Respite care	Minimum of 50 h per month of care is needed No cash benefit
Norway	Care wage (*Omsorgs-lønn*)	No	Below average pension credits. Post-care-giving pension. Contract.	Usually limited to 3–10 h weekly Exceptional use (burdensome care)
Slovenia	Home care assistance or family attendant	No	Pension credits Unemployment benefit Parental insurance Paid social contributions	Carer must be unemployed or working part time
Slovak Republic	Care allowance	Yes		May be accumulated with paid work up to 2 times the national subsistence minimum
Sweden	Carer's salary (*Anstälda anhørige*)	No	Full social protection Contract	Exceptional use
UK	Carer's allowance	Yes	Pension credits Supplement benefit for children Increased social benefits	Minimum threshold of care given is 35 h weekly Carer cannot be in full-time education (more than 21 h weekly of education)

Source: Reproduced with authorization from Huber et al. (2009): 83

Another dilemma policymakers may face is between providing relatively unregulated cash benefits (i.e. where little proof is required on how the money is spent) that may be seen as an empowerment tool for users. It may also have administrative advantages by saving on paperwork and inspections. However, it can also facilitate the creation of informal markets for the provision of care. This may well be one of the factors behind the growth of undocumented carers in the aforementioned cases of Italy, Austria and to a certain extent Germany (Da Roit and Le Bihan 2010). Even though the benefits may be small in value in their national context, existing wage gaps may make them attractive to migrant carers. On the other hand, some of the constraints such as excluding the employment or payment of close relatives may result in a reduced benefit take-up as preferred care options such as care provided by the spouse are excluded. This might be one of the reasons for the low take-up of Direct Payments by older people as in the case of England, for example (Glendinning 2008).

Cash benefits may also risk trapping caregivers and in particular women in a socially precarious and many times unwanted care role. Referring to the concept of familialism as mentioned earlier, critics of cash for care argue against these policies as a move towards a 'refamiliarisation' of care (see Kröger and Silipa 2005), i.e. a move towards the retrenchment of the role of the state which may harm families and in particular women. This trend occurs within the context of 'an increasing demand for caring labour and a shrinking supply of those who have traditionally provided it' (Ungerson and Yeandle 2007).

It remains however a complex issue, since cash-for-care benefits also represent the recognition of the role and importance of informal carers and may contribute to the improvement of their social status and well-being, as some of these benefits also entitle informal carers to pension credits or sickness insurance. However, given the strong gender dimension attached to the issue of cash for care, gender mainstreaming concerns seem to be conspicuously absent from the design of these benefits.

Another point against the provision of cash benefits to family carers relies on a much more nearsighted argument: that of (supposed) economic efficiency. Under this reasoning, close relatives should be precluded from receiving cash benefits since this would suggest paying for care that they would likely do anyway. This policy stance, however, risks overburdening carers even more and may lead to the further reduced availability of carers in the future.

(b) Providing Services to Carers

Although cash benefits can play a critical role for carers, it can also be argued that it is not the best way to alleviate their burden since it does not preclude the carer from performing his/her tasks to support the care recipient.

The intensity of their care tasks may preclude carers from enjoying sufficient leisure time, and the provision of long hours of care at home of the care recipient could easily isolate carers from their social environment. As a result of feeling

Table 12.4 United in diversity – limited availability of respite care across Europe

Country		Year	Available beds or beneficiaries in percentage of the 65+ (%)
Denmark	[a]	2007	0.3
Germany	[b]	2007	0.1
Ireland	[a, b]	2004	0.2
Netherlands		2003	1.4
Norway	[c]	2006	0.1
Spain	[a, b, d]	2006	0.1
Spain (day-care centres)	[a, b]	2006	0.7
Switzerland	[b]	2006	1.4
Sweden		2006	0.6
UK		2005/2006	0.6

Source: Statistics Denmark (StatBank), Statistics Norway (StatBank), IMSERSO, CBS (Statline), Federal Ministry of Health (Germany), The Information Centre (Social Care Statistics), Department for Health and Children (Ireland), Swiss Federal Statistical Office and the National Board of Health and Welfare (Sweden)
Notes: [a]Number of places
[b]May include people younger than 65
[c]Age group is 67 and older
[d]Information is not available for all regions

socially excluded, many carers experience feelings of isolation, psychological distress including anxiety, depression and/or loss of self-esteem. The findings from a number of studies in the UK show that carers have more difficulties accessing primary care and may be more prone to suffer from ill health (Ross et al. 2008; Schulz and Martire 2004; Pinquart and Sorenson 2003; Navaie-Waliser et al. 2002; Vitaliano et al. 2003).

Social and health services targeted for family carers themselves are therefore equally important if many times overlooked. Respite care allows informal carers to take a break from their care duties, thus reducing the risk of burnout and improving their chances of maintaining sound mental health. Still, the availability of respite care is low across Europe, even in countries which have otherwise a relatively high provision of care services, as it may require a greater degree of flexibility in the delivery of care by providers (Table 12.4). Even when available, the take-up of respite care may be reduced because of lack of information, because of relatively high costs or because family members may find the temporary placement in a short-term institution to be too disruptive for the care recipient, particularly those with dementia.

The relevance of respite care and preventive health care measures may become even more higher as carers age and especially if older people are to become the main carers of their older counterparts. According to a study carried out in the UK (Doran et al. 2003), a substantial number of carers were aged 85 or older; more than half of these were providing at least 50 h of care a week; and one-third of these heavily burdened carers rated their health as 'not good' – a picture that may become more common with demographic ageing. For middle-aged carers – the so-called pivot generation – the challenge is how to conciliate caring responsibilities for their own children and their dependent older people. One of the consequences could be an increase in absenteeism from work or presenteeism – being at work even though one is sick. The latter could be associated with the lack of appropriate leave arrangements for carers that conciliate informal care with employment.

(c) Providing Care Leaves to Carers

According to the recent OECD publication (2011: 124), a greater proportion of companies offer care leave to their employees in Scandinavian countries and in Poland (60% on average), while a much smaller fraction is found in Southern Europe (around 25%). Some of the reasons include the fear of not being promoted; work would not permit it as well as not wanting to appear as an unreliable colleague. A survey in the Netherlands illustrated how only a small proportion of people had made use of leave to care for other family members: most people taking time off for an emergency took annual leave or leave accrued in lieu of pay and a small number (about 5%) reported ill themselves to justify taking emergency leave (Portegijs et al. 2006). Respite care is not the only service likely to impact positively on informal carers. Day-care centres may also ease the burden of care on family members and so can other home care services. However, there remains a huge variety in access across Europe, and even within regions of a country. For instance in 'northern European countries, Spain or the United Kingdom, municipalities are in charge of organising respite care particularly in the case of day-care and in-home respite, which leads to large local disparities in access and availability' (OECD 2011: 129) (Fig. 12.3).

As discussed above, in Northern Europe where the provision of home care services is higher, more family members seem to be able to provide informal care by limiting it to less demanding tasks (instrumental activities of daily living such as household chores) and thus limiting the feeling of overdependence of older relatives on their family for care – Figure X. Therefore, to some degree, both the amount and type of services offered by the formal sector will influence the type of care needed by the care recipient from his/her relatives. Indeed the most recent empirical evidence suggests that the availability of home care services may reshape the type of informal care provided towards less burdensome domestic help (Bonsang 2009) (Fig. 12.4).

There is a strong case for conciliating support for informal carers while investing in formal care services, for 'if anything the evidence points to family carers providing rather more hours of care when formal services are provided as well' (OECD 2005: 45). However, recent policy developments show contradicting signs on this matter. In the Netherlands, the concept of 'usual care' has been introduced in the assessment

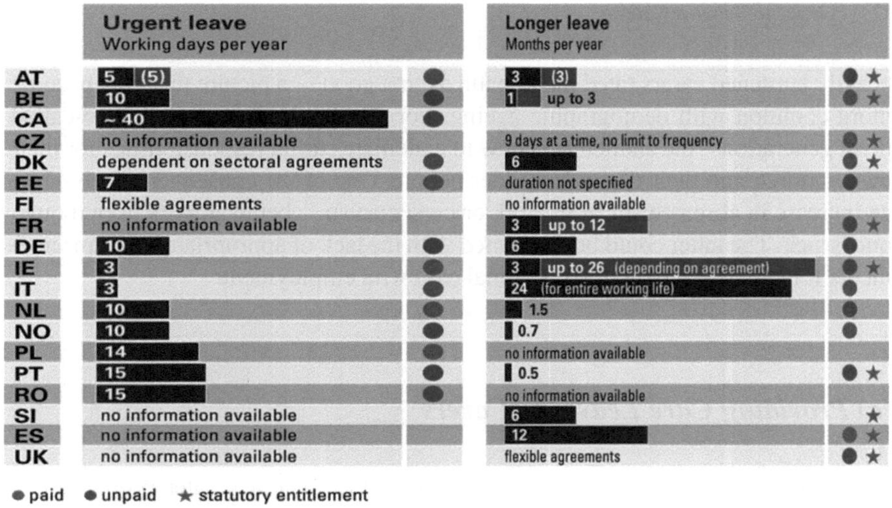

Fig. 12.3 Overview of care leaves in Europe: united in diversity (Source: Statistics Denmark (StatBank), Statistics Norway (StatBank), IMSERSO, CBS (Statline), Federal Ministry of Health (Germany), The Information Centre (Social Care Statistics), Department for Health and Children (Ireland), Swiss Federal Statistical Office and the National Board of Health and Welfare (Sweden), Council of Europe (2009) 'Reconciliation of work and family life', retrieved from Family Policy Database at [www.coe.int/familypolicy/database], MISSOC tables (2009), retrieved from European Commission Website, National sources, Department of Labour, New Zealand, Website: http://www.dol.govt.nz/PDFs/research-parental-leave-international.pdf)

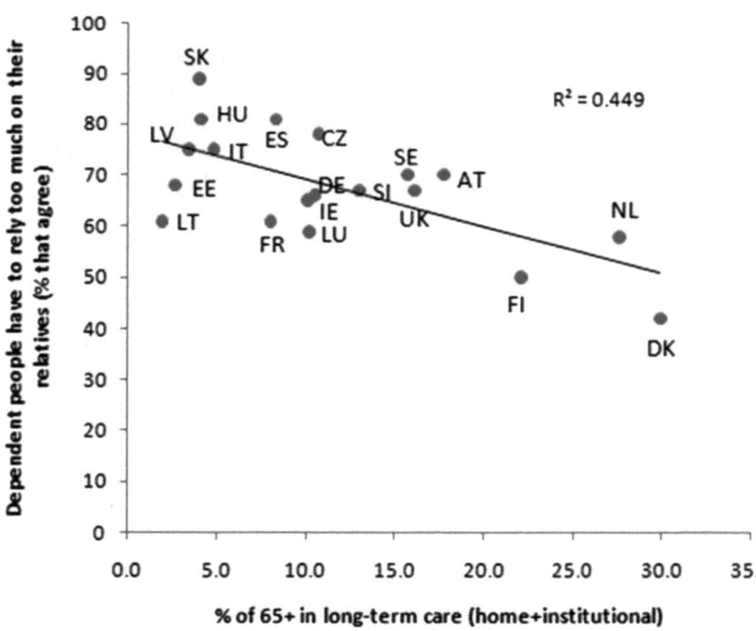

Fig. 12.4 Overburdened carers? Correlation between agreeing that 'dependent people have to rely too much on their relatives' and public expenditure on LTC (Note: $N = 19$. r^2 significant at a $p < 0.05$) (Source: Own calculations based on Eurobarometer 2007; Huber et al. 2009)

of eligibility for home care services, which effectively implies that those closest to the person affected – most likely the partner and/or children of the dependent – are expected to provide the necessary care. Pijl and Ramakers remark that the 'provision of unpaid care by relatives was becoming a formal expectation of the agencies that allocate support to care users' (Pijl and Ramakers 2007). The policy trend observed in some countries towards targeting services to those more in need of care (e.g. in England and Sweden) may also leave some tasks to be carried out by informal carers alone. Aside from their exclusion from the labour market, there remains the equally distressing exclusion from their community and social networks which can be highly detrimental to their mental health in particular. This is particularly the case for migrant carers who as well as living far from their home environment are most often also socially excluded in the country where they currently live.

Several carers' associations across Europe have themselves established websites and hotlines that help carers navigate through the complexity of care systems. ICT-based services have the potential to increase informal carers' quality of life, the quality of care provided as well as to improve family caregiver's social inclusion and integration into the labour market. A number of ICT-based initiatives exist to contribute to improving the quality of care through the caregiver – mainly in the form of ICT-based training, information or professional support from a call centre. Such services may seem rather simple and obvious but nonetheless may play an important role in skilling family caregivers and preparing them better for their – often unexpected and sudden – duties. ICT-based services to support family caregivers and privately employed care assistants at emotional level and with their caregiving tasks have the potential to render an important contribution to improve carers' quality of life. In addition, training and information support may have an impact on the quality of care provided to the dependent older person. Andrea Schmidt et al., for example, point to the Swedish initiative *Anhörigstödsportalen (Family Care Support Portal)* that allows family caregivers to keep an electronic diary, send messages to family care support centre staff directly and keep themselves informed about support activities in the municipality on a regular basis. Also, the service allows them to make a booking request for a respite care stay of the older person, thus contributing to an increased participation of caregivers, for example, in the labour market (Schmidt et al. 2011).

Less burdensome care could also help mitigate the possible trade-off between care and employment faced by informal carers. Supplementing informal care with formal care services at home could thus prove to be the best way of striking a balance between fulfilling the employment goals of the Europe 2020 Strategy which aims to have 75% of the population aged 20–64 in employment, while ensuring that informal care remains available. While juggling employment with caring responsibilities can be daunting, remaining in paid work can also have a positive impact on carers as it provides income and pension rights, helps to maintain social networks, offers a temporary relief from their caring role, enhances self-esteem and offers the opportunity to share concerns with colleagues in a similar situation.

Conclusions

Public policies are a main driver of the provision of informal care, shaping not only the availability but also the intensity of care provided by informal carers in Europe. Given the high degree of substitutability between formal and informal care for some levels of care need, informal care bridges the gaps in the provision of formal care. However this should not necessarily imply complete substitutability between the two, for home care services can act as a supplement to informal care and actually allow for more people to be engaged in informal care albeit in less demanding care tasks.

Public policies may also impact informal care through the provision of cash benefits that are very often seen as a way of reinforcing the role of the family as providers of welfare. Furthermore, depending on the restrictions attached to the use of cash benefits as well as the availability and affordability of other care options, cash benefits might also contribute to the creation of grey markets of care. This might be changing the profile of informal caregiving in the south of Europe as the role of relatives as caregivers has given way to care provided in-house by migrant carers.

Although public policies are of high relevance, they remain nonetheless one of several factors impacting informal care, together with demographics and living arrangements of older people. In fact, the current picture of informal care may be in a state of flux driven precisely by changes in demographics, living arrangements and the labour market participation of women of working age that today make up a substantial part of informal carers. While it is difficult to predict the exact profile of informal carers in the future, it appears highly probable that on average they will be older, possibly already retired and themselves facing health problems. Spouses or friends may replace daughters or daughters-in-law of working age as the main caregivers.

Although governments have gradually recognised the critical role played by carers, current policies may not be particularly well suited to accommodate for changes in the profile of informal carers. While cash benefits may be used by households to acquire care services in the market to relieve carers from more burdensome care tasks, it is not altogether clear that providing cash has resulted in the development of formal care services. Moreover, many of the care benefits provided directly to carers seem to be tailored to carers of working age, or even explicitly limited to those below 65 years of age. Respite care – which allows carers to maintain their mental health or access mainstream health care services, which are fundamentally important for caregivers that are themselves already old – remains marginal across Europe. In conclusion, there seems to be a potential mismatch between the design of policies that are in place today to support carers and the potentially changing landscape of informal caregiving in the future.

References

Anttonen, A., Sipilä, L., & Baldock, J. (2003). Patterns of social care in five industrial societies: Explaining diversity. In A. Anttonen, J. Baldock, & J. Sipilä (Eds.), *The young, the old, and the state* (pp. 167–177). Cheltenham/London: Edward Elgar.

Bettio, F., Simonazzi, A., & Villa, P. (2006). Change in care regimes and female migration: The 'care drain' in the Mediterranean. *Journal of European Social Policy, 16*, 271.
Bolin, K., Lindgren, B., & Lundborg, P. (2008). Informal and formal care among single-living elderly in Europe. *Health Economics, 17*, 393–409.
Bono, E., Del Sala, E., & Hancock, R. (2009). Older carers in the UK: Are there really gender differences? New analysis of the individual sample of anonymised records from the 2001 UK. *Census Health and Social Care in the Community, 17*(3), 267–273.
Bonsang, E. (2009). Does informal care from children to their elderly parents substitute for formal care in Europe? *Journal of Health Economics, 28*(1), 143–154.
Da Roit, B., & Le Bihan, B. (2010). Similar and yet so different: Cash-for-care in six European countries long-term care policies. *The Milbank Quarterly, 88*(3), 286–309.
Doran, T., Drever, F., & Whitehead, M. (2003). Health of young and elderly informal carers: Analysis of UK census data. *British Medical Journal, 327*, 1388. Available at: http://www.bmj.com/cgi/reprint/327/7428/1388
Dykstra, P. A., & Fokkema, T. (2011). Relationships between parents and their adult children: A West European typology of late-life families. *Ageing & Society, 31*, 545–569. Cambridge University Press.
Esping-Andersen, G. (1999). *Social foundations of post-industrial economies*. Oxford: Oxford University Press.
Eurobarometer. (2007). *Health and long-term care in the European Union* (Special Eurobarometer 283). European Commission. Available at: http://ec.europa.eu/public_opinion/archives/ebs/ebs_283_en.pdf
European Commission, ECFIN. (2009). *The 2009 ageing report: Economic and budgetary projections for the EU-27 member states* (2008–2060) (European Economy, No 2/2009). Brussels. Available at: http://ec.europa.eu/economy_finance/publications/publication14992_en.pdf
Glaser, K., Tomassini, C., & Grundy, E. (2004). Revisiting convergence and divergence: Support for older people in Europe. *European Journal of Ageing, 1*, 64–72.
Glendinning, C. (2008). Increasing choice and control for older and disabled people: A critical review of new developments in England. *Social Policy & Administration, 42*(5), 451–469.
Himmelweit, S. (1999). Caring labor. *The Annals of the American Academy of Political and Social Science, 561*, 27–38.
Huber, M., Rodrigues, R., Hoffmann, F., Gasior, K., & Marin, B. (2009). *Facts and figures on long-term care – Europe and north America*. Vienna: European Centre for Social Welfare Policy and Research.
Jensen, C. (2008). Worlds of welfare services and transfers'. *Journal of European Social Policy, 18*(2), 151–162.
Jochimsen, M. A. (2003). *Careful economics. Integrating caring activities and economic science*. Dordrecht: Kluwer Academic Publishers.
Kemp, P. A., & Glendinning, C. (2006). Introduction. In C. Glendinning & P. A. Kemp (Eds.), *Cash and care: Policy challenges in the welfare state*. Bristol: Policy Press.
Kröger, T., & Silipa, J. (2005). *Overstretched European families up against the demands of work and care*. Oxford: Blackwell.
Leitner, S. (2003). Varieties of familialism: The caring function of the family in comparative perspective'. *European Societies, 5*(4), 353–375.
Navaie-Waliser, M., Feldman, P. H., Gould, D. A., Levine, C., Kuerbis, A. N., & Donelan, K. (2002). When the caregiver needs care: The plight of vulnerable family caregivers. *American Journal of Public Health, 92*(3), 409–413.
OECD. (2005). *Long-term care for older people*. Paris: OECD.
OECD. (2011). *Help wanted? Providing and paying for long-term care*. Paris: OECD.
Pijl, M., & Ramakers, C. (2007). Contracting one's family members: The Dutch care allowance. In C. Ungerson & S. Yeandle (Eds.), *Cash-for-care in developed welfare states* (pp. 81–103). Basingstoke: Palgrave Macmillan.
Pinquart, M., & Sorenson, S. (2003). Associations of stressors and uplifts of caregiving with caregiver burden and depressive mood: A meta-analysis. *Journals of Gerontology: Psychological Sciences & Social Sciences, 58B*, 112–128.

Portegijs, W., Hermans, B., & Lalta, V. (Eds.). (2006). *Emancipatiemonitor 2006* [Emancipation Monitor 2006]. Den Haag: Sociaal en Cultureel Planbureau/Centraal Bureau voor de Statistiek. English summary available at: http://www.scp.nl/english/publications/summaries/9037702864.html

Reher, D. S. (1998). Family ties in western Europe: Persistent contrasts. *Population and Development Review, 24*(2), 203–234.

Robine, J. M., Michel, J. P., & Herrmann, F. R. (2007). 'Who will care for the oldest people in our ageing society? *British Medical Journal, 334*, 570–571.

Rodrigues, R., & Schmidt, A. (2010). *Paying for long-term care. Policy brief of the European centre for social welfare policy and research.* Vienna: ECSWPR. Available at: http://www.euro.centre.org/data/1283437589_95069.pdf

Ross, M., Lloyd, A., Weinhardt, M., & Cheshire, H. (2008). *Living and caring? An investigation of the experience of older carers*. London: ILC-UK.

Schmidt, A., Barbabella, F., Hoffmann, F., & Lamura, G. (2011). *Analysis and mapping of 52 ICT-based initiatives for family caregivers, deliverable 2.3, draft report from the CARICT project – ICT-based solutions for caregivers: Assessing their impact on the sustainability of long-term care in an ageing Europe* (Contract Number IPTS-2010-J04–44-RC).

Schulz, R., & Martire, L. M. (2004). Family caregiving in persons with dementia: Prevalence, health effects, and support strategies. *The American Journal of Geriatric Psychiatry, 12*(3), 240–249.

Simonazzi, A. (2009). Care regimes and national employment models. *Cambridge Journal of Economics, 33*, 211–232.

Tolkacheva, N., Broese Van Groenou, M., De Boer, A., & Van Tilburg, T. (2011). The impact of informal care-giving networks on adult children's care-giver burden. *Ageing & Society, 31*, 34–51.

Ungerson, C., & Yeandle, S. (Eds.). (2007). *Cash-for-care in developed welfare states*. Basingstoke: Palgrave Macmillan.

Vitaliano, P., Zhang, J., & Scanlan, J. M. (2003). Is caregiving hazardous to one's physical health? A meta-analysis. *Psychological Bulletin, 129*, 946–972.

Chapter 13
Caught Between a Troubled Past and an Uncertain Future: The Well-Being of Asylum-Seeking Children in Sweden

Ulla Björnberg

Introduction

Drawing upon a study of the experiences of asylum-seeking children and their families in Sweden, this chapter examines how children cope with their life situations while awaiting their asylum decisions. What influences the well-being of asylum-seeking children caught up in a tension between experiences of past and present exclusion and expectations of improvement upon arrival in the host country? The analysis is based on qualitative interviews with 17 children (aged 9–18) and 17 parents (one parent for each child). The interviewed families had been waiting for a decision on their residence permit application for several months and sometimes even years. Utilizing concepts such as resilience, social capital, trust, and social recognition, the ways in which social networks might function as important resources fostering the well-being of asylum-seeking children and their parents are assessed. Possibilities for social networking among the interviewed children were found to be often constrained due to their specific social and legal situation in the host country. They were also undermined by their family circumstances and factors related to their past experiences and the challenges inherent in their everyday life during the waiting period. Concrete measures to support asylum-seeking families and their children in order to foster their well-being are suggested.

This chapter addresses the well-being of children who, at the time of the study, were in Sweden with their families as asylum seekers awaiting a decision on their residence permit application. At a general level, the overarching goal of the Swedish

U. Björnberg (✉)
Department of Sociology, University of Gothenburg,
P.O. Box 720, SE-405 30 Gothenburg, Sweden
e-mail: Ulla.Bjornberg@sociology.gu.se

A. Moreno Mínguez (ed.), *Family Well-Being: European Perspectives*,
Social Indicators Research Series 49, DOI 10.1007/978-94-007-4354-0_13,

policy towards asylum seekers and refugees is to promote their integration into the host society already at an early stage following their arrival in the country. The waiting period during the asylum process is to be made as meaningful as possible while also preparing the asylum seekers for the eventuality of having to return to their country of origin. At the same time that it is intended to strengthen asylum seekers' self-reliance, it then also keeps alive the risk of forced return, doing little to alleviate the emotional tensions and anxieties created by the circumstances that led the asylum seekers to leave their country of origin in the first place.

Studies about asylum seekers' experiences show that the local institutional context in the host country is perhaps the most influential factor affecting their well-being. Of crucial importance here are the resources that the individuals have at their disposal to guide and control their life situation, determining, in a word, the scope allowed for their agency and voice. Regulations and their implementation during the asylum process thus greatly influence the welfare conditions and the well-being of the asylum-seeking families (Ascher 2005).

This chapter is based on an ongoing study of the health and well-being of asylum-seeking children and their families in Sweden. While the overall aim of the study is to contribute to our understanding of what influences asylum-seeking children's well-being more generally, a special focus is laid on the interactions between local practices in the implementation of policies regarding the reception of children. The health and well-being of children are assessed both in the context of their immediate living conditions such as the family, the school, the material conditions, and the local environment, looking at these in relation to different policy levels. In view of the many aspects of the research problem, a multidisciplinary approach has been adopted to enable analysis of the way in which general structures influence actors nationally and locally, along with the children themselves.

This chapter draws in particular on one sub-study of the overall research project, consisting of qualitative interviews with 17 asylum-seeking families. At the time of the interviews, the families had been waiting for the decision on their residence permit for several months or even years. The children in the families were aged between 9 and 18. Eight of them were in their upper teens (aged 14–18), five in their lower teens (aged 12–13), while three were 9 years old. The interviewed families came from Afghanistan, countries of the Middle East, Iraq, Iran, and Uzbekistan. The interviews with the parents and the children were conducted separately, each lasting 2 h and taking place on two separate occasions. All in all, a total of approximately 4 h of interviews were recorded per individual and 8 h per family. Two interviewers were present for each of the families: one for the parent and another for the child.[1] With few exceptions, authorized and experienced interpreters were used. The interviews were open-ended, covering experiences before, during, and after the arrival in Sweden.

[1] The interviews were conducted by the author and Mirzet Tursunovic.

Well-Being

One of the main objectives of the study was to identify elements in the conditions of the children that contribute to their sense of well-being. The research into this question was informed by Article 24 of the Convention on the Rights of the Child, which emphasizes the right of children to protective conditions fostering their health. The main focus in this investigation was on how well-being was experienced by the children: what they regarded as good or bad for their well-being and how they coped with adversity during the waiting period.

Coping is linked to the period of transition, spanning the time from departing from the home country to the issuance of the residence permit or a deportation order. Transition in these cases means moving to a new set of conditions characterized by low predictability and high uncertainty. The transitional process itself can be described as a social state or phase of great ambiguity in which one's position, identity, and social belonging are no longer clearly defined. It is marked by experiences of social exclusion in the homeland, often accompanied by encounters with physical and psychological violence and significant circumscription of one's civil and economic rights. The tension between these experiences of exclusion and the expectations of improvement directed at asylum seekers after their arrival in the host country forms then the framework in which strategies for dealing with one's life situation need to be studied.

In the analysis that follows, concepts such as resilience, social capital, trust, and social recognition are used to better understand coping among asylum seekers. Resilience concerns the capacity of individuals and their families to resist adversities they experience as harmful to their psychological well-being. It is promoted by resources that increase one's operational capacity in the environment, most importantly social relationships. A supportive environment fosters greater resilience in the individual, which, in turn, contributes to improved capacity to cope with and master stress. While resilience is developed primarily in the family context, within the family system, it must also be analysed in the context of institutional rights and options availed to asylum seekers in the host country (Ungar 2008). As argued by Morrow (1999) and others, the extent to which children feel embedded in social networks, neighbourhoods, schools, and other formal organizations important in their everyday lives is related to their well-being. In this connection, the concept of social capital helps to understand the role of the social environment. Social capital is usually understood in terms of resources that can be of benefit to, or useful for, the individual (Field 2003). Coleman (1990) has defined it as the value that actors can derive from social structure, enabling them to realize their interests. As a resource, it functions as a personal asset that is constituted in families and local communities and depends on relations of reciprocity and trust.

A social network in itself, however, is not sufficient to create social capital; more than just a network of individual ties is required. The ties between individuals must be of a particular type: They must be reciprocal and trusting and involve positive emotion (Morrow 1999). Social capital thus comes about as a result of the quality of social relationships within a social group or community; only when the latter criterion, too, is filled can the social network provide social capital. From the perspective of an individual, also small networks may create potential for resilience if they are based on relations of trust and reciprocity and involve positive emotion. Social networks characterized by absence of trust, reciprocity, and positive emotions from their constitutive relationships do not function as social capital, regardless of their size. Through social relations based on trust and mutual recognition, a sense that the environment is understandable and manageable can be transmitted.

Based on her research on the health and well-being of young people, Morrow (2001) has suggested that social capital should be related to how young people view their social context in everyday life, with the extent to which they experience a sense of belonging in their social environment serving as a measure of the social capital they possess. Useful questions to ask would then include: How do young people perceive their neighbours, classmates, and other persons in their environment? How do they explain their reasons for perceiving these relationships in a certain way? For Morrow, social capital is useful:

> as a tool or heuristic device for exploring social processes and practices in the experiences of the social environments of the young, as a way to grasp their social resources or lack of them that are related to the acquisition of other forms of capital. (Morrow 2001, p. 757)

Morrow's thinking here is inspired by Bourdieu's work that conceptualizes social capital as an individual resource: Actors must actively perceive their networks as a resource in order to have them available to themselves as social capital (Bourdieu 1985). This capital, however, is not rooted in informal social networks alone; it also develops through more formal organizations and connections like community groups and collective resources created through schools and local associations, depending on the individual's access to these (exclusion or inclusion).

Given the ambiguity marking the situation of asylum-seeking children, trust, or the absence of it, forms an important element to focus on when examining their everyday life. Indeed, both *trust* and *social recognition* are of special significance as necessary preconditions for the cultivation and shaping of social interaction and social capital. Trust can be characterized as the set of:

> socially learned and socially confirmed expectations that people have of each other, of the organizations and institutions in which they live, and of the natural and moral social orders that set the fundamental understandings for their lives. In social interaction, a sense of normality is constructed through some tacit understanding of rules that make our world predictable, reliable and legible. (Barber 1983, pp. 164–165)

To feel comfortable and safe, one needs to minimize irregularity and follow the rules of interaction recognized by those involved in the social interaction. Trust plays an essential role in determining how individuals interpret the social interaction that they are part of (Misztal 1996). It is therefore an essential element of any social interaction capable of creating a sense of predictability and normality: Having trust in a person means confidence that those with whom one interacts will follow shared norms. In more formal contexts, trust thus implies that the applied rules are transparent and fair. The ability to see that, again, is quite clearly of vital importance in the special situation faced by asylum-seeking adults and children.

Another aspect on trust concerns risk management in one's choice of action. Luhmann (1988) has defined risk in terms of the extent to which our present behaviour impacts future possibilities: "Risks...emerge only as a component of decision and actions. They do not exist by themselves. If you refrain from action you run no risk. It is a purely *internal* calculation of *external* conditions which creates risk" (Luhmann 1988, p. 100). The presence of trust, in reducing the risk related to situational uncertainty, is thus a necessary condition for building social relationships and social capital.

Trust is also connected to *social recognition* among the persons involved in the social interaction. Social recognition takes place when the individual is met with symbols, gestures, or talk signifying positive value and an invitation to reciprocity. It is about being made visible, and thus the opposite of being made invisible, for example, by harmless inattention or general lack of interest by others who may see one as socially insignificant. At the same time, to avoid the risk of being held in negative regard, the individual can also make a conscious choice to remain socially invisible (see Heidegren 2009).

Social recognition is closely connected to self-esteem and social identity. It is to act while attributing positive value to others. What this implies is that the subject commits to acting in a moral way, showing regard for the others. In socially recognizing the other in the interaction, the subject thus no longer ignores or neglects the other party. Through this process, social recognition becomes part of the project of building trust. Trust and social recognition thus become elements of emotional capital that can be drawn upon in social interaction. In its basic form, trust means having confidence in one's own ability to anticipate the actions of those with whom one interacts; it is a matter of double confidence – confidence in others and in oneself (Barbalet 2008).

As this study of asylum-seeking families demonstrated, trust and social recognition come about as a result of one's experiences of social interaction. At the same time, they are also a condition for one's desire to interact. It is therefore of vital importance that the question of trust and recognition be properly addressed by those in charge of processing and deciding on asylum applications and by those first coming into contact with asylum seekers – and not only to be able to better identify reasons for granting asylum in deserving cases, but also to demonstrate to asylum seekers, especially when they are children, that they are socially recognized as individuals in their own right. Asylum seekers need to appear trustworthy in their interactions with the reception officers, caseworkers, and handling officers but also with local and state authorities on whom they depend for provision of services and benefits. They find themselves in a situation where they must be able to present convincing asylum claims while the criteria for the acceptance of these claims often remain unclear to them. Both the children and the adults studied for this chapter stressed the need to have their reasons for migration believed. Yet, since migration officers must carefully scrutinize all the information and testimonies provided in support of the asylum application, the process can but take on some elements of apparent distrust. The perception of not being regarded as trustworthy then gives rise to insecurity and lack of predictability in social relationships, both in everyday interaction with others and in more formal interaction with authorities.

Results

Free and Safe but Anxious

The transition period for the asylum-seeking families and children included in this study was fraught with different kinds of adversity. It meant the loss of resources, social capital, and trust that one was accustomed to relying on in the home country. Nevertheless, both parents and children expressed that their arrival in Sweden had brought a sense of security and relief. The children described feelings of freedom and a release from the anxiety and stress that had marked their experience of the constraining and threatening living conditions at home.

Amir,[2] aged 16, explained what well-being meant to him:

> [It means] to feel free here. We didn't feel free in Iraq. We were closed in all the time. We couldn't go outside, we couldn't go to school, we had no friends. But here it's different; we feel free.[3]

Yet, effects of the traumatic experiences lingered, impacting the asylum seekers psychological and physical well-being. Symptoms such as depression, anxiety, sleeplessness, and stomach and headaches were reported. The sense of insecurity linked to events in previous life diminished after a while, but in the course of the protracted asylum process, the newly found sense of security was eventually replaced by feelings of uncertainty and unpredictability regarding the future. In the research literature, this transformation is often connected to "the trauma of return" (Brekke 2004): For many refugees, the prospect of having to return back home causes the future to be identified with the past, often traumatic experiences. This was exemplified by the following asylum-seeking parent:

> Because of this stress you feel sick even though you are not sick…. The stress has been cut into two halves, and one half of it remains…. The first half, that's the stress we left behind in Iraq – the killings, their threats to punish my son. Now my son is safe, nobody can kill him; now we don't feel unsafe and that uncertainty is no more. But then we have this other half [of this stress] that's left and feels threatening to us: that we might be denied permission to stay here. They might not want Iraqis in here. We don't have a residence permit, my husband is not here, and my relatives, they are not here, either; I am worried about them. This is the other half of my anxiety.

The threat of being forced to return blocks the motivation to manage the new circumstances of one's everyday life in the host country. The situation has also been described using the concept of liminality, or a position in between two statuses: While no longer in the old country, one nevertheless remains outside of the new society without the right to work, with limited access to health care and other resources important in everyday life, and, not least, without an official social security or personal identification number enabling one to assume an active role in the host society (Brekke 2004).

---

[2] All interviewee names have been changed.

[3] The quote is from another sub-study within the project (Ascher and Mellander 2010).

Material Deprivation and Social Inclusion

Almost all of the families studied had experienced material deprivation. The children had lived in economically deprived circumstances for a prolonged period, given the length of time they had been waiting for their asylum cases to be decided. This, in turn, meant that their possibilities for expanding their range of social activities had remained restricted, with the children unable to afford spending free time with friends. As a result, they expressed themselves having a sense of otherness in many dimensions of daily life. Overcrowded living conditions and the necessity to repeatedly change accommodation were common experiences that added to the difficulties of making friends and socializing.

Some children's experiences also included exploitation by other adults in the vulnerable conditions of their passage from the home country to Sweden. These experiences combined to create in them distrust in other people. The children's own and their parents' experiences of dealing with the Swedish Migration Board, in turn, gave them a sense of being mistrusted about their reasons for wanting to stay in the country.

The effect of such experiences is often mitigated when the children start attending school. In the school environment, children can develop a sense of being included, taking part in activities that normalize and bring structure to their everyday life. All of the children in the study spoke appreciatively about being at school, commenting positively about teachers and how teaching and learning differed from what they were used to in their home country. When asked about their experiences of school, most of the children mentioned that the teachers were kind, that they did not use physical punishment like in schools at home, and that they explained things instead of forcing pupils to learn them by heart. The different school system, however, was also a source of worry among parents and children in view to the possibility of having to return to the home country and the risk of lagging behind in what was expected of pupils back there.

Social Networking in Neighbourhoods and in Schools

As already noted, trust is an important dimension in a salutogenic perspective, forming a necessary condition for establishing social contacts and a sense of safety while waiting for the asylum verdict. Social networking with one's schoolmates may be regarded as a particularly influential factor in this regard. Among the asylum-seeking children studied, however, there seemed to be a little going on by way of expanding one's social relations among the classmates. Judging from their own descriptions of the social landscape at school, there seemed to be small cliques of individuals keeping to themselves, with no more than occasional socialization between them. Many asylum-seeking children in Sweden are first enrolled in a preparatory class where they learn Swedish and receive some basic education on other fundamental topics; these classes also serve as an introduction to the Swedish school system.

Class sizes are very small, and the children attending the classes all share the same basic life situation. This more intimate context made it also easier for the asylum-seeking children in this study to make friends; as they themselves reported, these classes were the most important social context for them in which to make friends. Laila (aged 15), for instance, who had one close friend at school, stated that "If we had first met in a normal class, we might not have become such close friends, because we both felt marginalized. Here [in Sweden] you have to trust people more; to have someone to trust is very important".

All the asylum-seeking children attending the preparatory class had similar experiences even when they were not from the same country. They all told about the important role the preparatory class at school played in terms of their ability to make friends: friends, moreover, with whom they were able to stay close and continue being friends even later when moving on to a regular class.

The children also reported spending time primarily with other immigrant children at school, regardless of whether they were from the same country or not. As Kaden (aged 15), for example, described it:

> My school is an immigrant school. There are some Swedes there, too, but I don't have any contact with them. Sometimes it happens that some Swedes come along [with us]...but still there is no real contact. I feel better with other immigrants.... The Swedish guys seem so cold towards one another.

Statements like Laila's and Kaden's indicate that asylum-seeking children, and immigrant children more generally, may have very little trust in others. Both Laila and Kaden felt anxious about making mistakes, about not speaking properly and not wearing the right clothes. Laila claimed that she did not in fact need any more acquaintances since, in her view, these could also be potential enemies: "At first I wanted to have more friends, but now I feel happy with how things are. I try not to make more enemies". The reason why she did not have more friends, she explained, was that there were no arenas where she could make friends outside school. She was involved in a film project at her school, but this involvement had not resulted in more friendships. Laila also avoided speaking her own language with other pupils sharing the same language, due to dialectical differences: "They will laugh at you [when you speak]", she explained.

Laila further mentioned that she was careful not to be involved in conflicts with other children at school, explaining her deliberate strategy: "If you stay calm and don't aggravate things, then you avoid conflicts". According to her, she socialized with a few other children with whom she always hung out at school. In general, everybody was nice, nobody was mean, and nobody had a higher status, in her opinion, "even when they think they have a higher status". This "high status", for her, was displayed by the fashionable clothes worn. All in all, the cases of Laila and Kaden then illustrate the important role that risk management has in regulating social interaction: By avoiding interaction beyond a narrow circle of trusted friends, they both strived to limit their risk of being held in negative regard.

The social contacts that the asylum-seeking children in this study cultivated at school did not, however, extend to free time and leisure activities. Moreover, most of the children had hardly any friends and acquaintances in the neighbourhoods where they lived. Their attitudes towards these neighbourhoods were also markedly suspicious or indifferent. There was ambivalence about how to relate to people living in their area that had its roots in the children's experiences as asylum seekers. For some, this experience translated into feelings of outright mistrust. Kaden was one example: In both his own and his parents' view, the youths living in their neighbourhood were drug users. As Kaden put it: "I see them every day.... They are always high on something...and they carry knives, too". Kaden had to be back home by eight in the evening, as his parents did want him to be out late at night. He spent most of his non-school hours with his parents. The parents, to be sure, did encourage him to go out more, but since he did not have any friends where he lived, he stayed mostly at home, even though in principle he would have liked to spend more time outside in his neighbourhood. His sense of embeddedness in the local neighbourhood was fairly weak, suggesting itself as both a cause and a consequence of this situation.

The lonely children in the study group also had lonely mothers (and fathers). It was typical of both the mothers and the fathers participating in the study that they tended to either just wait out their time in the place where they lived, without venturing to create social contacts there, or remain openly suspicious or even afraid of people familiar with their situation.

As these examples show, lack of trust and fears about negative recognition were thus significant factors contributing to the asylum-seeking children's aversion to forming new friendships in their local environment.

Practical Help and Support

The asylum-seeking children in the study group were also asked about exchange of gifts and support with classmates and friends at school. None of them reported doing either of these. Sonia (aged 15), for example, stated that she did not want to exchange help with anyone because, in her eyes, any help was extended to her out of pity, and she did not want to be pitied. "There are many who want to show that they have compassion for you, but it is better that they don't come", as she herself put it. She had nothing against gratitude for help received, but felt strongly about being pitied, which to her meant not relating to her as a person in her own right.

According to Sonia, her parents were suspicious about people around them in the neighbourhoods where they stayed (they moved frequently) as they did not want others to know about their situation as asylum seekers. Sonia and her family were in a difficult position: They had applied for a residence permit several times but had had their asylum application rejected each time, and now they remained in the country pending the decision of a Europe-wide court to which their case had been appealed. To survive, the family had to rely on helpers, and it had become stuck in a situation of asymmetric dependency. Sonia's parents had accumulated debts to people they had met through their church activities, something that for them was a highly sensitive matter. Their social situation was thus characterized by a pendulum movement between exclusion and inclusion. The social network surrounding the family was linked to the church where they had found their helpers. For Sonia, this semiformal social support system had created increased trust in the Swedish society in general: “Here you can find people who care about you”, she stated, while in her home country “nobody cares, especially if you are not wealthy”. As a result, she felt a certain freedom and greater self-confidence in her new circumstances.

Emotional Support

The separate studies undertaken within the overall research project have clearly showed the most important source of resilience for the asylum-seeking children and their parents to be the family. In the interviews for this chapter, the strong interdependency relations within families were expressed in different ways. The parents talked about their great responsibility to protect the children from worries about lack of resources in everyday life: Freeing children from the burden of such concerns was perceived as their main parental task in the circumstances (cf. Eastmond 2010). The children believed their parents to know what was best for them and that the parents’ decisions were for their own good. At the same time, the children, for their part, tended to feel responsible for the well-being of their parents. Some of them had a close relationship with their parents, claiming to be able to talk with them about their worries and concerns. In those cases, they could find temporary relief from their thoughts and feelings of exclusion at not being able to socialize on equal terms with their classmates. Laila, for example, had great trust in her mother and her close friend. She could talk openly with both of them about matters that caused her anxiety. She talked with her mother about her fears about having to return to her home country, but also about missing it deeply. It helped her to talk about such things, although, as she herself put it, “it is like taking a pill: it calms you down but after a while the worries return”. Sometimes she was struck by a sudden fear that she would lose her mother; this, her mother thought, was probably owing to the fact that they were so alone in the new country. Hardly any of their relatives were there with them; they were all scattered around the world. Attending school had nevertheless helped alleviate this fear of Sonia’s.

On the whole, the children were unwilling to talk to others about the problematic situation of their families. One stated reason for this was that talking, by bringing fears out in the open, only heightened their anxieties by making the problem seem more formidable and real. Another reason, according to the interviewed children, was that parents (usually mothers) should be protected from their children’s problems. Jemina (aged 15), for instance, whose family was in a particularly vulnerable situation, stated that she felt unable to talk to anyone about her worries and problems, whether it be her mother or her close friend. Instead, she kept everything to herself without even wanting to talk about her feelings and concerns. When asked whether this was because she thought that her mother was already encumbered by so many worries and she did not want to disturb her even more, or whether it was because she simply did not like to talk about her feelings or worries in general, Jemina responded: "It's both; I just think that it's best for me not to talk". Her reluctance to share her feelings and thoughts was not, however, because she thought she would not find a sympathetic ear. On the contrary, she believed that her mother actually wanted her to talk about them; she simply preferred to keep it all inside herself. In addition to her mother, her sister and grandparents who lived with the family, she also had a brother, none of whom she wanted to open up to. She did, however, express that she would have liked to have someone to share her thoughts with. When asked how she managed this inner conflict of hers, she explained: "I write, at nights" (she suffered from sleeping problems and stomach aches). Her wish was to learn music or acting, as she thought that that way she could act out her problems instead: "I want to get it out of me", she confessed.

Among the asylum-seeking children in the study, Sonia had a similar dilemma. She did not speak with anyone in her family about their situation. While she did much to support her mother, she nevertheless felt unable to open up to her; like Sonia, she simply preferred not to talk. There was also a school nurse that she said she trusted and knew she could visit anytime, but she only went to see her once. Both Jemina's and Sonia's families were in a precarious situation, and they both feared that talking about their problems might only make them seem bigger. Yet, what also lay behind their unwillingness to talk was a basic problem of trust – or, rather, insecurity about the extent to which they could trust others. Sonia and the other children in the more vulnerable families studied were highly sensitive to the difficult situation faced by their mothers who were lonely, very worried about their future, and frequently depressed. The children were aware of their mothers' dependency on them, which inspired deep loyalty in them. In order to be more supportive to their mothers, they then discounted their own needs. Yet, when asked about it, they spoke of their positive expectations for the future, with an immediate future that promised to deliver their much-longed-for residence permits. At the same time, they all tried to avoid thinking and talking about their past and future, opting instead to make themselves invisible to reduce the risk of being held in negative regard. Among the many bystanders failing to recognize this situation of theirs were the authorities at the Swedish Migration Board: Only few of the children in this study had ever been interviewed or directly addressed by any of them.

Relationships with Kin

A recurrent theme in the interviewed children's stories was the children's relationships with their extended families that were generally quite attenuated. Some of the children maintained some form of contact with their cousins living in Sweden, while most of them had only sparse contact with relatives back home. Laila, for instance, called her father, who had divorced her mother many years ago and stayed behind in her country of origin, "every now and then". In Sweden she and her mother lived with an aunt. She also stayed in contact with her grandmother in Canada, talking to her on the telephone about once a month. In addition, she sometimes chatted with two cousins (children of her aunt) who, too, lived in Canada.

Also the parents in the study tended to have few or infrequent transnational family contacts. This situation may, however, have been temporary, coming about as a result of factors such as guilt for having left close kin, problems linked to the uncertainties of the future, and practical difficulties encountered while waiting for the asylum decision. The general impression gained from the interviews was that the children followed a pattern similar to their parents but that they were also constrained by limited access to means of communication. At the same time, some of the families were deeply embedded in local networks of close kin. One of the mothers interviewed (Leena, aged 40) expressed appreciation for the strong relationships with and support from relatives that she felt her family could enjoy even in Sweden. The family lived with an uncle who also provided her and her husband with job opportunities. Theirs was a migrant family that, through multiple family reunifications, had been brought to close contact with most of its kin networks in both Sweden and some other parts of the world. The family maintained no social relations outside these networks; they had no contacts with native-born Swedes and saw no reason to extend their relationships to them, either. The close network of relatives around them brought trust and a sense of confidence in the future in their lives. The children in this and similar families included in the study were fairly well connected with peers at school and with friends and close kin in the home country.

The Role of Formal and Semiformal Institutions

Asylum-seeking parents and children in Sweden are under the authority of the Swedish Migration Board and the lawyers assisting them with their asylum application. These institutional actors basically settle the future of the families they work with. Contacts with officers and caseworkers at the Swedish Migration Board and the lawyers on whom the families studied were highly dependent for their accommodation and financial support thus obviously played a major role in their lives. The asylum seekers' descriptions of their relationships with the Migration Board officers conveyed a sense of uncertainty and lack of control they experienced in their interactions with authorities even more broadly. This experience was exacerbated by the long waiting periods and a lack of transparency regarding the relevant rules and rights. The asylum seekers found their contacts with the officers in charge of their individual cases to be frequently ambiguous, causing insecurity and mistrust. Mistrust in particular seemed an inherent feature of the asylum process, with the asylum seekers having to convince the authorities of the merit of their asylum claim and of their need and qualification for support and benefits. Some parents reported their children to have been upset by the questions they were posed about what the parents had stated. In these cases, the children had felt that they had to confirm the stories told by their parents. On the other hand, the Migration Board was also perceived as helpful for the asylum seekers. Some of the interviewed parents spoke appreciatively of the support they had received, although the availability and quality of this support seemed to depend on the person of the immigration officer or the lawyer assigned to their case.

Also church-based organizations had been found helpful; they had assisted several of the asylum-seeking families studied by donating food and clothing. In contrast to the authorities, the people working for these organizations were perceived to have time for the individual asylum seekers and in general seemed to have shown a more helpful attitude. None of the interviewed asylum seekers had turned to immigrant associations for socializing, however; according to their statements, they felt "unsure" about the people working for these associations.

Conclusions

Among the asylum-seeking families studied, family bonding provided a strong source of resilience for both the parents and the children, in particular in families with many adversities to cope with. Uncertainty about the future was usually accompanied by a desire to appear independent and self-reliant vis-à-vis the environment. The mothers' commitment to their children provided them with emotional capital that they could draw upon in everyday life, translating into an atmosphere of protection and sustenance of a sense of safety and belonging. Building emotional capital within the family was thus used by mothers as a way to develop resources for coping with past insecurity and uncertainty about the future. The high degree of dependency and reliance on the family as a source of resilience nevertheless put new pressure on family members, given how keen they were to protect one another from their worries and how responsible they felt for the well-being of one another. Worries, psychologically straining memories, and closure against the environment could then combine to create a vicious circle. While parents and children felt responsible for each other's well-being, the ambiguous interdependency that this sentiment gave rise to could be experienced as a burden by the children, who often felt a need to suppress their own needs of emotional support vis-à-vis their mothers or friends, thus compromising their own well-being. The findings of the study thus suggest a close linkage between emotional capital and social capital but also the complexity of this linkage: While giving emotional support might bring relief to both the support giver and the receiver, the reciprocity of emotional support can also give rise to mutual dependencies that entail significant emotional costs.

Both the children and the parents in this study kept a low social profile, expressing an attitude that, in their situation, this was "better" for them. This attitude can be interpreted as linked to the interviewed asylum seekers' lack of a sense of trust and to the uncertainty they felt about their status, reflecting, in turn, their ambiguous situation as individuals caught in between two statuses.

The asylum seekers' disconnection from their social environment can be understood through the concepts of social capital, social recognition, and trust. "Social capital" highlights the value of social relationships in which trust and reciprocity are important emotional elements – relationships which enable individuals to give and take resources under conditions of equality and mutual dependency. The period of transition in which the asylum-seeking families were caught at the time of this study brought with it uncertainties, ambivalence, and asymmetric dependencies affecting their lives. To engage in reciprocal exchange of resources presupposes that one can expect a more balanced exchange to develop within a certain time frame. In this situation, it is thus important for both parties to be able to prove self-reliance and independence.

This study suggests that there seems to be a basic lack of trust among asylum-seeking adults and children, which prevents them from building social capital during the transition period to refugee status. Not cultivating social relationships, however, can also be looked upon as a matter of self-protection. Keeping a low profile functions a resilience strategy helping to reduce the risk of experiencing shame and humiliation in the straitened economic circumstances and poor housing conditions typical of the asylum seekers' situation upon arrival in the host country.

Based on the interviews conducted for this study, mistrust seems like a built-in part of the organization of the asylum process and is mostly associated with the inquisitive nature of the asylum determination procedure. The asylum seekers' position is frequently one of dependency, where the absence of trust by others and lack of social recognition influence their sense of self-confidence. Needs testing in particular is often associated with a feeling of negative social recognition, especially when the rules are not transparent and are applied differently from case to case.

At the same time, institutions such as schools, churches, voluntary associations, and healthcare agencies can also play an important role in helping asylum-seeking parents and children receive social recognition and trust. In this fashion, they, and other similar institutions and organizations, can function as important sources of resilience for asylum seekers. The staffs of formal institutions can be considered as social capital for the families to utilize. Starting school, for example, is usually of very high importance for both the children and their parents in precisely this sense. In different ways, all of the children interviewed for this study expressed trust in their teachers. Similarly, also parents demonstrated high levels of trust in teachers and in the school system more generally.

Based on the findings from this study, we might then conclude that social networking is not a "natural" process but, instead, an intricate project with many constraining elements. Another important observation is that the dynamics of the social interactions discussed above can create a vicious circle, aggravating a socially exposed position to the point of social exclusion. Both in the context of the migration policy in Sweden and more generally, the findings from this study thus highlight the importance of finding new ways to support asylum-seeking families and their children. The strategy of integration into the host society already during the waiting period should be made more responsive to the applicants' needs. One concrete way to do this could be by improving communication about the school system (cf. Tursunovic 2010). In addition, support making it possible for children to take part in leisure activities would predictably have important effects in improving their general well-being, thus helping to reduce stress in their families as well.

Acknowledgements The study on which this chapter is based was funded by the European Refugee Fund. The author wishes to thank her colleague Mirzet Tursunovic for all his help in conducting the interviews for the study.

References

Ascher, H. (2005). Rapes in war: Effects on mother-child relations. In H. Andersson, H. Ascher, U. Björnberg, M. Eastmond, & L. Mellander (Eds.), *The asylum-seeking child in Europe* (pp. 101–111). Gothenburg: Centre for European Research at Gothenburg University (CERGU).

Ascher, H., & Mellander, L. (2010). Asylsökande barns tankar om hälsa. In H. Andersson, H. Ascher, U. Björnberg, & M. Eastmond (Eds.), *Mellan det förflutna och framtiden. Asylsökande barns välfärd, hälsa och välbefinnande* (pp. 207–243). Gothenburg: Centre for European Research at Gothenburg University (CERGU).

Barbalet, J. (2008). Tillitens emotionella bas och dess följder. In Wettergren, Å., Starrin, B., & Lindgren, G. (Ed.), *Det sociala livets emotionella grunder* (pp. 57–77). Malmö: Liber.

Barber, B. (1983). *The logic and limits of trust.* New Brunswick: Rutgers University Press.

Bourdieu, P. (1985). The social space and the genesis of groups. *Theory and Society, 14*(6), 723–744.

Brekke, J. -P. (2004). *While we are waiting: Uncertainty and empowerment among asylum-seekers in Sweden* (Report 2004:10). Oslo: Institute for Social Research.

Coleman, J. (1990). *Foundations of social theory.* Cambridge, MA: Belknap Press of Harvard University Press.

Eastmond, M. (2010). Gäster i välfärden? Föräldraskap i asylprocessen. In H. Andersson, H. Ascher, U. Björnberg, & M. Eastmond (Eds.), *Mellan det förflutna och framtiden. Asylsökande barns välfärd, hälsa och välbefinnande* (pp. 87–109). Gothenburg: Centre for European Research at Gothenburg University (CERGU).

Field, J. (2003). *Social capital.* London: Routledge.

Heidegren, C. -G. (2009). *Erkännande.* Malmö: Liber.

Luhmann, N. (1988). Familiarity, confidence, trust: Problems and alternatives. In D. Gambetta (Ed.), *Trust: Making and breaking cooperative relations* (pp. 94–109). New York: Basil Blackwell.

Misztal, B. A. (1996). *Trust in modern societies: The search for the bases of social order.* Oxford: Polity Press.

Morrow, V. (1999). Conceptualising social capital in relation to the well-being of children and young people: A critical review. *The Sociological Review, 47*(4), 744–765.

Morrow, V. (2001). Young people's explanations and experiences of social exclusion: Retrieving Bourdieu's concept of social capital. *International Journal of Sociology and Social Policy, 21*(4/5/6), 37–63.

Tursunovic, M. (2010). Skolan i de asylsökande barnens vardag. In H. Andersson, H. Ascher, U. Björnberg, & M. Eastmond (Eds.), *Mellan det förflutna och framtiden. Asylsökande barns välfärd, hälsa och välbefinnande* (pp. 141–171). Gothenburg: Centre for European Research at Gothenburg University (CERGU).

Ungar, M. (2008). Resilience across cultures. *British Journal of Social Work, 38*(2), 212–235.

Chapter 14
Empowerment, Well-Being and the Welfare State: Family Social Work in Spain

Antonio López Peláez and Sagrario Segado Sánchez-Cabezudo

Introduction

Research on family well-being focuses on three key issues: firstly, the social and economic context, specifically the existing welfare state model; secondly, the characteristics of the families themselves, analysing key issues such as children, power, money, work, leisure or housing; and a third key issue, the cultural imaginary about family, success and failure, its evolution and to what degree family narratives empower or disempower families to achieve a dignified life in advanced democratic societies. Two of the negative consequences of explanations grounded in clichés or pseudo-reasoning are that they reproduce existing power relations and relegate to the realm of the unthinkable or unmentionable relevant dimensions of social life (Bourdieu and Wacquant 2005). Both topics are particularly important when analysing family narratives: narratives that give meaning to families and the strategies they use to achieve their goals in all spheres of life.

Research on families and family well-being in today's complex societies must not overlook social policies specifically targeted at these groups or social intervention programmes implemented by social workers. Particularly in southern European countries, the family is the last barrier to social exclusion, while family social work seeks to empower and recover families at serious risk of social exclusion. Since 2006, we have developed a line of research on family social work that encompasses three dimensions: firstly, the analysis of the characteristics of Spanish families through their narratives (Del Fresno 2011); secondly, problems deriving from social exclusion processes currently taking place in Spain, Nicaragua and Guatemala (in these two Latin American countries, we have developed a social intervention

A. López Peláez (✉) • S. Segado Sánchez-Cabezudo
Department of Social Work of the National Distance Education University (UNED), Universidad de Educación a Distancia, Madrid, Spain
e-mail: alopez@der.uned.es; ssegado@der.uned.es

A. Moreno Mínguez (ed.), *Family Well-Being: European Perspectives*, Social Indicators Research Series 49, DOI 10.1007/978-94-007-4354-0_14,

programme in indigenous communities aimed at peace education and reducing violent behaviour within the family) (López Peláez 2010b); and thirdly, the design of social intervention programmes to improve social integration by groups of families at risk of social exclusion (Segado Sánchez-Cabezudo 2011).

In this chapter, we present some of the results of our research. We first analyse the main paradoxes of our societies which influence our ability to live with dignity and achieve our aspirations. We then present the theoretical orientation that has guided our intervention projects, namely, empowerment. Finally, based on the experience we have gained through our projects, we discuss the elements that should be included in a key stage of any family intervention project: the assessment process. In short, our aim is to complement other theoretical approaches presented in the chapters of this book by delving deeper into a key issue, namely, how to take the step from describing a reality to actually transforming that reality using a properly designed method of assessment. In this process of constructing social well-being, social work plays a key role (Featherstone 2011).

From the Invisible Family to the Helping Family: Paradoxes of Welfare Societies

In our environment, the family enjoys good health as a social institution, but is also described as an institution that is permanently in crisis. Clearly, this is a paradoxical situation. While the family remains the most highly valued institution in the Latin countries of southern Europe, these countries have the lowest birth and marriage rates (Del Fresno 2011). While it could be said that we value the family, we are increasingly less willing to form one. Perhaps this particular situation can be explained from the perspective of Bourdieu as we are embedded in a conceptualisation that renders the family invisible as an institution, posits extreme individualism, exalts the symbolic mechanisms of personal competence and describes the family as a burden or constraint, as well as social policies (thereby advocating the abandonment of social policies based on the notion of citizenship and legitimising only purely charitable support measures, that is, returning to the social models that existed prior to the industrial revolution).

This theoretical model renders us powerless because it degrades our capacity for social interaction and promotes the dismantling of the welfare state. However, the dynamics of the Enlightenment are based on a contrary legitimacy (Bronner 2007). Against the individual is the citizen, who in order to exercise his or her rights demands that the state and institutions be structured in such a way as to allow them to exercise their freedom. First, by placing limits on the arbitrary exercise of power and, secondly, by establishing a context in which citizens, because they are in good health, possess knowledge, enjoy freedom and have a livelihood, can compete and pursue their goals in an environment made up of free citizens whose rights are guaranteed by law.

It is precisely the concept of empowerment, interwoven with Sen's notion of freedom and capabilities, which underlines the inadequacy of the neo-liberal approach. Because we are relational beings, our well-being is also relational. The family is the basic institution in which we are socialised and where we internalise the idea of justice, altruism, legitimacy and cooperation, as Boszormenyi-Nagy and Krasner (1986) insightfully noted within the strict limits of family intervention. The family plays a crucial role in the life of all individuals. The concern for reaching the maturity required in social interactions, whether for our own personal fulfilment or to attain family and group goals (including those related to the work setting), has highlighted the growing need to understand what exactly happens in family dynamics, and analyse the proper techniques for developing dynamics that will permit individuals to strengthen their skills, recover their competences and ultimately help them in achieving their personal life trajectories and well-being.

Nonetheless, it would be naïve to think that simply because we are social, family-oriented animals that constantly interact with others, we are experts in relating to others. Indeed, although we are aware of the mistakes we make and conscious that these errors have an impact on our life trajectories, we are unable or do not know how to change our behaviour. Failure is often justified in a technical, "mythical" sense: we explain what happens to us by appealing to causes of a different and sometimes inconsistent nature than the phenomena that happens to us or that we produce. Moreover, it is often the manner in which we explain the phenomena that leads us to err—something which is very evident in the field of social relations with vast offering of self-help books to learn to relate to others, to cope with failures, deal with a job layoff, mend a relationship, improve our employability or any other problem that we may face.

Since the origins of family research in the field of social work, one of the concerns of social workers has been to gain insight into personal and family behaviours that have been internalised through a complex process of socialisation and which must be redirected with the aid of professional intervention. In short, our theoretical frameworks, our typifications of reality and the stereotypes that we classify and on which we base our thought provide us guidelines to orient social interaction but also constrain, limit and condition us. Each of us is immersed in a given linguistic, cultural and relational universe governed by established patterns of behaviour, modes of interpretation and strategies to cope with problems.

We find ourselves immersed in complex explanations of reality, what we might call the cultural and technological traditions in which we operate. These explanations comprise a set of theories that, while not scientific in the strict sense, guide our behaviour. The majority of us live according to such theories simply out of habit or inertia. This is, then, the *first paradox*: although we know the external world, the physical reality that surrounds us, we are often not conscious of the theories in which we live and move and which in turn move us. That is, although we are constantly theorising, we do not realise that we are immersed in theories. We identify our way of viewing and explaining reality with the natural order of things. For this reason, the motto of the Enlightenment (*sapere aude*) brilliantly formulated by Kant shows us the way: break free of tradition and rigorously examine the physical reality and social reality, as well as the power structure characterising a society at a given historical moment.

In the families we interviewed, and in those that participated in our intervention project, we have observed this paradox: explanations and behavioural patterns are accepted as part of nature, as something obvious, and are not contrasted against their outcomes. Ways of thinking and behaving that promote social exclusion and foster violent behaviour within families are reinforced and regarded as the natural order of things. A social worker's first task, therefore, is to establish a different relational model that enables individuals to reflect on other ways of behaving and thinking and thus break free from deeply embedded habits.

The *second paradox* we encountered during our social intervention projects is what we call the myth of individualism. This is an explanation of behaviour and our life that only takes into account our individuality. Family and society are perceived as something that is provisional, a mere playground for our decisions. Although this is a hotly debated topic in philosophy and contemporary sociological theory, in our intervention projects we have seen to what extent this individualistic concept of life has been internalised. This has two consequences: first, it prevents us from properly analysing our social reality such as processes of exclusion, which are also social; and secondly, it incapacitates people: if we do not take social relations into account, we will be unable to cope with life's challenges. Indeed, as we have seen in our social intervention projects, many people have once again turned to their families as their only recourse for survival as a result of the economic crisis that began in September 2007.

We define ourselves as autonomous beings and individuals when we find ourselves immersed in social structures. All people are attentive observers of the reality that surrounds them and need the proper information to survive. To this end, they use a language in which they have been socialised, codes of behaviour and a theoretical scheme that permits them to frame the events, make sense of the facts and act in a particular way to consciously or unconsciously pursue their aims. We are individuals, but we are primarily social animals since before birth we have been accepted or rejected in our environment, we are born into a family unit, within a given society, and we are raised in a language and reach maturity after a long process of socialisation. In a certain sense, each of us faces a life of solitude (an individual path). Yet it is also true that from the very first moment life is social, it is defined by others, and that without the gaze of those others, without language and without expectations and goals which are always social (although we can later modify them in a process of active reformulation), we are unable to understand our identity since our likes and dislikes, our behavioural patterns, beauty, order and disorder, crime and conflict, failure and success are defined by the society to which we belong.

Individualistic explanations that do not take into account our social reality are nevertheless very appealing in our mass society. Apparently, in thinking that each of us makes our decisions alone (i.e. what we consume or in any area of life), we forget that we form part of a larger, mass society characterised by repetitive, induced behaviour and that our lifestyles are to a great extent shaped by advertising. To put it in Heideggerian terms, we forget that we have forgotten. If we call oblivion memory, how can we become aware of our situation? If we do not objectify our situation, we will believe that an induced decision is an individual one, thus losing our capacity for critical thought—our ability to objectify the origin of our behaviour.

Individualism merges with postmodernism and neo-liberalism to give rise to a new social Darwinism. In this context, we do not accurately analyse the influence of structural factors in determining our life trajectories and everything, from job success to basic relational skills to having an emotionally balanced life, becomes a personal matter, an individual responsibility. Processes of social exclusion become personally chosen trajectories, and the consequence is clear: guilt is projected on the individual, regardless of the structural factors that impede upward social mobility. In the context of the current economic crisis, which originated in the sub-prime mortgage fraud of October 2007, the shortage of capital worldwide has forced numerous companies to close that were functioning well and whose workers and managers were fulfilling their obligations. Yet an external situation, which was not their responsibility and beyond their control, caused companies to declare bankruptcy and workers to lose their jobs.

How can this be explained from an individualistic perspective, or from a discourse based on extreme neo-liberalism in which the market is presented as a system that automatically reorganises itself and where good management is rewarded with success understood in individual terms? Indeed, several authors have demonstrated the link between postmodern culture and the stratification of individuals, groups and countries in this new technological environment: "This whole global (…) postmodern culture is the internal and superstructural expression of a whole new wave of (…) military and economic domination" (Jameson 1991: 18–19). For this reason, many propose a new politics of postmodernism: "the new political art (if it is possible at all) will have to hold to the truth of postmodernism, that is to say, to its fundamental object—the world space of multinational capital—at the same time at which it achieves a breakthrough to some as yet an unimaginable new mode of representing this last, in which we may again begin to grasp our positioning as individual and collective subjects and regain a capacity to act and struggle which is at present neutralized by our spatial as well as our social confusion" (Jameson 1991: 120–121).

The *third paradox*, which is closely related to the above, is as follows: we are relational beings, but we do not cultivate social relationships. Throughout our professional experience in the field of social intervention, we have found an increasingly larger number of people lacking basic relational skills—people who are not only technologically illiterate but also illiterate in terms of relations. We have detected these characteristics chiefly in younger people who are not able to evaluate and adopt the behavioural patterns needed to integrate themselves into a given social environment. Thus, a *new syndrome* is on the rise: *relational illiteracy* (López Peláez 2009). The behavioural patterns of previous generations have long been lost, and in a context defined by individualism, the pursuit of profit and individual experiences, little room has been left for cultivating personal relationships targeted at personal fulfilment.

The relational models reflected in video games, television, film and literature often do not provide guidelines for developing strategies that permit us to accept our own or others' errors, tolerate frustration with our own life experiences in a reasonable manner (from the difficulties of finding a job to the limitations of old age), or build links based on solidarity, honesty, loyalty and mutual support. This loss of relational skills in advanced societies is related to the socialisation of violent or criminal behaviour in both the First and the Third World and is a serious barrier to social integration. For this reason, one of the key strategies for re-socialising people who come from the world of violence, terrorism, the mafia or war such as children soldiers in countries of Africa is aimed at designing group dynamics where these individuals can relearn patterns of behaviour that permit them to abandon their former life model.

The paradox of individual conscience, that of each of us, which needs others to be oneself, to develop as individuals, in short, the apparent contradiction between being unique and being social animals at the same time, was already present in the first reflections about the social nature of human beings. Innate selfishness and the pursuit of survival give way to altruism and friendship as the most appropriate survival strategy and permit us to develop as individuals. We cannot survive unless our way of life and that of others (who are part of us as well) do not survive as the innate altruism of parents towards their children shows. In this sense, our research highlights the power of the empowerment approach, which brings us to a fundamental issue: the capacity of individuals and families to confront reality from their own power, a power that must be regained, enhanced and actualised. In this sense, social ties are based on reciprocity, mutual support, loyalty and a functionally necessary altruism that is necessary for us to develop as individuals and to ensure, in biological terms, the continuity of the species. However, in the neo-liberal discourse that permeates our societies, all things related to the interaction with others or mutual interdependence are branded as "the social bond [which] arises elementally from a sense of mutual dependence. All the shibboleths of the new order treat dependence as a shameful condition (…) Almost without thinking we accept the contrast between a weak, dependent self and a strong, independent self. However, like the contrast between success and failure, this opposition flattens out reality. The truly self-reliant person proves to be by no means as independent as cultural stereotypes suppose" (Sennett 2009: 147).

In short, rather than an individualistic view, we must recover a vision more in tune with our reality as social beings, a vision in which altruistic reciprocity and interaction with others occupy their rightful place. We are trained to join the labour market, we are socialised through a discourse in which objectives are defined in terms of competition, control, individual experience and success, but we forget that emotions, knowledge and personal development are an essential element of our interaction with others. Interaction cannot be defined solely in terms of control or domination, but must also be conceived of in terms of equality, friendship or complicity. As Epicurus said, "of all the things which wisdom provides to make us entirely happy, much the greatest is the possession of friendship". The pragmatic interest that is present in our relationships does not have to be defined in opposition to altruistic interest: our actions always await the response of others, and when that response is supportive and beneficial to those who are communicating, we access the realm of friendship (Lledó 1995: 120).

Well-Being and Family Social Work

Any analysis of family well-being must bear in mind that well-being is a dynamic and aspirational concept contextualised in a concrete social environment. In this sense, it is important to analyse the strategies required to achieve a level of well-being that is characteristic of what is known as the area of social inclusion. As a scientific discipline, this is precisely the scope of action of social work. In a context such as the one we have described in the previous section, evaluating the negative consequences of our lifestyles and developing strategies to enhance our capabilities must be a priority of social policy. For this reason, in what follows, we explore the empowerment approach in social work as it allows us to examine in greater depth one of the factors that is most detrimental to the well-being of families: deskilling, that is, the powerlessness to cope with their lives both theoretically (as they do not asses their situation adequately) and in terms of their behaviour (patterns of interaction that impede recognising opportunities and facing problems).

Social work is primarily a scientific discipline (López Peláez 2010a) that allows us to evaluate our environment with rigour and method, and based on an adequate description of opportunities and problems, to design and implement a social intervention project that permits achieving the objectives that are set. From the very beginning of the discipline, families were considered a relevant object of study (as demonstrated in "social case work"), a focus that has ultimately become a specific sub-discipline known as family social work. When analysing a key topic such as family well-being from the perspective of social work, we must address several issues. First, social policies that permit families to attain a given level of well-being that is quantifiable in terms of benefits or available services. Second, the heterogeneity of families in cosmopolitan societies and the diversity of personal, family, group and community life trajectories, which have given rise to new demands and made it necessary to redefine social policies—policies which in turn promote or constrain certain family models. Third, the theoretical models or cultural imaginary in which we are embedded—models that give meaning to our aspirations and projects, and which to a large extent enable us to cope with our circumstances and transform or perpetuate them.

In this regard, we must examine all the major challenges faced by families and individuals in today's context (Collins et al. 2007), as well as the narratives and discourse of the families themselves regarding their problems and opportunities if we are to develop strategies that promote change and empower families according to their own potential (Hook 2008). Family social work investigates and discusses families, the most appropriate models and techniques, the characteristics of professional practice, its ethical orientation and the consequences of the theories we use.

As we saw in the previous section, we currently find ourselves in a context of growing individualism where traditional family-based support networks are eroding, to which we must add the effects of the economic crisis and tensions over welfare state funding and benefits (particularly in Europe and North America). From our point of view, it is necessary to once again emphasise the importance of capacitating people, giving or giving them back power over their own lives, but from a perspective that goes beyond the limitations of the theory of rational action. We must take into account communication, the building of bonds and the analysis of capabilities to empower them, an approach that is clearly linked to Amartya Sen's theory of justice (2010). In contrast to the somewhat nostalgic and pessimistic description of the consequences of "liquid links" (Bauman 2009), it is important to reconsider the benefits of self-reinforcement as the aim of both personal and family trajectories. In this sense, the empowerment theory allows us to redefine the objectives and methodology of social intervention to promote active citizenship in which individuals confront the future with better skills through a process of personal and family strengthening. This new way of facing reality through increased autonomy and critical thinking is linked to the basic objectives of social work. Above all, it permits families to attain higher levels of well-being because it abandons the welfare perspective and focuses on empowering the subject (the individual and the family), thus ensuring that the process of change and improvement will be sustainable in the future.

In our opinion, the concept of empowerment must be the cornerstone of family-centred programmes. Empowerment begins with the belief that families deserve respect, have strong positive attributes, can change their lives and are resilient. Therefore, providing assistance involves facilitating families' access to their power, not giving them power (Kaplan and Girard 1994). In the field of social work, the principles of empowerment have been applied to families in several ways: family health (Bowman 1983), family strengths (Littlejohn-Blake and Darling 1993; Schumm 1985), family functioning (Olson et al. 1983), nurturing families (Satir 1988) and resilient families (Hook 2008).

In the field of family social work, empowerment is defined as a process of mutuality and cooperation by which the family, its individual members and the social workers themselves achieve greater awareness and increase their power through a process in which goals are set and work is done to achieve them. It is important to highlight the notion of "process" in this definition. Here, process refers to participation by the family and the social worker through a constructive discourse in which the experiences of all the members involved are used to assess the reasons, justify, accept or reject. Throughout this process, decisions to act are made as a result of the "insight" gained. The goal is that families adopt a critical position that enables them to negotiate and act in ways that are meaningful for their purposes, values and feelings, rather than for the purposes of others that have been assimilated in a non-critical way. Learning in this manner leads people to gain greater control over their lives, to become socially responsible individuals and, above all, to make clearly thought-out decisions that connect their motives to the actions they take. This transformational process of "learning" focuses on areas in which families need to acquire skills or knowledge to be healthy. In this sense, empowerment views family problems as the result of underdeveloped skills or as the need to learn new skills.

The empowerment approach overcomes a classic ideological dilemma that has accompanied social work throughout its history (Lee 1989). On the one hand, there are those who give priority to the work itself rather than the "causes", that is, they hold that social work must focus chiefly on social change as a means of achieving a fairer society. In contrast, others give priority to the work itself rather than the "function", that is, they attach greater importance to the design and use of techniques that foster individual change. As we have seen in our social intervention projects since 2006, the empowerment approach merges both proposals because it considers them to be complementary and necessary to achieve a satisfactory outcome. Moreover, empowerment introduces a further element in this dilemma that ultimately serves to dismantle it: the criterion for selecting which issues to work on is not determined exclusively by the "cause" or the "function", but by the family's *needs* or *deep desires*.

The Empowerment Approach: Making Family Well-Being Possible

Family well-being can be analysed from three perspectives: at the personal level (the individuals that comprise the family unit), at the level of interpersonal relationships, and the community level. In a similar way, family social work based on empowerment is targeted at three levels of intervention: personal, interpersonal and community or political. Social workers must take all of these levels into account simultaneously since excluding any one of them is an important predictor of the lack of success.

Chart 14.1 Levels of Intervention from the Empowerment Perspective

Personal: On the personal level, empowerment has been defined as a process by which the social worker and client focus on activities "that aim to reduce their powerlessness (or access to power itself) that has been created by negative valuations based on membership in a stigmatized group" (Solomon 1976: 19). This type of empowerment occurs when there is less feeling of powerlessness and aspects are enhanced such as self-esteem, self respect, self-worth and self-efficacy, one's own sense of competence, mastery, empathy and relationships of mutuality, the ability to identify and use information to identify and cope with difficulties, the ability to seek internal and external resources and the capacity to use them to one's own and the family's benefit effectively, flexibility, hope, a certain degree of confidence that the future will bring satisfaction, strengths and skills to effect changes, and the ability to seek and accept help (Gitterman and Germain 2008; Miley et al. 2007: 87; Lee 2001).

(continued)

Chart 14.1 (continued)

Interpersonal: Interpersonal empowerment is the ability to act for a specific purpose by mobilising the energies, resources and strengths of each person through a mutual relationship.

Positive and affective relationships both within the family and in the private realm of individuals stimulate development in several ways. They fulfil the needs of families at various levels and promote the integrated development of children's sense of self, resulting in the establishment of authentic relationships with others (Kilpatrick et al. 2000). When such positive relationships are lacking within the nuclear family, individuals are usually able to find someone within the extended family such as teachers, neighbours, associations or individuals within their community with whom to establish this type of relationship (Hook 2008).

At the interpersonal level, it strengthens the inner consistency of the family, regular routines, parental coherency and participation by family members in family activities (Bowlby 1973).

Community or Political: At the community or political level, the situation of families that are the object of social work has led us to the realisation that we must work to restore health not only within these families, but in the community and society at large (Hook 2008). Empowerment is a process of community action aimed at securing human rights and social justice for groups in situations of poverty and exclusion. Through this process, the community, and the families that form it, enhance their participation, negotiation and organisation to influence policy decisions that affect them as a way to achieve well-being (López Peláez 2010a, b). When social workers assist members of a family in accessing community resources, the opportunities for empowerment, that is, access to and the maintenance of power, will continue to exist even long after the social worker has intervened. The better the resources and connections that they have developed, the greater the success of the community where the family lives and the family's ability to cope with the multiplicity of problems that arise (Solomon 1976). Lessons on social and community empowerment, in addition to the lessons of oppression, are first learned in one's family. Indeed, "these are lessons that never leave us. Children are astute observers and they discern emotional environments built on strength, contribution, opportunity, mutuality, cooperation and respect from those built on weakness, limitation, deficiency, domination and lack of respect" (Bula Wise 2005: 49).

Source: The authors

In both social work practice and the field of theoretical discussion, as well as in the practical experience, we have gained through our recent social intervention projects that a key issue arises: whether to consider the *subject* of the problems and opportunities (the person, family, group or community) as the *subject* of change or as a *passive object* of change. In our case, the empowerment approach led us to design questionnaires and methods of intervention based on the ability of families to acknowledge their opportunities and cope with their problems as subjects of change. This entails transforming the vision of the social worker as a scientist who diagnoses a patient with no technical ability that passively accepts the diagnosis, to a professional scientific activity which assesses the capabilities and potential of the individual, family, group or specific community so that they become subjects of their process of change. Accepting the knowledge, assessment and proposals regarding behaviour in the first person allowed us to achieve better results. Moreover, it transformed social intervention into a process that was *sustainable over time*, as those involved become responsible for continuing the dynamics once the worker has finalised his or her work.

In this sense, if we examine the traditional views associated with the diagnosis of problems, we find that social workers analyse the inability of people to cope with events that oppress them. Although social workers may differ in terms of the methods of analysis they, how they define problems, and the intervention strategies they implement to overcome them, all agree that people need help because they have a problem. In this way, the individuals or families that receive assistance according to these approaches are defined from the beginning in a different manner than those who do not have such problems. Social work literature abounds with information about problems of dysfunctionality, maladaptation, victimisation and powerlessness, and yet the information about the strengths, capacities and power of clients seems to be relegated to the background (DuBois and Miley 2005: 26).

At the social level, we believe that this pathology and problem-centred approach may be one of the reasons for the ineffectiveness of current social work practices in Spain. By diagnosing the problem in this traditional sense, people, families, groups and communities are situated on the dark side of the continuum that separates capacity from incapacity, thus reaffirming their exclusion and sense of powerlessness. Increasingly, however, the social work discipline in both Spain and the rest of the world attaches greater importance to a context-based assessment focusing on capacities, strengths and power rather than weaknesses, problems and pathologies (Bula Wise 2005; Collins et al. 2007; De Robertis and Pascal 2007; Greene 2008; Hepworth et al. 2010; Lehman and Simmons 2009; López Peláez and Sánchez-Cabezudo Segado 2010; Shulman 2009; Yanca and Johnson 2008).

From the perspective of empowerment, family social work is guided by a set of core principles that are repeated regularly in works by renowned social work researchers who support, investigate and put into practice the empowerment approach (Bula Wise 2005; DuBois and Miley 2005; Gutiérrez and Lewis 1999; Hepworth et al. 2010; Lee 2001; Miley et al. 2007; Mondros and Wilson 1994; Simon 1994; Zastrow 2004). As these principles constitute the core of both practical and theoretical applications, it is essential that social workers internalise and apply them in professional practice. When social workers are successful in doing so, professional practice becomes a natural event that is guided at every step of the way and not left to the mercy of chance or improvisation. These principles do not aim to solve a momentary problem/need: the need is simply the starting point for undertaking work that will transform families. In this case, the goal is not only to resolve the oppressive situation in which families find themselves, but provide them with the skills, abilities and strategies required to achieve the well-being they desire in their lives. In this sense, the principles of empowerment in social work practice are:

1. Start from personal strengths and capacities
2. Interculturality
3. Three-dimensional diagnosis
4. Foster linkages between power, resources and capacities
5. Reciprocity and mutuality
6. Shared power
7. Cooperation and mutual support
8. Social justice

Assessment: A Key Phase in Fam3ily Social Work

Throughout our social intervention projects in the family social work field, we have confirmed the importance of what may be termed the first phase of any project: assessment. If the situation of families is not assessed properly, the objectives of the intervention and the commitment between the social worker and the family cannot be clearly established, impeding us to design and develop activities aimed at enhancing the family's well-being. Descriptive analyses of the sociological development of families, well-being, the welfare state or factors that influence processes of social exclusion should also take into consideration how to revitalise families, shape social policies and intervene professionally to promote social inclusion. In this sense, research on family well-being must be multidisciplinary, while including the perspectives typical of social work. In what follows, we present an assessment model that we designed based on our own practical experience, and which highlights key aspects of family well-being.

From a methodological standpoint, the assessment process is the most important phase in social intervention projects to ensure that families and the members that comprise it are protected. However, assessment policies and manuals vary from country to country. In the United States, for example, the chief trend is to use scientifically validated, objective measures (Holland 2007). In Europe, particularly in England and Wales, quantitative and qualitative assessments are more common as outlined in the Framework for the Assessment of Children in Need and Their Families (Department of Health 2000). In Spain, the information gathered in family assessments is eminently qualitative (Rodriguez and Luengo 2003), with different protocols used depending on the regions where the assessment is made, although validated questionnaires with objective measurements of the families are being employed on an increasing basis.

Processes of change in individuals, families or communities are very costly. It is therefore important to base intervention on assessments that will provide the best guarantee of success. In order for assessments to be valid and useful, as well as the decisions that are taken according to them, they must be based on logical reasoning and inferences grounded in the available evidence (Meyer 1993). Family involvement is essential. It is not the job of the social worker to make value judgements or ensure families that a specific outcome will occur. The aim of the assessment process is to guide families in achieving their own potential as individuals, strengthening family relationships and aiding them to take an active part in the process towards change and empowerment.

To properly assess the family unit from this perspective, it is necessary to use the following criteria: (a) environmental/contextual factors should be considered as important as individual factors; (b) systems that are external to the individual, group or community involved can be identified as targets for change; (c) we must clearly emphasise and explain that we work "with the user" and not "on the user" based on the idea of power sharing or "power with"; (d) we should focus on the strengths of the people with whom we work, and maintain that (e) diagnoses are something external to people, something performed by a professional with "expert" knowledge about the situation. We must not forget that in the field of social work, the people with whom we work are the primary experts on their situation.

In this decision-making process based on available evidence, social workers must make well-founded choices from the beginning of the intervention process. Some of these choices will revolve around issues of great importance in the process (Lopez and Segado 2010a): deciding where and when to address the family situation, the type and duration of the intervention, when to work on specific events or on feelings that may arise, and when to work with verbal or non-verbal material. Assessment can be carried out even in especially controversial areas. For example, estimating the damage that can be done if one or more family members remain in the household, making decisions about when a child should be separated from his or her family, if it is safe for the child to return home, or if the child should live elsewhere on a permanent basis.

In what follows, we briefly present the assessment model that we have had the opportunity to design, implement and modify over the last 4 years. Often, one of the most important problems confronting social workers in professional practice is the lack of a suitable map or guidelines to orient their intervention at each stage of the process. Social workers must be equipped with a set of references, explanations and a repertoire of techniques to address each stage of the process. In both social case work and family social work with groups and communities, reference manuals establish a series of stages or phases in the intervention process. We describe in detail the characteristics that the assessment process of intervention projects should include, distinguishing between four phases: the preliminary phase, the initial phase, the intermediate phase and achieving commitment.

Preliminary Phase of the Assessment Process

From the perspective of empowerment, communication between the social worker and the family should be framed within the notion of "power sharing" or "power with". To contextualise the relationship in this framework, both parties must work to build an authentic relationship based on empathy that gives rise to respect and trust, two essential conditions for creating a safe, collaborative environment to undertake the work. However, social workers must take extreme caution when beginning the assessment process. We cannot ignore that in interpreting the actions of families, we use both everyday language and the jargon of the profession to denote representations of reality—representations that exist in part but are also invented. In designating such representations, in using a given concept or a word to define them, we attach an added meaning, which is, in some way, intentional. Given that all human beings have needs, values, feelings and a mediated or biased perception of their environment as a result of their life events, and given that social workers are human beings, it should be assumed that they will also be affected by these factors. Social work professionals must therefore ensure that they take the appropriate measures so as not to sway the evaluation process. At the same time, they must take into account the biases that are already present in the family's understanding of its own dynamics. For this reason, we have analysed the cultural paradoxes in which we are immersed in the first sections of this chapter. In each case, social workers must examine their own biases as well as the prejudices and biases already operating within the family involved in the intervention and its cultural environment.

To achieve this aim, a series of processes and tasks are carried out (Table 14.1) at two levels: an analysis of the social worker's own biases and an analysis of the biases that shape the self-perception of the family to avoid making biased assessments. In a first stage, social workers must (a) establish a channel of communication in consonance with the practice of empowerment that is underpinned by two fundamental elements, empathy and authenticity; (b) reflect on and use language that will strengthen and transform the power of the family members; and (c) observe themselves and their own life trajectories through the lens of the principles of empowerment. In a second stage, they must (a) collect all the background information available on the family and (b) examine the cultural imaginary and the main patterns of interpretation and guidelines of behaviour in the family's immediate environment.

Initial Phase of the Assessment Process

As we saw above, the preliminary phase of the assessment process provides the social worker with a physical, cognitive and emotional context before making contact with the family. After contextualisation, the time comes to start working face to face with the family. From the moment of the first contact, there are three rules that mark the relationship between the social worker and the family: interaction, mutuality and reciprocity.

The assessment process involves collecting data and gaining deeper knowledge about the family's functioning. In the first or initial interviews, a clear record is obtained of the family's strengths, resources, problems and needs, aspects that must be given priority are determined, and which interventions to put in practice are decided upon. Assessment has several objectives: (1) determine the level of family functioning; (2) assess the strengths and needs of the family; (3) explore the environment,

Table 14.1 Family assessment from the empowerment perspective: the preliminary phase

	Tasks	Techniques/skills	Objectives
Preliminary phase Before the social worker enters into direct contact with the family, a series of processes and tasks must be developed	*Prepare a channel of communication* in consonance with the practice of empowerment Training in a *language that stren-gthens* and is capable of mobilising families' power *Self-analysis of the worker* according to the principles of empowerment Collect all the *background information* available about the family	*Empathy*: This is the vehicle by which the worker becomes emotionally significant and is therefore capable of influencing the lives of others *Authenticity*: This involves "opening up" and sharing feelings, opinions and ideas with the members of the family Acknowledge and not confront *obstacles to communication*	Create a safe and collaborative environ-ment to undertake the work. This begins long before the first contact between the worker and the family Equal relations of power between the worker and the family Identify barriers to communications in order to anticipate aspects that must be overcome or worked on if possible

Source: The authors based on Bula Wise (2005), DuBois and Miley (2005), Gutiérrez and Lewis (1999), Lee (2001), Miley et al. (2007), Rappaport and Hess (1984), Zastrow (2004), Rapp (1998), Saleebey (2006), Weick (1992), Sulman (1991), Hepworth et al. (2010), Raines (1996), and Berman-Rossi (1993)

specifically individual, interpersonal, cultural and community factors; (4) analyse areas for change; (5) collaborate with the family in deciding which interventions to implement; and (6) achieve a commitment.

Changes in patterns of interaction (limitations and communication patterns) and family functioning (roles and tasks) are sought at the individual and family level, but these changes must also be targeted at the interactions the family has with its closest environment, that is, relatives, friends, co-workers, leisure companions and the community. The degree of change arises from the direct relationship between the family's needs and the goals and skills of the social worker. The complexity of the change also varies: it can be as simple as modifying behavioural patterns or as complex as reworking the entire family system.

The most important feature of this phase is the emphasis on structuring the intervention around resources, strengths, capacities and achievements. It is surprising to find that a deeper than expected understanding of the family unit is often gained through this knowledge. In addition to identifying these factors, it is also necessary to assess the needs/problems of the family unit and each of its members. Family problems are often manifestations of unmet needs, that is, the poor match between such needs and the available resources. Frequently, they are desires that are deeply rooted in the individual or family which motivate behaviours that may not be essential for survival, but are essential in achieving greater individual and family well-being. Families usually do not identify them as needs or deep desires, but only think they have "problems" (Hepworth et al. 2010). The process of translating complaints and problems into needs and desires is usually of great help to families who remain focused on or blame others for their problems and are unable to see or conceive of such problems as "their specific needs".

Translating problems into needs involves an enormous challenge for families, but is the mechanism that ignites the process of change and the path towards well-being. An important cognitive distinction must be made between (1) formulating problems as needs that must be met and (2) thinking that we are plagued by problems, that we are the makers of problems, that problems are inherent to our existence, or even that "we" are the problem. Often, families that seek help or are referred by other services have exhausted their strategies to cope with adversity or simply do not have the resources to do so. It is very frustrating to see that even though one has fought to the point of exhaustion, problems not only remain unresolved but, in many cases, have worsened or new ones have arisen.

Ensuring that both the family and its members acknowledge and internalise what they call "problems" are actually needs is a revolutionary process. When they identify their needs and desires, they no longer feel stigmatised and begin to see that the problems may not be something inherent in their lives. By accepting that they have legitimate needs and desires, they will find it easier to identify and negotiate the goals they want to achieve in their lives in conjunction with the social worker and greatly increase their motivation to work towards these goals. Identifying needs provides families and family members a *new identity* as agents with power to make changes. The outcome is the same whether changes are formulated as a cognitive shift by the individual or if they are formulated in terms of power, that is, the processes of oppression to which these families are subjected.

From a cognitive standpoint, there is a shift from an external locus of control[1] ("*I always have problems and I cannot do anything about them*", "*everything I do turns out wrong*", "*the truth is that I must be the problem*") to an internal locus of control ("*I have needs and desires in my life and with the collaboration and assistance offered to me I will work to achieve them*"). From the viewpoint of processes of oppression, reflecting on one's own and the family's needs could lead to the abandonment of oppressive dynamics that grips families in need. "For forty years my work has been driven by this sentence: families living in a situation of extreme poverty and exclusion have to make their own contribution". In this assessment phase, Lee (2001) points to the need to explore these "manifestations of oppression". Such manifestations of oppression are not only found in the environment, but in the subjects themselves: people come to internalise very negative views of their abilities and capabilities. In the same vein, Freire (1970: 48) suggests that individuals must confront the reality of the dual nature of their own consciousness, discover their inner oppressor and become aware of the actual situation in order to be free and develop. In this sense, and from the perspective of empowerment, translating problems into needs is key to giving families the power to change and finding satisfaction in a collaborative intervention process (Table 14.2).

Intermediate Phase of the Assessment Process

We must deepen our knowledge about the family relations at all levels of the system to identify the dynamics that impede them from achieving a state of well-being. Families usually interact with the following systems (Hepworth et al. 2010): (a) the nuclear family and the extended family; (b) social networks such as friends, neighbours, co-workers, members of associations, clubs or cultural groups; (c) public institutions such as educational and recreational institutions, legal services, health care (general, mental, etc.), social services, employment, economic security; (d) personal access to services including doctors, dentists, hairdressers, waiters, mechanics, bank employees, landlords (if renting); and (e) spiritual/religious belief system.

The aim of this phase is to understand how these systems interact in given situations involving the family. Indeed, the recognition of patterns of family interaction both internally and externally and at all levels is the cornerstone of systems theory applied to family social work (Carlson et al. 1991). The term "pattern" refers

[1] The locus of control is a personality trait proposed in social learning theory. See Rotter and Murly (1965). The locus of control is measured according to the capacity of control and self-control, that is, to what extent subjects are capable of self-control when faced with social situations or, in contrast, their actions are influenced by such situations.

Table 14.2 Family assessment from the perspective of empowerment: the initial phase

	Tasks	Techniques/skills	Objectives
Initial phase In the first or initial interviews, a clear record is obtained of strengths, resources, problems and needs. Priority needs and the interventions to be implemented are determined	The *first contact with the family:* This is an assessment process in which data is gathered and deeper knowledge about family functioning is gained The *initial interview:* The initial interview will not unveil some latent and important family issues, but will reveal the family's initial predisposition. The social worker will begin to gain knowledge of family interaction patterns	*Achieve a commitment* that involves a therapeutic alliance between the social worker and all members of the family *Specify the concerns* and work to be implemented to show that they are not private matters affecting only one member of the family but the entire family unit *What attempts have been made to change and what changes do they want to make in their lives?* As the family discusses the efforts tvhey have made so far, aspects in need of change emerge more clearly and are not mere conjecture. This discussion will give rise to proposals for change and offers of services by the social worker that must be agreed upon at a future time *Mutually identify resources, strengths, needs/problems, and factors of oppression*	Create an environment where family members can safely talk about themselves and other members of the family Secure respect and collaboration. Ensure that the family understands the work that will be done Initiate feedback among members of the family. Often this is the first feedback families have shared in a long time and is a symbolic starting point of great importance Families seeking assistance should view themselves as experts of their own life trajectories and situations. This process gives families the authority and control they deserve over their own affairs Instil the vision among the family that they are not oppressed by "problems" but rather have "needs" or "deficiencies"

Source: Authors based on Bula Wise (2005), Hepworth et al. (2010), Kirst-Ashman et al. (2002), Lee (2001), Sánchez Urios (2006), Thomlison (2007a, b), Satir (1967), Collins et al. (2007), Rooney (2009), Miley et al. (2007: 148), Cowger (1996), Cowger et al. (2006), Vosler (1990), Freire (1970: 48), and Saalebey (2004)

to behaviours that occur repeatedly and are therefore predictable. Patterns are habits and families find security in them. Such patterns may be harmful to both individual members or the family as whole, but family members are often not aware of such patterns or their possible adverse effects. This lack of awareness leads to inertia and the perpetuation of these patterns. This process of deepening our knowledge of family relations concludes when goals are identified.

The formulation of objectives begins with a need or a desire expressed by the family, or in the case of families who do not request assistance on a voluntary basis, it involves adapting to an objective or objectives set by someone outside the family system. As mentioned above, although the needs manifested by families who come voluntarily will not necessarily determine the objective or objectives of the intervention, such manifestations will certainly be valuable for pre-selecting the objectives.

In the case of involuntary clients, the objectives are established by the social services that have referred them or by court order. In general, families who come on a non-voluntary basis consent to the process in a passive manner because "someone says they need help". On many occasions, however, they are not willing to accept the service (Shulman 2009). One of the aspects of intervention that causes greatest disconformity among clients is the lack of agreement regarding the objectives that have been set for them based on their deficiencies or pathologies. When consensus is not reached on the objectives, families again become immersed in perceptions of powerlessness and are placed on the side of powerlessness and marginalisation (Rooney 2009). Yet from the perspective of empowerment, the message must be sent to the family that they have much to say on the subject, that their needs will be heard, and that they will work together to put all the available resources at their disposition, meet their needs and achieve the goals that have been imposed on them, while making it clear that they have the right to not share them (DeJong and Berg 2001). When acting according to the principles of empowerment to define objectives, the involuntary family that comes with the idea that the needs imposed on them are not their own ("*I don't have any problems, it must be my husband since he's the one who does drugs*") is likely to acknowledge that they do indeed have needs and that having needs is legitimate. Moreover, the belief that these needs can be satisfied will surely serve as a source of motivation to undertake the work.

When voluntary families must define their objectives, the perception that the family has of the social worker is one based on trust. Yet even for these families, the motivation and emotional involvement needed to set objectives and work towards them must stem from the belief that by working together they can alleviate or resolve their concerns and needs (Meyer 2001). Under the empowerment perspective, social workers adopt a mediating role. They do not have power or authority over the objectives to be set, nor do they play a passive role. Instead they act as guides who achieve a balance between their role as qualified professionals and that of another member of the family who is collaborating in the process (Table 14.3).

Table 14.3 Family assessment from the empowerment perspective: the intermediate phase

	Tasks	Techniques/skills	Objectives
Intermediate phase Deeper knowledge is gained of the family's internal and external relations. This is an essential requirement to orient the intervention work in an appropriate manner	*Deepen understanding of the relations:* This involves identifying patterns of family interaction at both sub-levels and supra-levels	*Use of maps and graphic tools:* Family Time Line. Maps or tables of social networks. The culturegram	Guide the family in unders-tanding their patterns of interaction and how some of these patterns may be sustaining dysfunctionality and oppression The maps and graphic tools are developed mutually between the family and the social worker to permit both parties to gain a greater understanding of the relational processes that are taking place
	Identify the objectives of the work: Initially, broad objectives can be formulated. At a later point in time, other more specific objectives can be set in order to achieve the general objectives formulated at the beginning of the process	*Use of standardised questionnaires:* Structural interviews. Questionnaires targeted at the strengths of families: the Family Functioning Style Scale (FSSS) and the Family Resources Scale (FSR) Use of specific, standardised questionnaires to measure empowerment: interviews, participatory observation methods, scales on personality categories and attitudes indicative of empowerment, vignettes to measure personal and political empowerment. Questionnaires to measure empowerment in school-age children and a Family Empowerment Scale The importance of *cultural diversity* put into practice: Clarifying roles and options for family members to participate in the process. Knowing family perceptions, identifying their needs and desires. Use of the culturegram	Assessing cultural diversity allows family members to be heard and at the same time increase family involvement in the work Establish the characteristics of family dynamics and the areas in which the family as a whole and each of its members can work on their empowerment

Source: Authors based on Shulman (2009), Rooney (2009), DeJong and Berg (2001), Weinberg (2006), Meyer (2001), Hudson and McMurtry (1997), McGoldrick et al. (1999), Holman (1983), Bula Wise (2005), Collins et al. (2007), Montalvo et al. (1998), Tracy and Whittaker (1990), Congress (1994), Szapocznik et al. (1991), Peñalva (2001), Dunst et al. (1994), Dunst and Leet (1986), Kieffer (1984), Maton and Rappaport (1984), Zimmerman and Rappaport (1988), and Gutiérrez and Ortega (1991)

Table 14.4 Family assessment from the empowerment perspective: the commitment phase

	Tasks	Techniques/skills	Objectives
Commitment	*Make a commitment*	*Oral or written:* When the commitment is made in writing, the family becomes more involved in the process. Families also have the opportunity to reflect on and add content	Determine the type of need, delimit roles and responsibilities Identify and delimit the dimensions that must be strengthened throughout the intervention

Source: The authors based on Germain and Gitterman (1996), Thomlison (2007a, b), and Lee (2001)

Achieving a Commitment in the Assessment Process

Achieving a commitment is the final phase of the assessment process and will lead the way to the following phases of the family social intervention project. The key element of this phase is the commitment that the family makes with the social worker to undertake all the tasks that have been designed based on the results of the initial evaluation. However, social workers must be wary when families make the commitment as they often expect the social worker to solve their problem. In this sense, social work professionals should remain vigilant and reject this role. Instead, they must help the family to sustain their power as agents of change with the capacity to decide about their lives. The objectives that have been set out and recorded in the contract must be realistic; vague and unrealistic objectives are impossible to achieve. The contract should include an agreement on the nature of the need/problem in transactional terms, contain realistic goals and provide a detailed explanation of how to reduce stress levels and enhance coping strategies within and outside the family (Germain and Gitterman 1996). Likewise, the contract should specify "both the practitioner's role and the family's role in the intervention. Expected gains, benefits and other outcomes that may occur are also clearly explained, as well as the costs and time" (Thomlison 2007b: 85). The contract can be made in writing. When this is the case, it is of great help if the user provides content and both parties remain open to possible changes depending on how the work evolves (Table 14.4).

Conclusions

From the perspective of empowerment, family social work is targeted at helping families and their members to overcome obstacles that prevent them from achieving a state of well-being based on their own capacities and power to become "subjects" of their life trajectories (and not just "objects" that are assisted by social policies). From this perspective, survival is not pursued, but life experiences and overall health. The current situation of families in Spanish society calls for new theoretical and practical models to cope with new demands. Empowerment involves training, as well as the acquisition and development of skills and abilities. It is a way of viewing life that pursues coping with life events naturally and moves away from the "you can always do a little more" or "I'm not able to" to focus on acknowledging one's own personal power and self-knowledge as a way to discern what we really want in our lives and how to achieve our goals in a healthy manner. This is because the survival skills families have developed in conditions of exclusion, despite being an extremely valuable tool to cope with the stressful or negative events taking place in their lives, are not a way of life.

In this sense, empowerment allows individuals to recognise self-imposed constraints and limitations that are products of our cultural environment and our family trajectories. It also serves to highlight our potential and allows us to transform ourselves from objects to active subjects, come in closer contact with our reality as citizens of an advanced democracy who participate in collective decision-making processes about our common future. The well-being of families is closely linked to their ability to be subjects of their lives and cultivate their capacities to confront the challenges and opportunities of a changing environment.

The analysis of family life conditions and the economic and social policies that need to be developed to foster their well-being must also take into account the methodologies of social intervention. Through them, we can help families (as subjects that can change their lives) to regain their ability to face challenges and opportunities, and to live as citizens in our contemporary democracies. By doing so, families will be able to cross the border that defines social inclusion, that is, by truly exercising their condition as citizens and transforming their rights into capacities (Sen 2010). As we have shown in this chapter, in order to achieve these aims, it is essential to establish an evaluation process through which families make a commitment to themselves and the social worker to become the subject of their own dynamics of change.

References

Bauman, Z. (2009). *Amor líquido. Acerca de la fragilidad de los vínculos humanos*. Madrid: FCE.

Berman-Rossi, T. (1993). The tasks and skills of social workers across stages of group development. *Social Work with Groups, 16*(1–2), 69–81.

Boszormenyi-Nagy, I., & Krasner, B. (1986). *Between give and take*. New York: Brunner/Mazel.

Bourdieu, P., & Wacquant, L. (2005). *Una invitación a la sociología reflexiva*. Buenos Aires: Siglo XXI.

Bowlby, J. (1973). *Separation: Anxiety & anger*. London: Hogarth Press.

Bowman, P. J. (1983). Significant involvement and functional relevance: Challenges to survey research. *Social Work Research, 19*, 21–26.

Bronner, S. (2007). *Reivindicación de la Ilustración*. Pamplona: Laetoli.

Bula Wise, J. (2005). *Empowerment practice with families in distress*. New York: Columbia University Press.

Carlson, J., Sperry, L., & Lewis, J. (1991). *Family therapy: Ensuring treatment efficacy*. Pacific Grove: Brooks/Cole.

Collins, D., Jordan, C., & Coleman, H. (2007). *An introduction to family social work*. Belmont: Thomson Brooks/Cole.

Congress, E. P. (1994). The use of culturegrams to assess and empower culturally diverse families. *Families in Society, 75*(9), 531–540.

Cowger, C. D. (1996). Assessment of client strengths. In D. Saleeby (Ed.), *The strengths perspective in social work practice* (pp. 69). Boston: Allyn y Bacon.

Cowger, C. D., Anderson, K. M., & Snively, C. A. (2006). Assessing strengths: The political context of individual, family, and community empowerment. In D. Saleeby (Ed.), *The strengths perspective in social work practice* (4th ed., pp. 93–115). Boston: Allyn & Bacon.

De Robertis, C., & Pascal, H. (2007). *La intervención colectiva en Trabajo Social. La acción con grupos y comunidades*. Buenos Aires: Lumen Humanitas.

DeJong, P., & Berg, I. K. (2001). Co-constructing cooperation with mandated clients. *Social Work, 46*(4), 361–374.

Del Fresno, García. (2011). *Retos para la intervención social con familias en el siglo XXI. Consumo, ocio, cultura, tecnología e hijos*. Madrid: Trotta.

Departamento de Salud. (2000). *Framework for the assessment of children in need and their families*. At: http://www.dh.gov.uk/en/Publicationsandstatistics/Publications/Publications-PolicyAndGuidance/DH_4008144

DuBois, B., & Miley, K. K. (2005). *Social work: An empowering profession*. Boston: Allyn & Bacon.

Dunst, C. J., & Leet, H. E. (1986). *Family resources scale FRS*. Cambridge, MA: Brookline Books.

Dunst, C. J., Trivette, C. M., & Deal, A. G. (Eds.). (1994). *Supporting and strengthening families: Methods, strategies and practices*. Cambridge, MA: Brookline Books.

Featherstone, B. (2011). The current economic crisis in Ireland: Why social work needs to be part of the challenge to a discredited system? *Comunitania. Revista Internacional de Trabajo Social y Ciencias Sociales* [International Journal of Social Work and Social Sciences], *1*, 17–29.

Freire, P. (1970). *Pedagogy of the oppressed*. London: Penguin.

Germain, C. B., & Gitterman, A. (1996). Ecological perspective. In R. Edwards (Ed.), *Encyclopedia of social work, I* (pp. 816–824). Washington, DC: National Association of Social Workers.

Gitterman, A., & Germain, C. B. (2008). *The life model of social work practice. Advances in theory and practice*. New York: Columbia University Press.

Greene, R. R. (2008). *Human behaviour theory and social work practice*. New Brunswick: Transaction Publishers.

Gutiérrez, L. M., & Lewis, E. (1999). *Empowering women of color*. New York: Columbia University Press.

Gutiérrez, L. M., & Ortega, R. (1991). Developing methods to empower Latinos: The importance of groups. *Social Work with Groups, 14*, 23–43.

Hepworth, D., Rooney, R. H., Rooney, G., Strom-Gottfried, K., & Larsen, J. (2010). *Direct social work practice: Theory and skills*. Belmont: Brooks/Cole.

Holland, S. (2007). *Child and family assessment in social work practice*. London: Sage.

Holman, A. (1983). *Family assessment: Tools for understanding and intervention*. Newbury Park: Sage.

Hook, M. P. (2008). *Social work practice with families. A resiliency-based approach*. Chicago: Lyceum Books.

Hudson, W., & McMurtry, S. L. (1997). Comprehensive assessment in social work practice: A multi-problem screening inventory. *Research on Social Work Practice, 7*(1), 79–88.

Jameson, F. (1991). *El posmodernismo o la lógica cultural del capitalismo avanzado*. Barcelona: Paidós Estudio.

Kaplan, L., & Girard, J. (1994). *Strengthening high-risk families: A handbook for practitioners*. New York: Lexington Books.

Kieffer, C. H. (1984). Citizen empowerment: A developmental perspective. In J. Rappaport, C. Swift, & R. Hess (Eds.), *Studies in empowerment. Steps towards understanding and action* (pp. 9–36). New York: Haworth.

Kilpatrick, A., Kilpatrick, E., & Callaway, J. (2000). Object relations family therapy. In A. Horne (Ed.), *Family counselling and therapy*. Itasca: Peacock.
Kirst-Ashman, K., Hull, G., & Vogel, V. (2002). *Student manual for understanding generalist practice*. Pacific Grove: Brooks/Cole.
Lee, J. A. B. (1989). *Group work with the poor and oppressed*. New York: Haworth.
Lee, J. A. B. (2001). *The empowerment approach to social work practice. Building the beloved community*. New York: Columbia University Press.
Lehman, P., & Simmons, C. A. (2009). *Strengths-based batterer intervention. A new paradigm in ending family violence*. New York: Springer Publishing Company.
Littlejohn-Blake, S. M., & Darling, A. C. (1993). Understanding strengths of African American families. *Journal of Black Studies, 23*(4), 460–471.
Lledó, E. (1995). *El Epicureísmo*. Madrid: Taurus.
López Peláez, A. (2009). Analfabetismo relacional e inteligencia emocional: ¿un nuevo reto para las organizaciones en el siglo XXI? *Orthopedic Business Rewiew, 3*, 3–9.
López Peláez, A. (Ed.). (2010a). *Técnicas de diagnóstico, intervención y evaluación social*. Madrid: Universitas.
López Peláez, A. (Ed.). (2010b). *Teoría del Trabajo Social con Grupos*. Madrid: Universitas.
López Peláez, A., & Segado Sánchez-Cabezudo, S. (2010). Técnicas de diagnóstico, intervención y evaluación social: Fundamentos teóricos. In A. López Peláez (Ed.), *Técnicas de Diagnóstico, Intervención y Evaluación Social*. Madrid: Universitas.
Maton, K. I., & Rappaport, J. (1984). Empowerment in a religious setting: A multivariate investigation. *Prevention in Human Services, 3*, 37–72.
McGoldrick, M., Gerson, R., & Shellenberger, S. (1999). *Genograms: Assessment and intervention* (3rd ed.). New York: Norton.
Meyer, C. H. (1993). *Assessment in social work practice*. New York: Columbia University Press.
Meyer, W. (2001). Why they don't come back: A clinical perspective on the no-show client. *Clinical Social Work, 29*(4), 325–339.
Miley, K. K., O'Melia, M., & Dubois, B. (2007). *Generalist social work practice: An empowering approach* (5th ed.). Boston: Allyn & Bacon.
Mondros, J. C., & Wilson, S. M. (1994). *Organizing for power and empowerment*. New York: Columbia University Press.
Montalvo, B., Harmon, D., & Elliot, M. (1998). Family mobilization: Work with angry elderly couples in declining health. *Contemporary Family Therapy, 20*(2), 163–179.
Olson, D., McCubbin, H., Barnes, H., Larsen, A., Muxen, A., & Wilson, M. (1983). *Families: What makes them work*. Beverly Hills: Sage.
Peñalva, C. (2001). Evaluación del funcionamiento familiar por medio de la "entrevista estructural". *Salud Mental, 24*(2), 32–42.
Raines, J. C. (1996). Self-disclosure in clinical social work. *Clinical Social Work Journal, 24*(4), 357–375.
Rapp, C. A. (1998). *The strengths model. Case management with people suffering from severe and persistent mental illness*. New York: Oxford University Press.
Rappaport, J., & Hess, R. (1984). *Studies in empowerment. Steps towards understanding and action*. New York: The Haworth Press.
Rodriguez, C., & Luengo, S. (2003). Un análisis del concepto de familia monoparental a partir de una investigación sobre núcleos familiares monoparentales. *Papers, 69*, 59–82.
Rooney, R. H. (2009). *Strategies for work with involuntary clients*. New York: Columbia University Press.
Rotter, J. B., & Murly, R. C. (1965). Internal versus external control reinforcement and decision time. *Journal of Personality and Social Psychology, 2*(4), 598–604.
Saleebey, D. (2004). "The power of place": Another look at the environment. *Families in Society, 85*(1), 7–16.
Saleebey, D. (2006). *The strengths perspective in social work practice* (4th ed.). Boston: Pearson Education.

Sánchez Urios, A. (2006). *Trabajo Social Microsocial: Intervención con Individuos y Familias*. Murcia: Diego Marín.
Satir, V. (1967). *Cojoint family therapy*. Palo Alto: Science and Behavior books.
Satir, V. (1988). *The new peoplemaking*. Palo Alto: Science and Behavior Books.
Schulman, G. (1999). Siblings revisited: Old conflicts and new opportunities in later life. *Journal of Marital and Family Therapy, 25*(4), 517–524.
Schumm, W. R. (1985). Beyond relationship characteristics of strong families: Constructing a model of family strengths. *Family Perspective, 19*(1), 1–9.
Segado Sánchez-Cabezudo, S. (2011). *Nuevas tendencias en Trabajo Social con familias. Una propuesta para la práctica desde el empowerment*. Madrid: Trotta.
Sen, A. (2010). *La idea de justicia*. Madrid: Taurus.
Sennett, R. (2009). *La corrosión del carácter*. Barcelona: Anagrama.
Shulman, L. (2009). *The skills of helping individuals, families, groups and communities*. Pacific Grove: Brooks/Cole. Cengage learning.
Simon, B. L. (1994). *The empowerment tradition in American social work*. New York: Columbia University Press.
Solomon, B. (1976). *Black empowerment: Social work in oppressed communities*. New York: Columbia University Press.
Szapocznik, J., Hervis, O., Rio, T., Behar, V., Kurtines, W., & Faraci, A. (1991). Assessing change in family functioning as a result of treatment: The structural family systems rating scale (SFSR). *Journal of Marital and Family Therapy, 17*(3), 295–310.
Thomlison, B. (2007a). Family assessment handbook. An introduction and practical guide to family assessment. *Thomson Brook/Cole Therapy, 17*(3), 295–310.
Thomlison, B. (2007b). *Family assessment handbook. An introduction and practical guide to family assessment*. Belmont: Thomson Brook/Cole.
Tracy, E. M., & Whittaker, J. K. (1990). The social network map: Assessing social support in clinical social work practice. *Families in Society, 71*, 461–470.
Vosler, N. R. (1990). Assessing family access to basic resources: An essential component of social work practice. *Social Work, 35*(5), 436–437.
Weick, A. (1992). Building a strengths perspective for social work. In D. Saleebey (Ed.), *The strengths perspective in social work practice* (pp. 18–26). White Plains: Longman.
Weinberg, M. (2006). Pregnant with possibility: The paradoxes of "help" as anti-oppression and discipline with a young single mother. *Families in Society, 67*(2), 161–169.
Yanca, S. T., & Johnson, L. C. (2008). *Generalist social work practice with families*. Boston: Pearson Education Inc.
Zastrow, C. H. (2004). *Introduction to social work and social welfare. Empowering people*. Belmont: Brooks/Cole.
Zimmerman, M. A., & Rappaport, J. (1988). Citizen participation, perceived control, and psychological empowerment. *American Journal of Community Psychology, 16*, 1–25.

Index

A. Moreno Mínguez (ed.), *Family Well-Being: European Perspectives*,
Social Indicators Research Series 49, DOI 10.1007/978-94-007-4354-0,

MIX
Papier aus verantwortungsvollen Quellen
Paper from responsible sources
FSC® C105338

If you have any concerns about our products,
you can contact us on
ProductSafety@springernature.com

In case Publisher is established outside the EU,
the EU authorized representative is:
Springer Nature Customer Service Center GmbH
Europaplatz 3, 69115 Heidelberg, Germany

Printed by Libri Plureos GmbH
in Hamburg, Germany